Digestive Disease Pathology

☐ VOLUME I

Digestive Disease Pathology

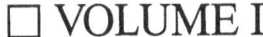 VOLUME I

Editors

Shaw Watanabe, M.D.

Chief for Epidemiology Division
National Cancer Center Research Institute
and Professor of Pathology
Keio University School of Medicine
Tokyo, Japan

Marianne Wolff, M.D.

Professor of Clinical Surgical Pathology
Columbia University
College of Physicians & Surgeons
New York, New York, and
Pathology Department
Morristown Memorial Hospital
Morristown, New Jersey

Sheldon C. Sommers, M.D.

Clinical Professor of Pathology
Columbia University
College of Physicians & Surgeons
New York, New York, and
University of Southern California
School of Medicine
Los Angeles, California

Springer-Verlag
Berlin Heidelberg GmbH

ISBN 978-3-662-11564-0   ISBN 978-3-662-11562-6 (eBook)
DOI 10.1007/978-3-662-11562-6

Library of Congress Catalog Card Number: 80-80334

MANUFACTURED IN THE UNITED STATES OF AMERICA

Contents

Contributors to Digestive Disease Pathology, Volume I

Hitoshi Asakura, M.D.
Assistant Professor, Internal Medicine
Keio University School of Medicine
Tokyo, Japan

Yasuyoshi Enomoto, Ph.D.
Chief Technician, Department of Pathology
Keio University School of Medicine
Tokyo, Japan

Hidemasa Ishikawa, M.D.
Department of Internal Medicine
Postgraduate School of Fukushima
Medical College
Fukushima, Japan

Kotaro Kaneko, M.D.
Department of Internal Medicine
Keio University School of Medicine
Tokyo, Japan

J. Lindeman, M.D., Ph.D.
Chairman, Department of Pathology
Stichting Samenwerking Delftse Siekenhuizen
Delft,
The Netherlands

C.J.L.M. Meijer, M.D., Ph.D.
Chairman & Director, Pathological Institute
Free University Hospital
Amsterdam,
The Netherlands

Soichiro Miura, M.D.
Internal Medicine
Keio University Hospital
Tokyo, Japan

Akira Morita, M.D.
Department of Internal Medicine
Tokyo Metropolitan Hiroo
Tokyo, Japan

Hiroshi Nagura, M.D., Ph.D.
Professor
Laboratory of Germfree Life
Research Institute for Disease
Mechanism and Control
Nagoya University School of Medicine
Nagoya, Japan

Masahiko Nakamura, M.D.
Department of Internal Medicine
Tokyo Electric Power Co. Hospital
Tokyo, Japan

Masaya Oda, M.D.
Assistant Professor, Internal Medicine
Keio University School of Medicine
Tokyo, Japan

Manuel Moutinho-Ribeiro, M.D.
Assistant Professor of Surgery
Department of Cirurgia 4
The Medical Faculty; Attending Surgeon
Hospital S. Joao
Porto, Portugal

Ricardo V. Lloyd, M.D., Ph.D.
Associate Professor of Pathology
University of Michigan Hospitals
Ann Arbor, Michigan

Mário Seixas, M.Sc., Ph.D.
Assistant Professor of Biophysics
Department of Biophysics
The Medical Faculty
Porto, Portugal

Manuel Sobrinho-Simões, M.D., Ph.D.
Professor of Pathology
Department of Pathology
The Medical Faculty and Hospital S. Joao
Porto, Portugal

Yukiko Sumi, M.D.
Assistant Professor
Laboratory of Germfree Life
Research Institute for Disease
Mechanism and Control
Nagoya University School of Medicine
Nagoya, Japan

Eiichi Tahara, M.D.
Professor
Department of Pathology
Hiroshima University School of Medicine
Hiroshima, Japan

Masaharu Tsuchiya, M.D.
Professor
Internal Medicine
Keio University School of Medicine
Tokyo, Japan

Yutaka Tsutsumi, M.D.
Assistant Professor
Department of Pathology
Tokai University School of Medicine
Bonseidai, Isehara-city
Kanagawa, Japan

J.P. van Spreeuwel, M.D.
Department of Internal Medicine
Division of Gastroenterology
University Hospital
Maastricht,
The Netherlands

P. van der Valk, M.D., Ph.D.
Pathological Institute
Free University Hospital
Amsterdam,
The Netherlands

Haruki Wakasa, M.D.
Professor
Department of Pathology
Fukushima Medical College
Fukushima, Japan

Hikaru Watanabe, M.D.
Chief
Division of Gastroenterology
National Sendai Hospital
Sendai, Japan

1

Differentiation of Gastric Cancer Cells: Analysis Using Immunohistochemistry and Mucin Histochemistry

Yutaka Tsutsumi

Most, even all neoplasms are known to show variable degrees of cellular differentiation, not only biologically, but also morphologically.[1] Thus, we pathologists can recognize the histological type of each tumor on the basis of morphological similarities to its normal or nonneoplastic counterparts. Carcinoma of the stomach, the most common cancer in Japan,[2,3] shows a variety of histological appearances, although it has been roughly grouped into two types, diffuse carcinoma vs. adenoplastic carcinoma.[4,5] The diffuse cancer is characterized by its scirrhous growth pattern and the occurrence of signet ring cells, a peculiar cancer morphology in the stomach. The histological heterogeneities of gastric cancer possibly reflect the fact that the gastric mucosa shows a bidirectional cell renewal pattern, (i.e., the generative (stem) cells differentiate upward to the foveolar epithelium and downward to the gastric gland).[6-9] The frequent occurrence of intestinal metaplasia in the aged gastric mucosa[2,10] makes the situation more complicated.

Studies of cell kinetics of normal gastric mucosa have proved that fundic gland cells (and endocrine cells) move in a stochastic flow system, while pyloric gland cells and foveolar cells move in a pipe line system.[6-9] Chief cells, parietal cells, and endocrine cells ultrastructurally show poorly developed junctional complexes, interdigitations, and necessarily connect to each other with a weak binding ability.[9] Thus, they can change their position with a random velocity as dissociative cells.[6,8,9] On the contrary, pyloric gland cells and surface epithelial cells ultrastructurally show well-developed junctional complexes and interdigitations, and necessarily connect to each other with a strong binding ability.[9] Thus, they change their position with a constant rate as associative cells.[7-9] Signet ring (diffuse type) cancer cells are typical of dissociative cells, whereas adenoplastic cancer cells belong to associative cells.[8,9]

Speaking of the histogenesis of gastric cancer, it has been pointed out that signet ring cell carcinomas often arise from the intact oxyntic mucosa, while adenoplastic carcinomas are intimately related to intestinal metaplasia of the gastric mucosa.[2,5,10] Nakamura et al specified the former as gastric-proper (or undifferentiated) type and the latter as intestinal (or differentiated) type.[5,11] Through the histological and mucin histochemical studies of minute mucosal cancer, Matsukura et al postulated that the incomplete type of intestinal metaplasia (devoid of Paneth cells) is more likely precancerous than the complete type (with Paneth cells).[12]

Functional and phenotypic expressions of human gastric cancer have been investigated concerning lysozyme,[13-15] secretory component (SC)[13] and IgA[13,16], pepsinogen II,[17,18] carcinoembryonic antigen (CEA),[16,19-21] α-fetoprotein (AFP),[21-23] human chorionic gonadotropin (HCG),[21,23,24] placental alkaline phosphatase (PALP),[21,25,26] mucins,[27-30] hormones,[31-34] and so on. We have also studied the expression of various histochemical markers of gastric epithelium in gastric cancer tissues.[35-40] These include mucin histochemistry for pyloric gland cells and goblet cells and immunoperoxidase staining for lysozyme, lactoferrin, SC, pepsinogen II, CEA, AFP, HCG, PALP, chromogranin, and five gastrointestinal hormones. Such a series of histochemical studies greatly contributes to investigating not only the histogenesis, but also the functional differentiations of gastric cancer or gastric cancer cells. In the present review, attempts were thus centered on clarifying the functional differentiations of gastric cancer cells by analyzing the expression of those markers.

MATERIALS AND METHODS

Surgically removed gastric tissues were routinely fixed in 10% formalin for 2–7 days and embedded in paraffin wax. Sections of 4 μm thickness from a representative site of cancer (mainly at the cancer–noncancer junction) were prepared for hematoxylin and eosin (H&E) staining, mucin histochemistry, silver methods for endocrine cells with light green counterstaining after Grimelius,[41] and Masson,[42] and immunoperoxidase method. The diagnosis of the histological type of cancer was applied corresponding to "the general rules of the gastric cancer study in surgery and pathology" of the Japanese Research Society for Gastric Cancer.[3,43] The typing was made on the basis of the predominance of histological varieties. An exception was as follows: scirrhous carcinoma mainly consisting of isolated small and immature-looking cancer cells with a small amount of intracytoplasmic mucin was included in signet ring cell carcinoma (sig), so that poorly differentiated carcinoma (por) means a solid carcinoma with a medullary growth pattern.

Mucin histochemistry: Alcian blue-periodic acid Schiff (AB-PAS), PAS with or without diastase digestion, and high iron diamine-alcian blue (HID-AB)[44] were employed. To detect mucins of pyloric glands and mucous neck cells specifically, Concanavalin A paradoxical staining (CPS) class III after Katsuyama and Spicer[45] was used. Briefly, diastase digested deparaffinized sections were oxidized in 0.5% periodic acid (PA) for 60 minutes, followed by the reduction in 0.3% sodium borohydride (SB)-1%NA$_2$HPO$_4$ solution for 3 minutes. The sections were then incubated with 0.1% Concanavalin A-phosphate buffered-saline (PBS) solution, pH 7.4 for 15 minutes, and, after rinsing in PBS, were dipped in 0.0005% horseradish peroxidase (HRP, Sigma type VI)-PBS solution. Finally, HRP was visualized by incubation in 30mg% 3,3′-diaminobenzidine tetrahydrochloride (DAB)-0.05M Tris-HCl solution, pH 7.6. Nuclei were counterstained with 1% methyl green buffered by veronal acetate at pH 4.0 or lightly with hematoxylin.

To identify N-acetyl neuraminic acid (NANA), mild periodate oxidation-Schiff (MOS) reaction by Katsuyama et al[30] was employed. The C8-9 vicinal hydroxyls of NANA are extremely susceptible to periodate oxidation. Thus, the periodate oxidation at an extremely low concentration (1 mM) and low temperature (0–2°C) and for a short time (5 minutes) in 0.05M acetate buffer, pH 5.5, provides a method for the selective demonstration of NANA. The MOS reaction after neuraminidase digestion was carried out as a control procedure.

To demonstrate O-acylated NANA (or O-acylated sialic acid), which is specific for gut goblet cell mucin especially of the large intestine, the sequence of PA-SB-PH-PAS after Culling et al[46] was employed. PH means potassium hydroxide. Oxidation by 0.5% PA was performed for 90 minutes, reduction by

TABLE 1-1
Primary Antibodies Used in this Chapter

Antigen	Animal Immunized	Final Dilution	Source
SC	rabbit	×200	Behringerwerke, AG, Marburg
lysozyme	rabbit	×200	DAKO Immunoglobulins, Copenhagen
lactoferrin	rabbit	×200	DAKO
pepsinogen II	rabbit	×500	Dr. K. Miki*
CEA	rabbit	×400	DAKO
AFP	rabbit	×200	DAKO
HCG	rabbit	×200	DAKO
PALP	rabbit	×200	Green Cross Co., Osaka
chromogranin (bovine)	rabbit	×200	Immuno Nuclear Co., Stillwater, MN
glicentin 49–69 (porcine)	rabbit	×500	Prof. N. Yanaihara**
glucagon 19–29	rabbit	×1500	Japan Immunoresearch Laboratores, Takasaki
PP (bovine)†	rabbit	×20000	Dr. R.E. Chance***
somatostatin	rabbit	×2000	DAKO Co., Santa Barbara, CA
gastrin (human)	guinea pig	×500	Prof. N. Yanaihara

* Department of Internal Medicine, University of Tokyo Faculty of Medicine, Tokyo

** Laboratory of Bioorganic Chemistry, Shizuoka College of Pharmacy, Shizuoka

*** Lilly Research Laboratories, Indianapolis

† pancreatic polypeptide

Concerning the specificity of antiglicentin 49–69 and antiglucagon 19–29 antibodies, see references 38 and 57.

0.3% SB in 1%Na$_2$HPO$_4$ was for 5 minutes, alkaline hydrolysis by 1% PH in 70% ethanol was for 10 minutes and the PAS reaction was performed in a conventional condition. Nuclei were lightly counterstained with hematoxylin. Negative control procedure was done, in which the step of PH was omitted.

Immunoperoxidase method: Immunohistochemistry was performed either with the indirect HRP-labeled antibody method after Nakane[47] or, for the study mainly in Parts 2 and 3, with the peroxidase-antiperoxidase (PAP) method after Sternberger et al.[48] Primary antibodies used are listed in Table 1-1 together with the animal immunized, final dilution and their source. A minor contaminating activity against alpha-chain of immunoglobulin in antiSC antibody was absorbed by mixing it with 1% normal human serum. The commercial antiCEA antibody contains a high antibody activity against nonspecific cross-reacting antigen (NCA).[49] The antiCEA was used with or without previous absorption by a perchloric acid (PCA) extract of human spleen, as described previously.[49,50] HRP-labeled Fab against rabbit IgG was prepared in our laboratory, and HRP-labeled antiguinea pig IgG was purchased from Miles Laboratories, Naperville, IL. Unlabeled secondary antibody and PAP complexes were obtained from DAKO Immunoglobulins, Copenhagen. Time of antibody incubation and rinsing in each step was 30 minutes. Endogenous peroxidase was inactivated by dipping sections in 0.5% PA for 10 minutes. For the purpose of coloration, the sections were incubated in the DAB solution for 5–10 minutes. Nuclear counterstaining was done with 1% methyl green or, in the case of the PAP method, with hematoxylin. For control immunostaining, the primary antibody was replaced by non-immune rabbit or guinea pig serum at a 1:200 dilution. Staining results obtained by the indirect immunoperoxidase and PAP method were fundamentally identical.

TABLE 1-2

Expression of Various Histochemical Markers in Nonneoplastic Gastrointestinal Tissues

	Stomach						Intestine	
				(Pseudo) Pyloric Gland	Intestinal Metaplasia			
	Surface Epithelium	Generative Cell	Fundic Gland		Incomplete	Complete	Small	Large
SC	−	N − G(+)	−	N − G(+)/−	+ (L≥U)	+ (L≥U)	+ (L>U)	+ (L>U)
Lysozyme	−	+	−	N+/− G +	PG+	P+	BG,P+	−
Lactoferrin	−	−	+/−	+/−	−	−	−	−
Pepsinogen II	−	+	+	+	PG+	−	BG+	−
CEA	+ (L<U)	−	−	−	+ (L<U)	+ (L<U)	+ (L<U)	+ (L<U)
Neutral mucin	+	+/−	MNC+	+	+/−	−	BG+	−
Sialomucin	N − G(+)/−	−	−	−	+	+	+	+
Sulfomucin	−	−	−	N- G+/−	+/−	−	−	+
CPS class III	−	−	MNC+	+	PG+	−	BG+	−
MOS	−	−	−	−	+	+	+	+/−
PA-SB-PH-PAS	−	−	−	−	+/−	+/−	+/−	+

−: negative

(+): weakly positive

+: positive

(+)/− or +/−: occasionally positive

BG: Brunner's gland

MNC: mucous neck cell

N: normal

G: gastritis, nonmetaplastic

L: lower layer

U: upper layer

P: Paneth cell

PG: pyloric gland

RESULTS

1. Histochemical Markers of Noncancerous Gastric Epithelial Cells

Table 1-2 shows the expression of various immunohistochemical and mucin histochemical markers in nonneoplastic gastric and intestinal tissues. Figures 1-1 and 1-2 illustrate representative features of the marker localization in nonneoplastic gastric mucosa with or without intestinalization.

Secretory component (SC), a key substance for secretory immunity, is a good epithelial marker for various exocrine tissues including intestinal, respiratory, pancreatobiliary, and genitourinary tracts as well as mammary, salivary, nasal, lacrimal, and sweat glands.[51] SC is produced by the epithelial cells and acts as a receptor for dimeric IgA on their basolateral plasma membranes.[52,53] Gastric mucosal epithelium under normal conditions, which means gastric mucosa with negligible inflammatory changes, is devoid of SC, probably owing to high acidity in the gastric lumen.[13,37,54] The high acid condition must be a "natural defense" of the gastric mucosa instead of secretory immunity.[13,54] However, cells in the generative zone, the junctional area between foveolar cells and gastric glands, turn weakly positive for SC when chronic inflammatory changes occur.[13,37,54] Infrequently, atrophic pyloric glands in the mucosa with chronic gastritis are faintly positive for SC. Intestinal metaplasia is immunohistochemically characterized by the prominent expression of SC, especially in Golgi areas of intes-

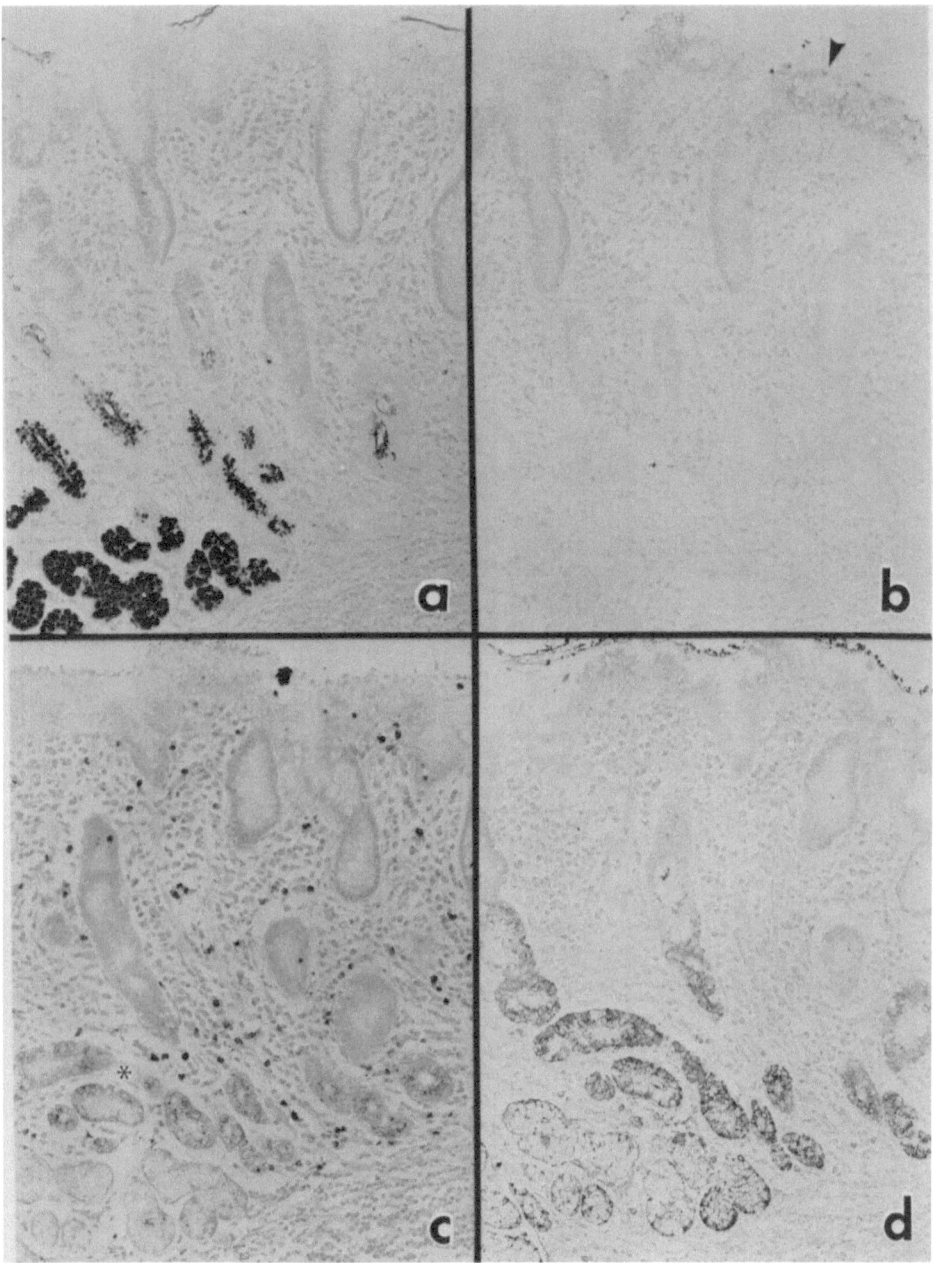

Fig. 1-1. Marker expression in nonintestinalized gastric mucosa. CPS class III (a) and indirect immunoperoxidase method for CEA (b), lysozyme (c) and pepsinogen II (d). Methyl green counterstain, ×120

CPS class III specifically stains pyloric gland cells where pepsinogen II is localized. Atrophic pyloric glands at the right side of each picture and cells of the glandular neck region (generative zone, asterisk) are positive for lysozyme. Mature pyloric glands at the left side are devoid here of lysozyme, which is also positive for granulocytes and histiocytes in the stroma. CEA, detected by antiCEA antibody after absorption with the PCA extract of spleen, is focally positive in the uppermost part of foveolar cells (arrowhead). Granulocytes and histiocytes are not stained with the absorbed antiCEA antibody.

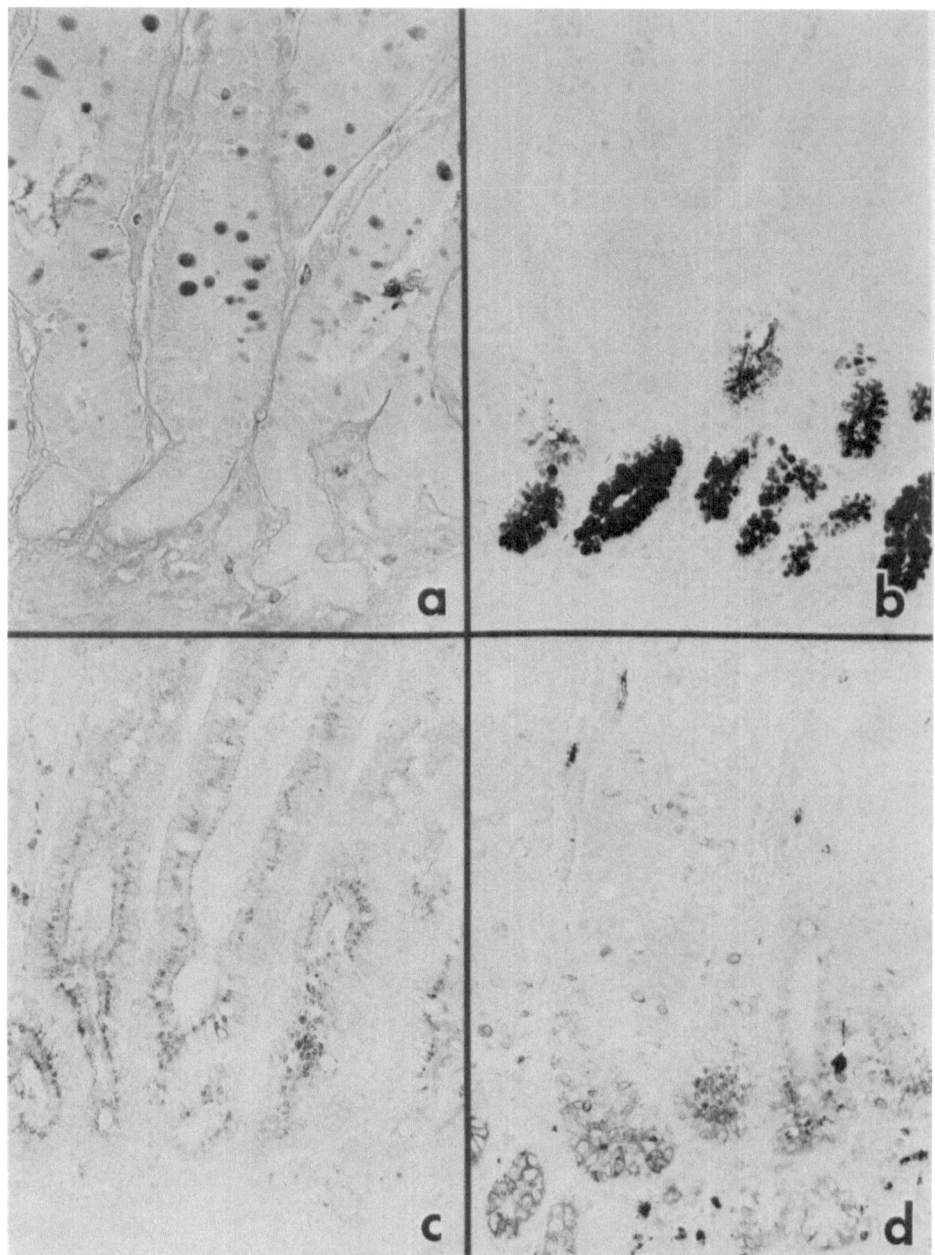

Fig. 1-2. Marker expression in intestinal metaplasia (incomplete type[12] or type B[57]). HID-AB (a), CPS class III (b) and indirect immunoperoxidase method for SC (c) and lysozyme (d). Methyl green counterstain, ×200.

Both sialomucin (blue) and sulfomucin (black) are seen in goblet cells. CPS class III and lysozyme are positive in atrophic pyloric glands remaining at the bottom of the mucosa. SC positivity is evident in intestinalized cells.

tinalized cells (Fig. 1-2c),[13,37,54] as seen in normal intestinal epithelium. A minority of intestinalized mucosal cells shows a polarity of the SC expression, as seen in normal intestinal epithelium,[53] i.e., SC immunoreactivity is stronger in cells in the lower half layer of the mucosa than in cells in the upper layer. But the majority shows strong immunoreactivity of SC throughout the intestinalized epithelium without the polarity.[54]

Lysozyme is a bacteriolytic enzyme, muramidase,[55] and is known to cooperate with secretory immunoglobulins.[56] In the small intestine and intestinal metaplasia of the complete type, Paneth cells are strongly positive for lysozyme, in addition to such inflammatory cells as neutrophils, eosinophils, and histiocytes.[13,35,55] Lysozyme is further localized in glandular neck cells at the generative zone of the gastric mucosa with minimal inflammation and pyloric gland cells, especially those showing atrophic changes (Fig. 1-1c).[13,35] Lysozyme immunoreactivity is also observed in the atrophic pyloric glands located at the bottom of intestinal metaplasia, (A and B of Tsutsumi et al[57]) (Fig. 1-2d) and in metaplastic pseudopyloric glands in the fundus.

Lactoferrin is an iron-containing bacteriostatic glycoprotein substance,[58] and is one of the major components of neutrophil granules.[59] Being similar to lysozyme,[55] lactoferrin is widely distributed in various exocrine glands such as salivary, nasal, bronchial, prostatic and lactating mammary glands and renal tubules.[51,58] In the stomach, pyloric gland cells and fundic gland cells except for parietal cells inconsistently show lactoferrin immunoreactivity.[35,60]

Pepsinogen II, an isozyme of gastric digestive enzyme, is consistently positive in pyloric glands including the glandular neck region (Fig. 1-1d), pseudopyloric glands, mucous neck cells, chief cells, and Brunner's glands.[17,61] Foveolar cells and intestinalized epithelia are negative for pepsinogen II.[17,61]

Carcinoembryonic antigen (CEA), an excellent tumor marker, was first described by Gold and Freedman in 1965.[62] Conventional antiserum against CEA including ours used in this study is known to contain antibody activities against several CEA-related substances and blood group substances.[49] The antigenicity of the latter, having antigenic determinants on sugar moieties, is destroyed mostly by the periodate treatment of sections, which was used for endogenous peroxidase inactivation in the present study. The most important CEA-related substance is a nonspecific cross-reacting antigen (NCA), which is present in neutrophils. Thus, the PCA extract of human spleen[50] was used for the elimination of antiNCA activity in the commercial antiCEA antibody. In this chapter the antigenicity recognized by the absorbed antiCEA antibody that does not stain neutrophils is regarded as "CEA" in a broad sense. Strictly speaking, however, "CEA" by this definition includes such CEA-related substances as NCA-2 and normal fecal cross-reacting antigen (NFCA).[49] Normal or metaplastic gastric mucosa has been shown to be positive with the antibody even after the absorption procedure, as reported previously.[37,49] CEA-related substances ("CEA" and NCA) are mainly present in the superficial mucosal part of the foveolar epithelium (Fig. 1-1b).[35,37,49] The antigenicity turns weaker after the absorption of the antibody. Goblet cells and cells in the generative zone are always negative for the antigens. The expression of the CEA-related substances is stronger in intestinalized gastric epithelium than in nonintestinalized epithelium.[35,37]

The AB-PAS procedure differentiates neutral mucin (stained red) from acidic mucin (stained blue or purple). The HID-AB procedure is useful to differentiate sialomucin (stained blue) from sulfomucin (stained black).[44] It is well known that normal human gastric epithelium such as foveolar cells, pyloric glands, mucous neck cells and Brunner's gland in the duodenum exclusively contain neutral mucin. When the foveolar epithelium shows a hyperplastic or regenerative change, however, it sometimes turns faintly alcianophilic. HID-AB staining further confirms the presence of a small amount of sialomucin in such altered foveolar cells. Atrophic pyloric

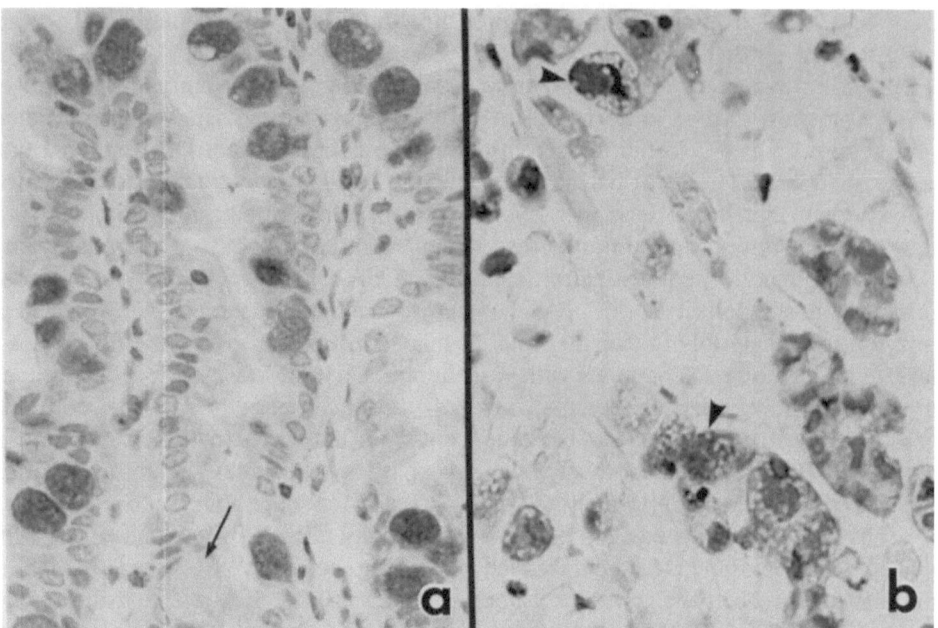

Fig. 1-3. PA-SB-PH-PAS reaction in goblet cells of intestinal metaplasia (a) and mucinous adenocarcinoma (b). ×480.
Goblet cells in some, but not all, intestinalized mucosa stain positive for O-acylated sialic acids. Arrow indicates a negative goblet cell. Mucin of signet ring cells in mucinous adenocarcinoma (arrowheads) mostly belong to the goblet cell type.

glands in inflamed antral mucosa or pseudopyloric glands in inflamed fundic mucosa are occasionally positive for sulfomucin.[35] The situation is the same in atrophic pyloric glands remaining at the bottom in intestinal metaplasia. Goblet cells in intestinalized glands are commonly positive for sialomucin, but sulfomucin-containing goblet cells are often noted in intestinal metaplasia of the incomplete type[12] (or types A and B of Tsutsumi et al (Fig. 1-2a).

CPS class III has been confirmed to be highly specific for mucins of pyloric glands (Fig. 1-1a) including those remaining at the bottom of intestinalized epithelium (Fig. 1-2b), pseudopyloric glands, mucous neck cells and Brunner's glands.[30,45,54,57]

Most of the goblet cells in the small intestine and intestinalized mucosa and some in the large intestine stain positive with the MOS sequence.[30,35] The PA-SB-PH-PAS sequence specifically detects mucins of all colonic goblet cells, some goblet cells in the small intestine and intestinal metaplasia of the stomach (Fig. 1-3a).[35]

Nonmetaplastic mucosal cells including hyperplastic or regenerative foveolar cells and sulfomucin-positive atrophic pyloric glands are equally negative for the goblet cell type mucins.

Negative staining results are to be obtained in all of the control specimens including those for immunoperoxidase staining incubated with nonimmune sera, for the MOS sequence followed by the neuraminidase treatment, and for the PA-SB-PH-PAS sequence with omission of the PH step. The same is true in the following Parts.

2. EXPRESSION OF HISTOCHEMICAL MARKERS IN GASTRIC CANCER CELLS

A total of 51 surgical specimens of gastric carcinoma of various histological types in-

TABLE 1-3

Gastric Carcinomas Histochemically Analyzed

	m	sm	pm˜	Total
sig	1	2	8	11
muc	0	0	5	5
pap	0	2	4	6
tub$_1$	3	3	3	9
tub$_2$	4	2	9	15
por	0	0	5	5
total	8	9	34	51

sig: signet ring cell carcinoma

muc: mucinous adenocarcinoma

pap: papillary adenocarcinoma

tub$_1$: well-differentiated tubular adenocarcinoma

tub$_2$: moderately differentiated tubular adenocarcinoma

por: poorly differentiated adenocarcinoma (with medullary growth pattern)

m: intramucosally localized early cancer

sm: early cancer invading into the submucosal layer

pm˜: advanced cancer invading into the proper muscle layer or into the serosa

cluding 17 early carcinomas (Table 1-3) were histochemically examined for SC, lysozyme, lactoferrin, CEA/NCA, CPS class III, MOS, and PA/SB/PH/PAS reactivities.[35] Three adenocarcinomas with lymphoid stroma were included in "tub$_2$" (moderately differentiated tubular adenocarcinoma). CEA/NCA means the immunoreactivity detected by an antiCEA polyclonal antibody without absorption with the PCA extract of the spleen. Results are summarized in Table 1-4.

SC and lysozyme were at least focally positive in more than 80% of cancer tissues. The frequency of positivity was principally independent of the histological typing, excepting for less SC immunoreactivity in mucinous adenocarcinoma (muc). Lysozyme can be regarded as a marker relatively specific for gastric epithelium, because intestinal epithelial cells other than Paneth cells and Brunner's glands are commonly negative for lysozyme. In H&E preparations of the gastric cancer tissues examined, no typical Paneth cell granules were seen. It is noteworthy that the expression of lysozyme was quite common even in adenoplastic or "intestinal-type" car-

cinomas (pap, tub$_1$ and tub$_2$). In a separate study, however, some crypt epithelium of either the small or large intestine was infrequently and inconsistently immunostained for lysozyme, and a very small number of lysozyme-positive cancer cells were identified in 11 of 28 adenocarcinomas (39%) of the colon and rectum (unpublished observation). Klockars et al[63] reported lysozyme-positive crypt epithelial cells in the lesion of ulcerative colitis.[60] Therefore, the significance of lysozyme as a gastric marker should be considered relative.

The demonstration of lactoferrin immunoreactivity in gastric carcinomas was quite inconstant. Only a few lactoferrin-positive cancer cells were detected in 18 of 51 carcinomas (35%) irrespective of histological typing. On the contrary, CEA/NCA or CEA-related substance(s) were positive in all carcinoma tissues, and the positive cells were generally plentiful. Poorly differentiated adenocarcinomas with a medullary growth pattern (por) were apt to show a lesser number of CEA/NCA-positive cancer cells. The positivity of CEA/NCA was noted on the plasma membranes in principle, whereas cancer cells showing a strongly positive cytoplasmic staining were not rarely encountered.

Intracytoplasmic mucins specifically demonstrated by CPS class III (for pyloric gland type) and MOS and/or PA/SB/PH/PAS (for goblet cell type) were positive in many cancer cells, again irrespective of histological typing. Mucins of the pyloric gland-type and goblet cell-type were fairly frequently detected in both diffuse and adenoplastic carcinomas. For the evaluation of MOS reaction, only intracytoplasmic staining was regarded as positive and positive staining of the surface coat of some neoplastic glands was neglected.

Mucinous adenocarcinomas were characterized by the constant occurrence of goblet cell type mucin. In other words, most signet ring cells in mucinous adenocarcinomas could be categorized as the goblet cell type, while a few small-sized cells containing neutral mucin and/or CPS class III mucin were also found in four of five tumors. The detection of PA/SB/PH/PAS reactivity in gastric

TABLE 1-4
Expression of Glycoprotein Markers and Mucins in 51 Gastric Carcinomas

		SC				Lysozyme				Lactoferrin				CEA/NCA		
		−	(+)	+	++	−	(+)	+	++	−	(+)	+	++	−	(+)	+	++
sig	11	1	3	7	0	1	2	6	2	6	5	0	0	0	0	3	8
muc	5	2	3	0	0	1	2	1	1	4	1	0	0	0	0	0	5
pap	6	1	2	2	1	2	2	1	1	3	3	0	0	0	0	1	5
tub$_1$	9	1	0	4	4	1	1	7	0	6	3	0	0	0	0	1	8
tub$_2$	15	2	4	7	2	1	2	6	6	10	5	0	0	0	0	4	11
por	5	0	2	1	2	2	1	0	2	4	1	0	0	0	1	3	1
total	51	7	14	21	9	8	10	21	12	33	18	0	0	0	1	12	38

		CPS Class III				PA/SB/PH/PAS				MOS			
		−	(+)	+	++	−	(+)	+	++	−	(+)	+	++
sig	11	2	4	4	1	10	1	0	0	4	4	3	0
muc	5	4	1	0	0	2	1	2	0	0	3	1	1
pap	6	3	2	1	0	5	0	1	0	3	1	2	0
tub$_1$	9	3	2	3	1	8	1	0	0	4	5	0	0
tub$_2$	15	3	6	3	3	14	1	0	0	7	6	2	0
por	5	4	0	0	1	5	0	0	0	3	1	0	1
total	51	19	15	11	6	44	4	3	0	21	20	8	2

−: negative

(+): positive in only a few cells

+: positive in a modest number of cells

++: positive in many cells

cancer was infrequent except for mucinous adenocarcinomas (Fig. 1-3b).

The present series included three adenocarcinomas with marked infiltration of small lymphocytes and plasma cells in the stroma. The cancer cells revealed constant morphological features showing a microalveolus, trabecular, or irregular small tubule-like arrangement with the formation of small lumina (categorized as tub$_2$ in this study).[64] The nuclear pleomorphism was not so marked. The formation of lymphoid follicles in the stroma and the infiltration of small lymphocytes inside cancerous nests were common, while necrosis of cancer cells was hardly seen (Fig. 1-4). The margin of invasion was well-demarcated, and the biological behavior was reported to be relatively less malignant.[64] Histochemical properties of the cancer cells corresponded to those of the pyloric glands.

Most tumor cells possessed intracytoplasmic neutral mucin with weak CPS class III reactivity. Lysozyme was positive in addition to SC and CEA/NCA. Surface coat-type mucin was occasionally seen along the lumen of cancerous tubules, but goblet cell-type mucin was hardly noted especially in the invading site.

A separate study has disclosed that IgG is predominantly shown in the plasma cells, and plasma cells containing IgM or IgA are minor components. With monoclonal antibodies, MB-1 and MT-1, from Bio-Science Products AG, Emmenbrücke, Switzerland, which are applicable to formalin-fixed and paraffin-embedded tissue, lymphocytes forming lymphoid follicles are mostly composed of B cells, while small lymphocytes scattered in the stroma and in cancer nests are largely T cells. It seems important to note that the morphology and histochemical features of cancer cells

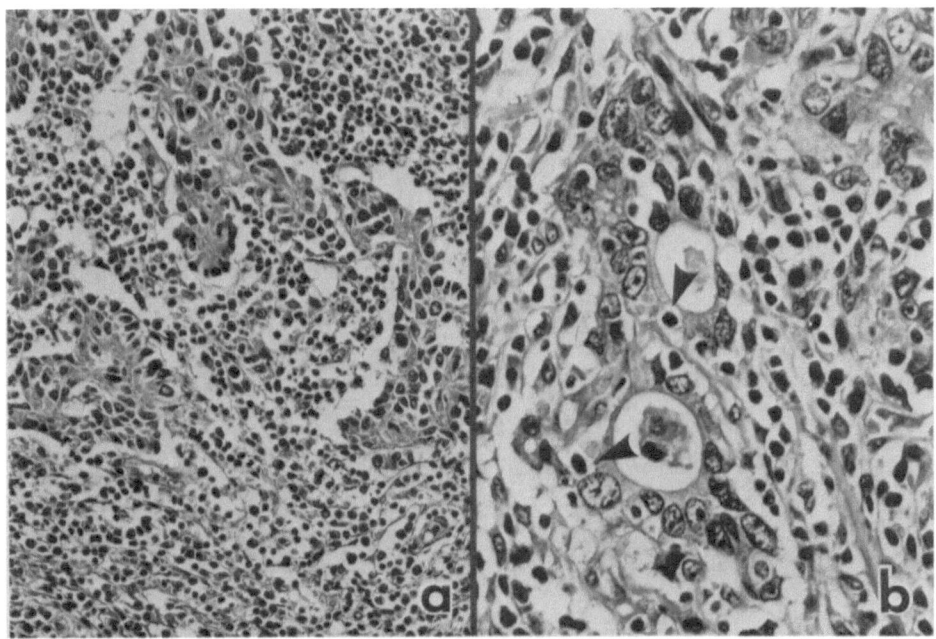

Fig. 1-4. Adenocarcinoma with lymphoid stroma. H&E, ×200 (a) and ×400 (b).
Cancer cells form a trabecular or abortive tubular arrangement. Marked stromal infiltration of lymphocytes and plasma cells is characteristic. The presence of intraepithelial lymphocytes (arrowheads) is a common finding.

of this special type are quite uniform, as seen in medullary carcinoma with lymphocytic infiltration of the breast.[65] In addition to the possibility of tumor immunity, the production of some factors chemotactic to lymphocytes and plasma cells (lymphoegresin)[66] by the specifically differentiated cancer cells should also be taken into consideration when we discuss the pathological significance of the lymphoid stroma.

In fact, the presence of "intraepithelial lymphocytes" (small T lymphocytes among epithelial cells) reflects an important function of nonneoplastic gastrointestinal mucosa.[54,67] We have reported the universal occurrence of "intraepithelial lymphocytes" in every colonic adenocarcinoma without evidence of tumor cell damage.[68] Additionally, the production of colony-stimulating and neutrophil chemotactic factor(s) has been clarified in poorly differentiated cancers with marked neutrophilic infiltration from a variety of primary sites.[69,70]

Table 1-5 summarizes the mode of mucin expression (the predominance of surface coat mucin, intracytoplasmic mucin or both) in the above 51 carcinomas. Nearly half (13/30) of the adenoplastic carcinomas showed the

TABLE 1-5

Predominant Type of Mucin in 51 Gastric Carcinomas: Surface Coat Type, Intracytoplasmic Type or Both

		Mainly SCM	SCM + ICM	Mainly ICM	Paucity of Mucin
sig	11	0	3	8	0
muc	5	0	0	5	0
pap	6	4	2	0	0
tub$_1$	9	6	3	0	0
tub$_2$	15	3	7	5	0
por	5	1	0	2	2
total	51	14	15	20	2

SCM: surface coat-type mucin

ICM: intracytoplasmic mucin

TABLE 1-6

Expression of Intracytoplasmic Mucins of Gastric and Intestinal
Type in 35 Gastric Carcinomas

		Intramucosal Lesion (m)				Invasive Lesion (sm⁻)				
		G	G+I	I	NS	G	G+I	I	NS	NL
sig	11	5	5	1	0	5	2	3	0	1
muc	5	0	4	1	0	0	4	1	0	0
pap	2	1	1	0	0	1	1	0	0	0
tub_1	3	1	2	0	0	0	0	0	0	3
tub_2	12	5	6	0	1	5	1	0	2	4
por	2	0	1	1	0	1	0	1	0	0
total	35	12	19	3	1	12	8	5	2	8

G: gastric type [neutral mucin and/or CPS class III mucin]

I: intestinal (or goblet cell) type [MOS and/or PA-SB-PH-PAS]

NS: not specified

NL: no lesion seen

predominance of surface coat-type mucin, while all diffuse carcinomas showed intracytoplasmic mucin. Five tub_2 adenocarcinomas predominantly with intracytoplasmic mucin included three adenocarcinomas with lymphoid stroma and two adenocarcinomas simulating an acinus-like arrangement.

Thirty-five carcinomas with intracytoplasmic mucin worth evaluating (ICM and SCMICM in Table 1-5) were further analyzed for the occurrence of mucins of the gastric or intestinal type. Neutral mucin (stained red both by the AB-PAS sequence and PAS after diastase digestion) and CPS class III mucin were regarded as gastric type, while PA/SB/PH/PAS and MOS reactions were regarded as intestinal (goblet cell) type. Results are summarized in Table 1-6 in which the reaction for the mucin in question was judged as positive even when only a few cells stained. About half of carcinomas of any histological type revealed an admixture of gastric and intestinal mucins. The dual expression of gastric and intestinal mucins was clearer in the mucosal lesion than in the submucosal or deeper lesion.

Comment: The division of gastric cancer into diffuse and adenoplastic types has been widely accepted so far because it allegedly reflects both biological behaviors and the histogenesis of the cancer.[4,5,11] The adenoplastic type is closely related to intestinal metaplasia, especially of the incomplete type,[12] while the diffuse type is believed to arise from nonintestinalized mucosa proper to the stomach.[5,11]

In the present study, however, the dual expression of gastric- and intestinal-type mucins was confirmed in gastric cancer cells irrespective of histological typing. Signet ring cell carcinoma occasionally contains cancer cells of the goblet cell type, while the demonstration of pyloric gland mucin in adenoplastic carcinoma is fairly common. Mucinous adenocarcinoma is predominantly composed of signet ring cells of the goblet cell type, and cancer cells of adenocarcinoma with lymphoid stroma, classified as tub_2, mainly show the properties of pyloric gland cells. Therefore, it is concluded that any type of gastric cancer possesses similar properties with regard to the bidirectional differentiation into gastric and intestinal type epithelial cells.[28,35,36]

As commented in the introduction, the most apparent cell biological difference between the two types is whether the cancer cell acts as a dissociative cell in a stochastic flow system or if it acts as an associative cell in a

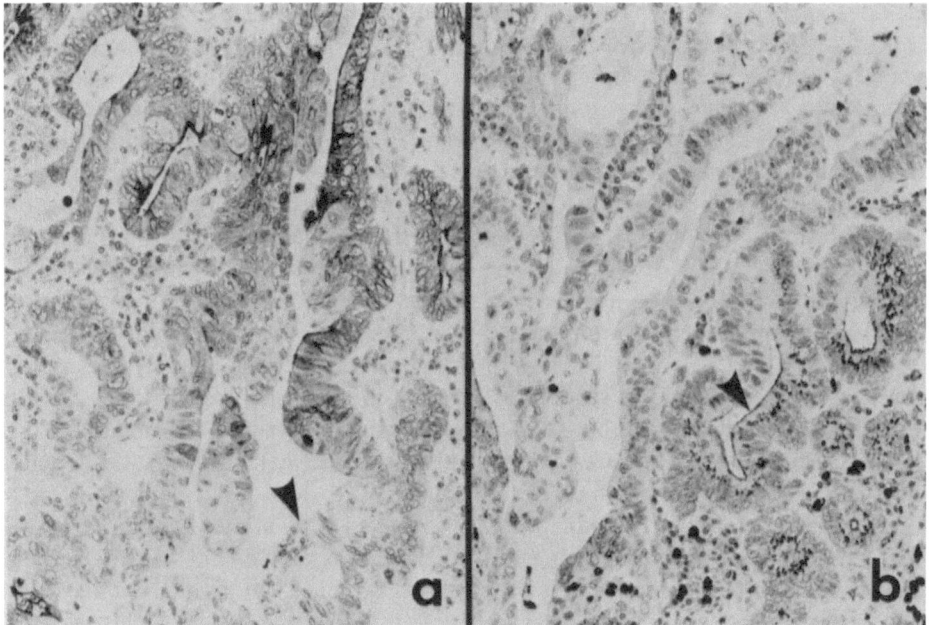

Fig. 1-5. Organoid marker expression in invasive tubular adenocarcinoma. PAP method for SC (a) and lysozyme (b). Hematoxylin counterstain, ×150.

Longitudinally arranged tubular area is positive for SC and negative for lysozyme, whereas the localization pattern is reversed in an associated gland-like area (arrowheads). The latter area is also reactive to CPS class III.

pipe line system.[8,9] In noncancerous gastric mucosa, the generative cells of intestinal metaplasia with remaining atrophic pyloric glands at the bottom (types A and B of Tsutsumi et al,[57] corresponding to the incomplete type),[12] differentiate bidirectionally upward to intestinal-type cells including goblet cells and downward to pyloric gland cells.[57] Accordingly, the similarity of the mode of differentiation among proliferative cells in gastric cancer of any histological type and generative cells in "incompletely" intestinalized mucosa is quite meaningful.

3. ORGANOID DIFFERENTIATION IN ADVANCED GASTRIC CANCER

The expression of the various histochemical markers in advanced gastric cancer is not necessarily discordant. Some degrees of organoid or polarized differentiation have been demonstrated in certain tumors. Several representative pictures of the organoid differentiation are shown below.

Figure 1-5 displays immunostaining for SC and lysozyme in a tubular adenocarcinoma. Cancerous epithelium is arranged in elongated and irregularly branching tubules associated with small glandular structures. SC immunoreactivity is mainly seen in the elongated tubular areas, while lysozyme is localized predominantly in the associated gland-like areas. The latter part is also focally positive for CPS class III reactivity. Although neoplastic goblet-like cells are absent, the morphological and histochemical features strongly suggest that the adenoplastic cancer cells imitate the "incompletely" intestinalized epithelium, which consists of strongly SC-reactive absorptive-type cells and lysozyme-positive atrophic pyloric glands at the bottom. A similar organoid differentiation has sometimes been observed at the invading site of other adenoplastic carcinomas, in which tumor cells protruding papillarily into cancerous lumina exhibit the properties of neutral mucin-containing surface epithelium or MOS-positive goblet-like cells, while tumor cells forming an associated gland-like structure and facing toward the interstitium reveal CPS class III reactivity, as described by Katsuyama et al.[30]

Regarding the differentiation toward Paneth cells in adenoplastic carcinomas, see below.

Figure 1-6 shows consecutive sections of adenocarcinoma (classified as tub$_2$) stained for HID-AB, lysozyme, SC, and CEA/NCA. The upper half is composed of both scattered goblet-like cells predominantly containing sialomucin (MOS reaction being also positive) and lysozyme immunoreactive cells with an abortive trabecular or tubular arrangement. In this area, CPS class III mucin is further identified (see Fig. 1-7d), but CEA/NCA is only focally and weakly positive in goblet-like cells. On the contrary, most cancer cells in the lower half show strong CEA/NCA immunoreactivity, but almost no mucin or lysozyme. SC is localized in both areas with stronger staining in the lower half. H&E stain does not discriminate morphologic differences between these two areas except for the presence of goblet-like cells in the former. The number of mitoses and the degree of nuclear atypia are nearly the same. Cancer cells in the former area may have characteristics of glandular neck cells differentiating toward the pyloric gland and goblet cells, while the latter area is solely composed of cancer cells differentiating toward surface-lining cells probably of intestinal absorptive type.

Figure 1-7 illustrates a high power view of the upper area of Figure 1-6. The cancer cells consist of both goblet-like large cells and small immature-looking cells. The goblet-like cells contain predominantly sialomucin and partially sulfomucin; they show a positive MOS reaction and weak CEA/NCA immunoreactivity. The small cells reveal neutral mucin with a positive CPS class III reaction. Lysozyme and SC are further localized predominantly in the small cells. The small cells are likely to have the properties of generative cells partially expressing pyloric gland nature. These histochemical findings indicate that cancer cells are capable of retaining their cellular characteristics, which they are destined to express even after the structural organization is completely lost. A similar phenomenon has been commonly encountered in mucinous adenocarcinomas or signet ring cell carcinomas with histochemical characteristics of goblet cell mucin. Namely, cancer cells reactive to lysozyme, SC, and CPS class III are often small in size and haphazardly intermingled with goblet-like mature signet ring cells.

Figure 1-8 illustrates a remarkable regional distribution of CEA/NCA and lysozyme in signet ring cell carcinoma.[35] The expression pattern of both markers forms a good contrast; CEA/NCA immunoreactive cancer cells are small in size, look immature and show numerous mitotic figures (Fig. 1-8c), whereas cells in the lysozyme-positive area reveal a fairly typical appearance of signet ring cells and scarcely show mitoses (Fig. 1-8d). The latter cells further focally display SC immunoreactivity, sulfomucin, and CPS class III reactivity, representing rather mature cells differentiating toward the pyloric gland. Almost no mucin is identified in the CEA/NCA positive immature cancer cells, which probably represents an actively proliferating component in the signet ring cell carcinoma. Infiltrating diffuse carcinomas with a scirrhous growth pattern are commonly composed of small-sized and immature-looking cancer cells with striking immunoreactivity for CEA/NCA. The concurrent occurrence of CEA/NCA and lysozyme, SC or CPS class III mucin in these scirrhous cancer cells is not infrequently seen.

Figure 1-9 shows a rather exceptional expression of lysozyme in goblet-like mature signet ring cells, which are also positive for CEA/NCA. The expression of CEA/NCA in goblet-like cancer cells is a very common phenomenon. Many of the signet ring cells in mucinous adenocarcinoma react positively to

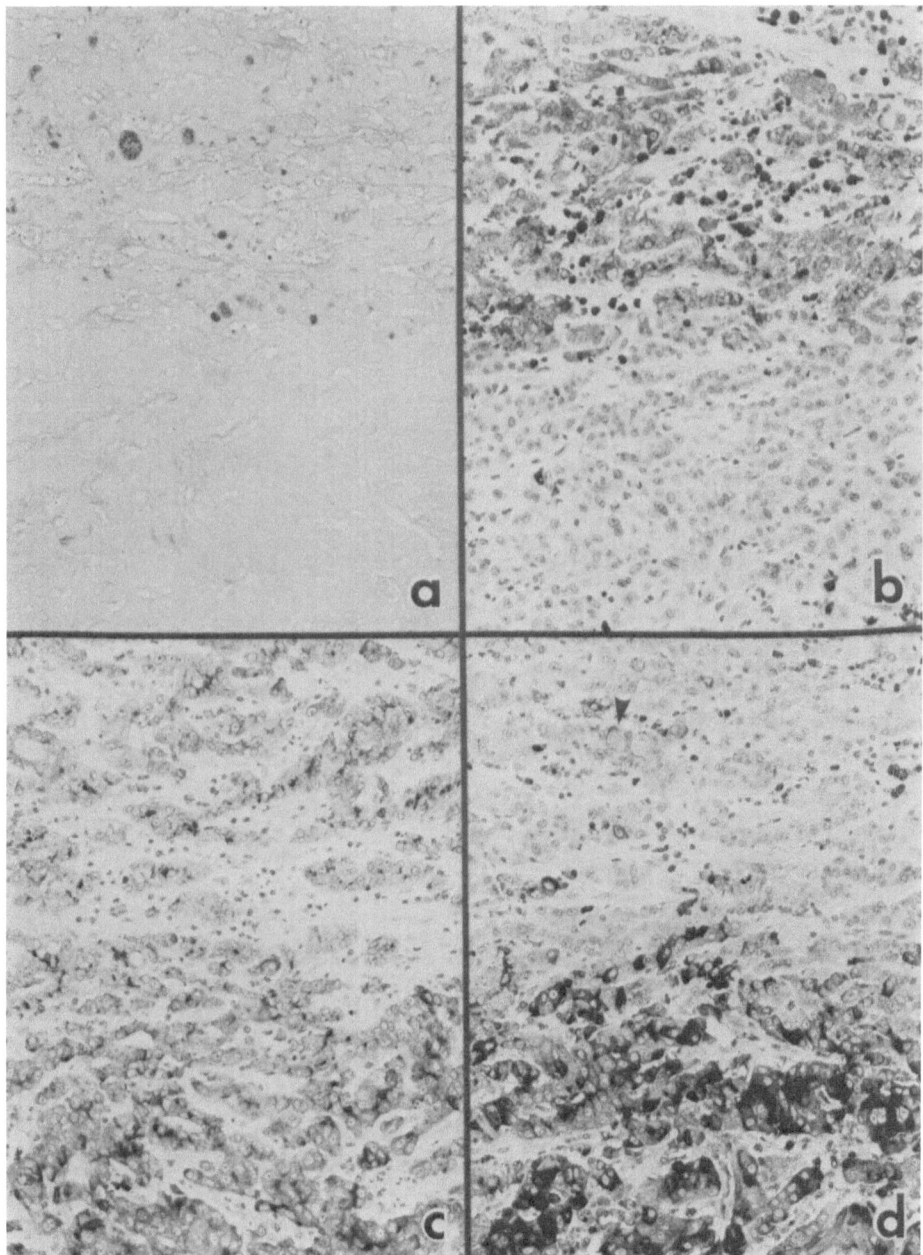

Fig. 1-6. Contrasted marker localization in rather poorly differentiated area of tub$_2$ adenocarcinoma. HID-AB (a) and PAP method for lysozyme (b), SC (c) and CEA/NCA (d). Hematoxylin counterstain (b–d), ×150.

Cancer cells in the upper half area are positive for lysozyme but negative for CEA/NCA except for a few goblet-like cells (arrowhead), in which acidic mucin (predominantly sialomucin) is demonstrated. The lower half is composed of cells strongly positive for CEA/NCA but unreactive to lysozyme and mucin. SC is detected in both halves with stronger staining of the latter.

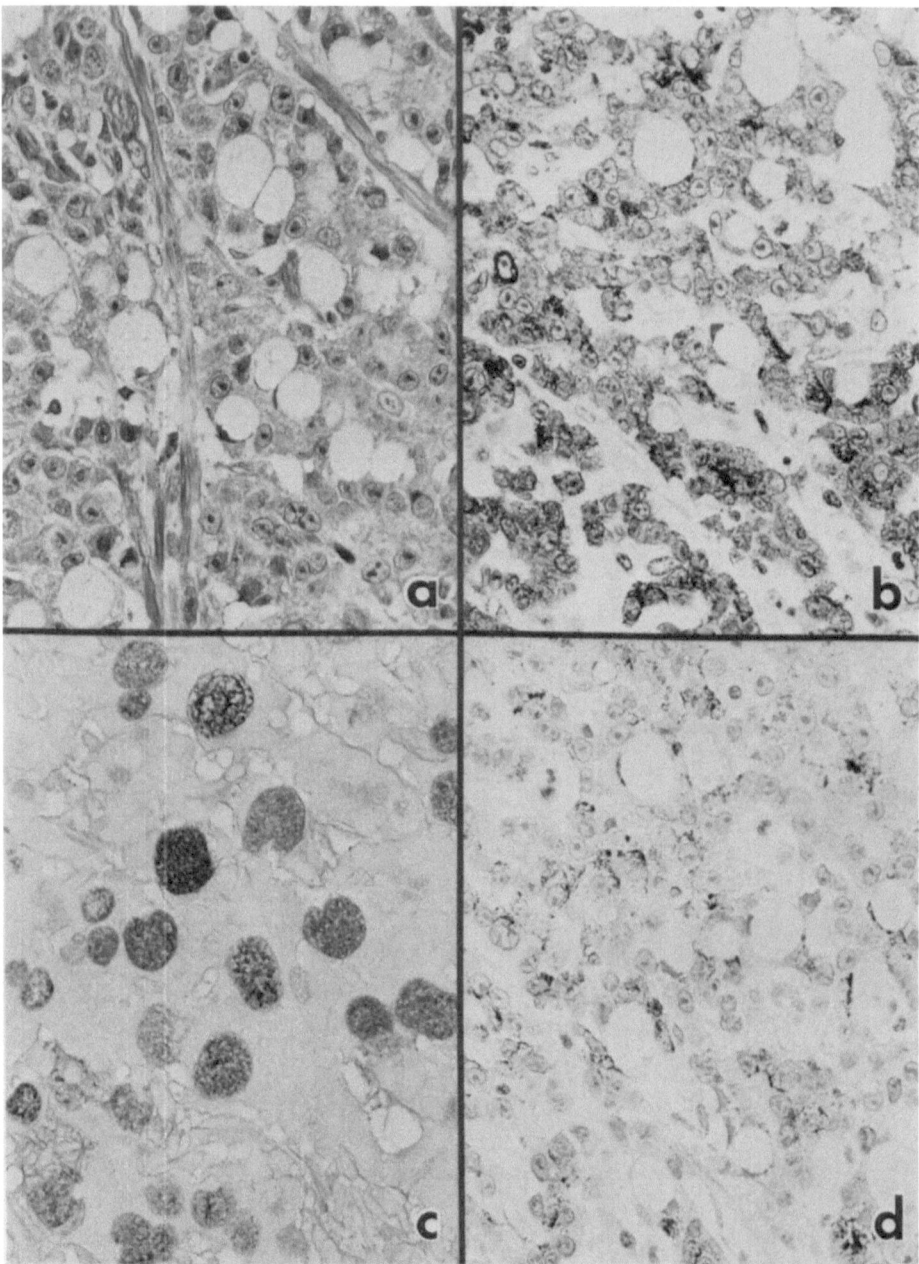

Fig. 1-7. Mixed differentiation toward goblet cells and pyloric gland cells in the upper half area of Figure 1-6. H&E (a), PAP method for SC (b), HID-AB (c) and CPS class III (d). Hematoxylin counterstain, ×400.

The tumor consists of both goblet-like large cells containing acidic mucin and immature-looking small cells with positive reactions to SC, lysozyme, and CPS class III. The former cells are also reactive to MOS. Even after the loss of structural organization, haphazardly differentiated tumor cells retain the nature of marker expression in their nonneoplastic counterparts.

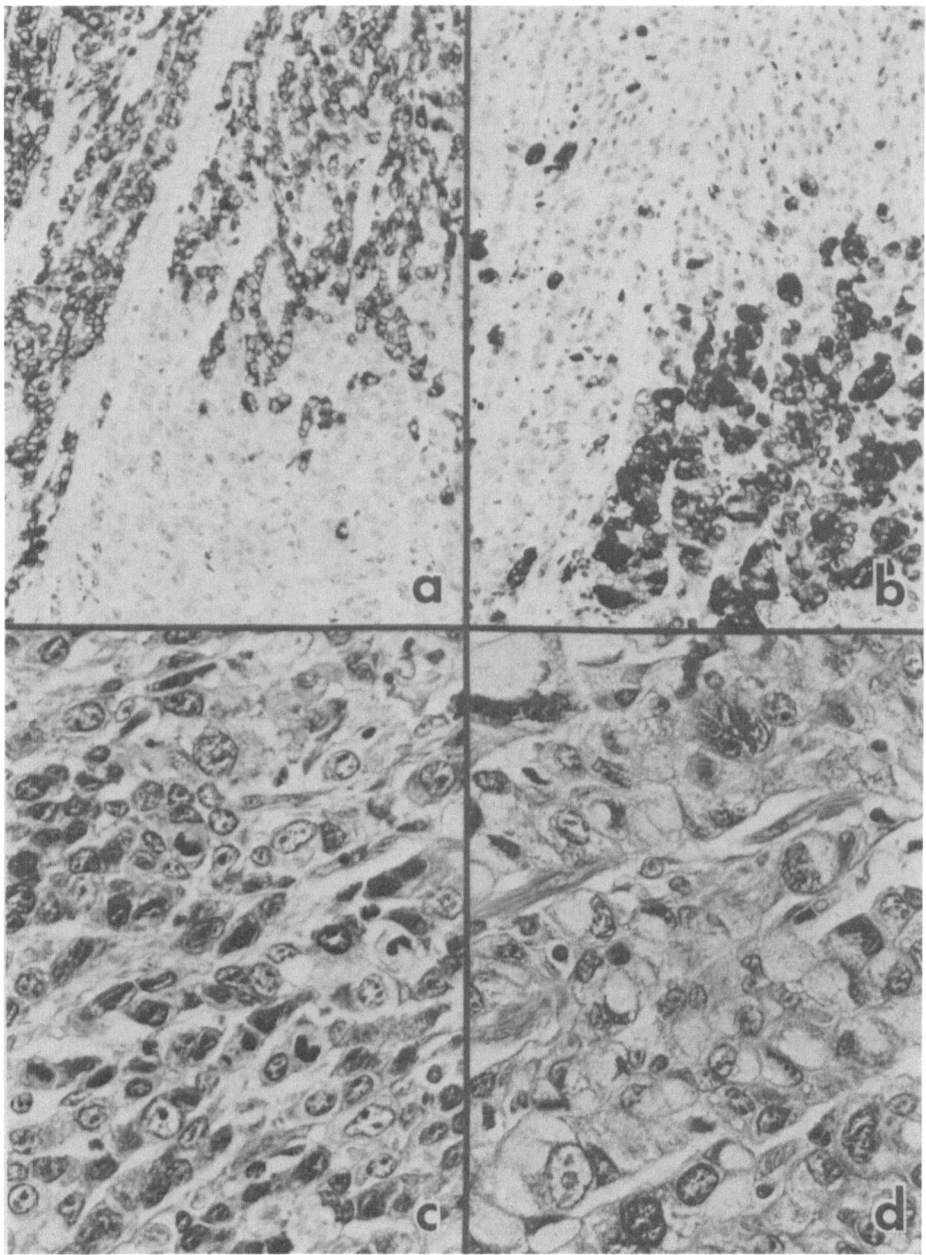

Fig. 1-8. Reciprocal distribution pattern of CEA/NCA (a) and lysozyme (b) and high power view of CEA/NCA-positive area (c) and lysozyme-positive area (d). a & b: PAP method with hematoxylin counterstain, ×150; c & d: H&E, ×480.

Cancer cells in the CEA/NCA-positive area are small in size and look immature, while the lysozyme-positive area is solely composed of fairly large signet ring cells with CPS class III reactivity. Mitotic figures are frequently noted in the former area.

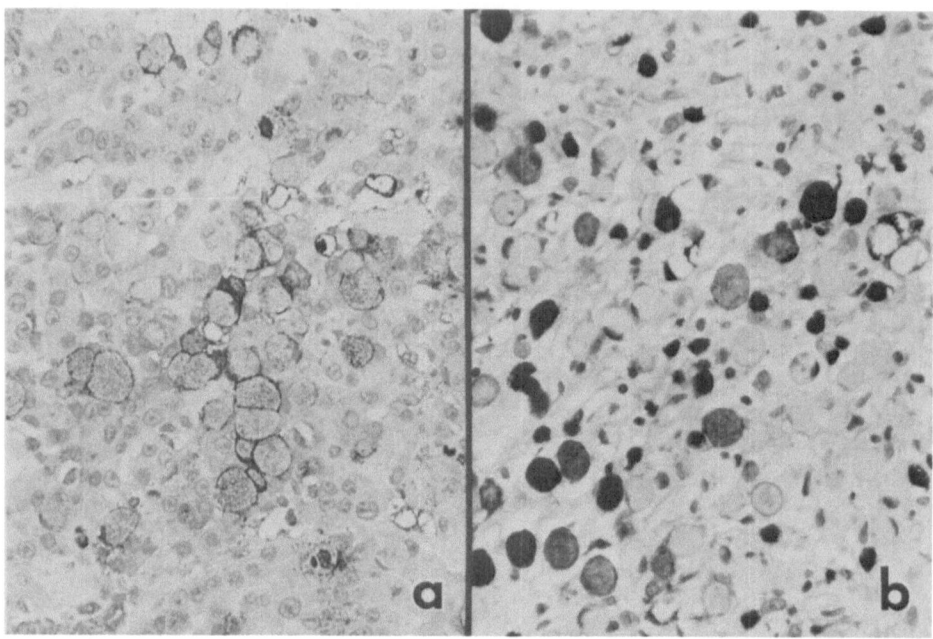

Fig. 1-9. Disorganized expression of CEA and lysozyme in mature signet ring cells of the goblet cell type. PAP method for CEA/NCA (a) and lysozyme (b). Hematoxylin counterstain, ×300.
  Mature signet ring cells, which are strongly reactive to alcian blue and MOS, are occasionally positive for lysozyme deep in their cytoplasm. CEA/NCA shows cell membrane staining. These marker expressions are unexpected, since nonneoplastic goblet cells lack both markers.

antiCEA antibody. However, this is also regarded as a deviation occurring during the neoplastic progression, since nonneoplastic goblet cells lack the antigen. Although such unexpected and disorganized expressions of the marker substances are one of the characteristic features of advanced cancer cells, the above-mentioned rather organized or polarized differentiations of cancer cells should be emphasized again.

4. ZONAL DIFFERENTIATION OF SIGNET RING CANCER CELLS IN THE MUCOSA

Here, peculiar zonal (lamellar or layered) differentiations shown by intramucosally located gastric cancer cells are described.[35,36] Careful observation of 40 intramucosal lesions from the above series disclosed a characteristic zonal (lamellar or layered) distribu-

tion pattern of the markers in some cancers. No mucosal lesions worth evaluating were left in 11 advanced carcinomas, especially of pap and por types. As shown in Table 1-7, lysozyme and CPS class III reactivities tended to localize in cancer cells occupying the bottom or lower half layer of the mucosa, whereas CEA/NCA and MOS reactivities had a tendency to be localized in cancer cells occupying the upper layer of the mucosa. Immunoreactive SC was found to be localized in cancer cells occupying either the lower or upper layer of the mucosa. It is apparent that the zonation pattern of the markers reflects well those seen in noncancerous gastric mucosa. The localization of SC in the lower layer of cancerous mucosa is likely to be a reflection of that attribute of nonmetaplastic gastric mucosa with chronic inflammation, while SC seen in the upper layer of the cancerous mucosa probably mimics the pattern in intestinalized epithelia with SC-negative pyloric glands at their bot-

TABLE 1-7
Zonal Differentiation of Gastric Carcinomas in the Mucosa

Marker Zonation	SC		Lysozyme Lower	CEA/NCA Upper	CPS,III Lower	MOS Upper
	Lower	Upper				
sig	11(3)	4(3)	1	5(2)	5(3)	6(2)	2(2)
muc	5(0)	0	0	0	0	1	0
pap	2(1)	0	0	1(1)	0	1(1)	0
tub$_1$	8(6)	2(2)	2(2)	4(4)	3(2)	6(5)	4(3)
tub$_2$	13(6)	3(2)	3(2)	6(4)	7(3)	6(3)	4(3)
por	1(0)	0	0	0	0	0	0
total	40(16)	9(7)	6(4)	16(11)	15(8)	20(11)	10(8)

( ): indicates the number of early carcinomas

toms. Early carcinomas more frequently showed the organized differentiation pattern than advanced carcinomas (Table 1-7). This fact suggests that less severely destroyed mucosal structures are required for the formation of the above-mentioned zonation pattern. The intramucosal zonation pattern, however, was seen only focally in most tumors judged positive. The exception included two of three early signet ring cell carcinomas, which clearly revealed the organized zonation pattern of the markers including SC, lysozyme, CEA/NCA and CPS class III mucin in any area of the mucosal lesion (Fig. 1-10). In addition, two of 22 adenoplastic carcinomas (tub$_1$ and tub$_2$ confined to the mucosa) also displayed the zonal distribution of lysozyme and CEA/NCA widely but not in every area of the cancerous mucosa, whereas the zonation of SC and CPS class III mucin was focal and abortive. Generally, the zonal differentiation shown by adenoplastic carcinomas was often partial (Fig. 1-11a). The expression of CEA/NCA in adenoplastic carcinomas was frequently so marked and exaggerated that all of the cancer cells stained strongly for the antigen (Fig. 1-11b). In a similar sense, we clarified the abnormal ultrastructural localization of CEA on the plasma membranes of individual adenoplastic cancer cells.[37]

To confirm the universality of the above-mentioned phenomenon seen in early signet ring cell carcinomas, an additional 50 tumors (38 mucosal cancers and 12 submucosally invading cancers) were analyzed both with the indirect immunoperoxidase method for SC, lysozyme, pepsinogen II, and CEA and with mucin histochemistry by AB-PAS, HID-AB, and CPS class III. CEA was visualized by a conventional antiCEA antibody previously absorbed with the PCA extract of human spleen. Results are summarized in Table 1-8. Representative pictures are shown in Figure 1-12, in which a rather well developed pyloric gland-like zone is observed in the lower half of the mucosa. Compare the width of CPS class III-positive zone of Figure 1-12b with that of Figure 1-10a.

Many signet ring cell carcinomas revealed a fairly constant zonation pattern of the marker expression as expected. The frequency and degree of the organized differentiation were not related to the degree of intestinalization in the surrounding mucosa, the site of cancer in the stomach, or to the age and sex of patients. The perfection of the organized differentiation was apparently dependent on the degree of persistence of noncancerous epithelial cells. Namely, in the lamina propria mucosae with well-preserved noncancerous epithelium, signet ring cancer cells differentiate quite well in a like manner to noncancerous cells. The zonal expression for CEA was most stable, then reactivities to lysozyme, CPS class III

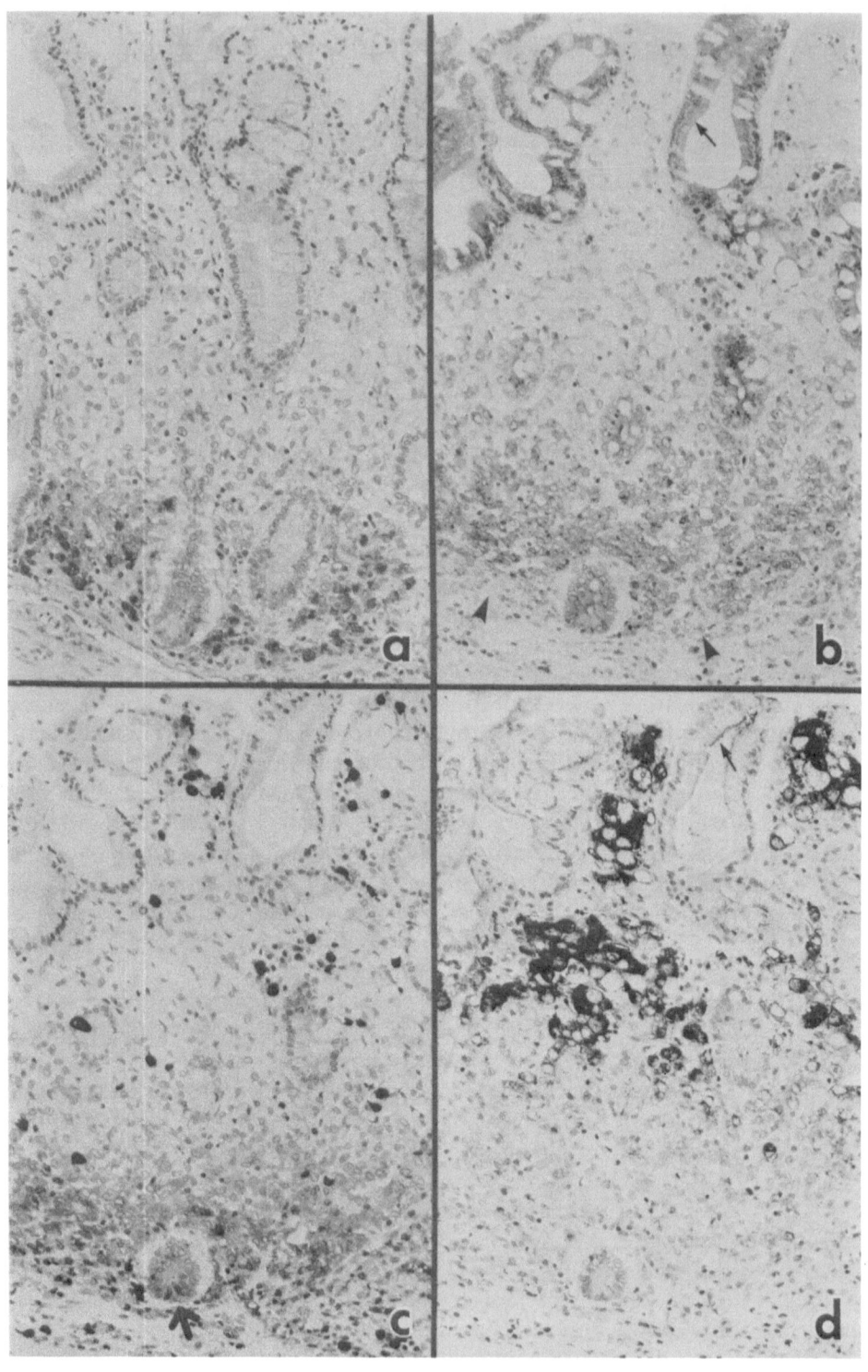

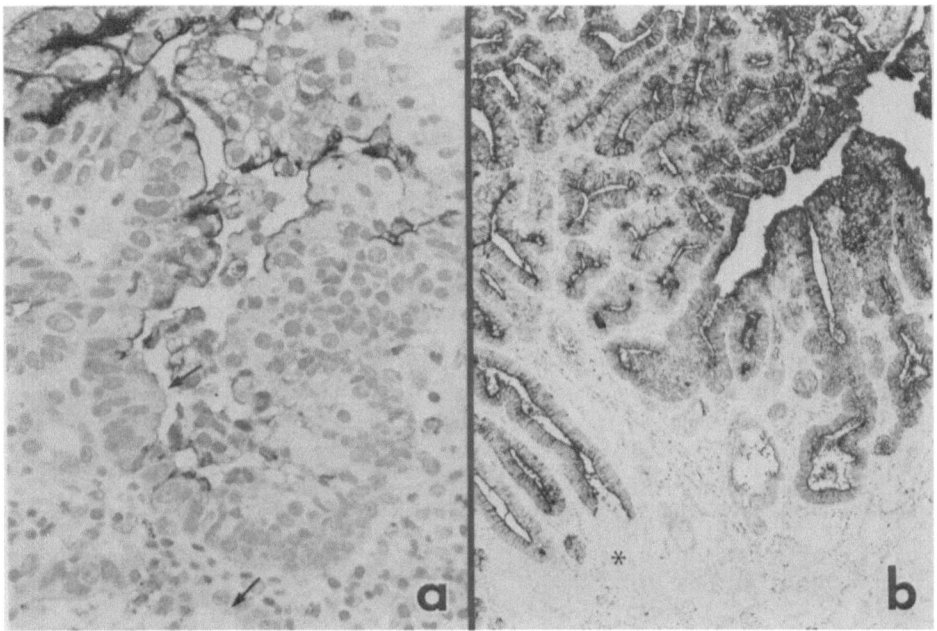

Fig. 1-11. CEA/NCA in adenoplastic carcinoma. PAP method with hematoxylin counterstain, ×300 (a) and ×60 (b).

Polarized expression of CEA/NCA is focally visualized in (a) where the antigen is localized on the apical plasma membranes of cells in the upper part of the cancerous tubule but cells in the lower part are negative (arrows). CEA/NCA is occasionally expressed so excessively in every adenoplastic cancer cell as to lose the polarized pattern (b). Asterisk indicates noncancerous pyloric glands remaining at the bottom of cancerous epithelium.

and SC followed it. Among the latter three markers, the width of the positive zone was broadest for SC and narrowest for CPS class III mucin, representing well the expression pattern in noncancerous epithelium. When carefully observed, cancer cells at the lowermost narrow zone of the mucosa were only weakly positive or even negative for SC (see Fig. 1-10), especially in the tumors with a wide CPS class III reactive zone. This certainly reflects the negative SC staining of mature pyloric gland cells in noncancerous mucosa.

CEA immunoreactivity in mature signet ring cells and submucosally invading immature-looking cells shown by the absorbed antibody was fundamentally identical to CEA/NCA immunoreactivity as detected by the

←—————————————————————→

Fig. 1-10. Typical zonal differentiation of signet ring cell carcinoma in the mucosa. CPS class III (a) and PAP method for SC (b), lysozyme (c) and CEA/NCA (d). Hematoxylin counterstain, ×150.

Layered distribution of markers is evident in any mucosal area of this signet ring cell carcinoma. Small-sized cells in the bottom layer are positive for CPS class III, SC and lysozyme, while CEA/NCA is strongly expressed in mature signet ring cells in the upper layer. SC is almost negative in the lowermost narrow zone (arrowheads) where CPS class III-reactive slightly larger-sized cells are distributed. SC-positive cancer cells may represent mitogenic cancer cells (see text). Intestinalized epithelia are positive for SC and CEA/NCA (thin arrows). Scattered cells strongly positive for lysozyme are granulocytes and macrophages in the stroma, and Paneth cells (thick arrow).

TABLE 1-8
Zonal Differentiation of Signet Ring Cancer Cells in the Mucosa: Analysis Using 50 Early Carcinomas

Marker	Zonation*	+++	++	+	−	Reversed**
SC	lower	10(3)	9(2)	13(2)	13(5)	5(0)
lysozyme	lower	17(4)	18(4)	10(1)	5(3)	0(0)
pepsinogen II***	lower	2(0)	9(3)	9(1)	27(6)	0(0)
CEA	upper	32(7)	13(4)	5(1)	0(0)	0(0)
CPS class III	lower	17(4)	13(1)	13(3)	7(4)	0(0)
sulfomucin	lower	5(4)	7(2)	8(1)	30(5)	0(0)

( ): indicates the number of "sm" cancer (total 12 cases)

* The zonal distribution of marker is seen in most (+++), less than two thirds (++), less than one third (+), or none (-) of areas of the mucosal lesion.

** The reversed pattern of SC is seen in five tumors, in which SC immunoreactivity is demonstrated in the upper layer of the mucosa.

*** Immunostaining of pepsinogen II was not done for three specimens.

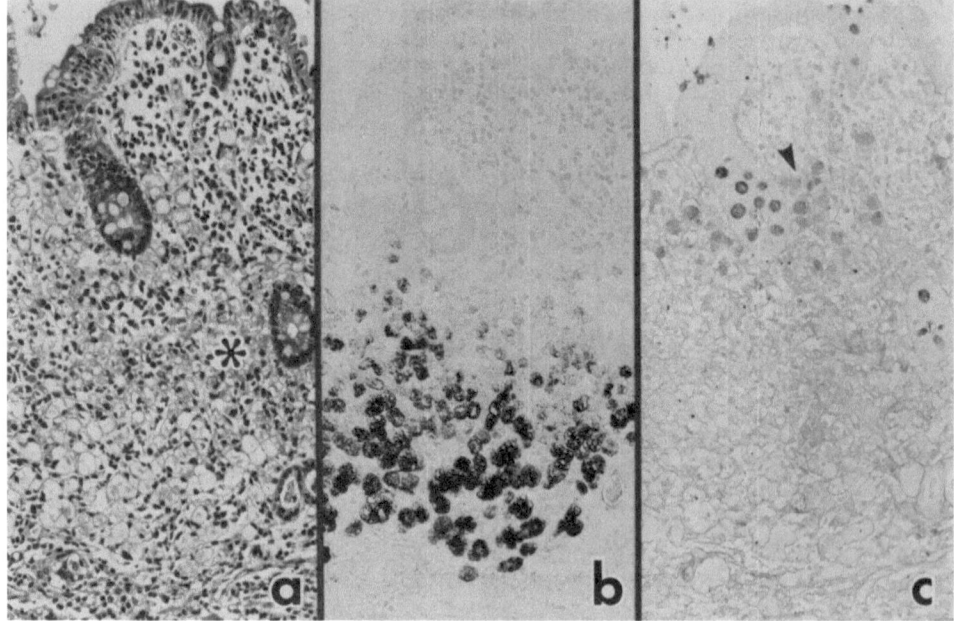

Fig. 1-12. Zonal differentiation of signet ring cell carcinoma in the mucosa. H&E (a), CPS class III with methyl green counterstain (b) and HID-AB (c), ×120.
　　Bidirectional differentiation of intramucosally occupying signet ring cells is evident. The lower half layer contains well matured signet ring cells of the pyloric gland type, while signet ring cells distributed in the upper layer are faintly alcianophilic (arrowhead) without CPS class III reactivity. The middle zone marked by asterisk is composed of small-sized immature-looking cells intermingled with CPS class III-reactive cells.

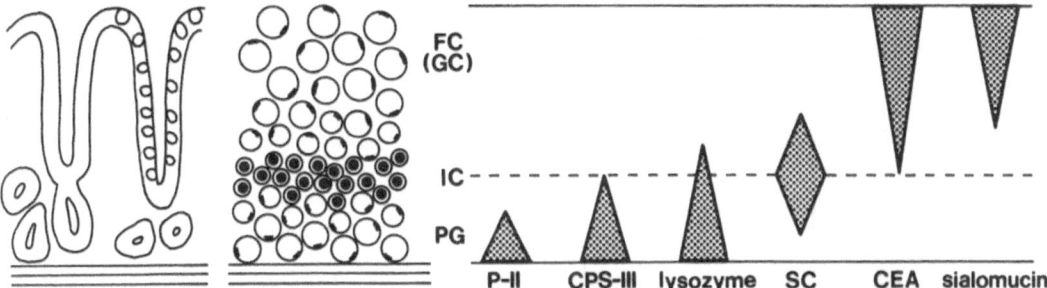

Fig. 1-13. Schematic representation of the zonal expression of markers in signet ring cell carcinoma in the mucosa.

FC(GC): signet ring cells of the surface epithelial cell type (occasionally goblet cell type)
IC: immature-looking cancer cells
PG: signet ring cells of the pyloric gland type
P-II: pepsinogen II

unabsorbed antibody, although some decrease of the number and staining intensity of positive cells was noted. The width of the CEA-positive zone in the "upper" layer varied from tumor to tumor: In some tumors, CEA was positive in most cells except for the lowermost narrow zone of the mucosa, while other tumors contained CEA-positive signet ring cells only in the uppermost zone. Less pronouncedly, the variation of the width of the positive zone was noted for SC, lysozyme, and CPS class III mucin. Thus, double positivity for CEA and SC, lysozyme or CPS class III mucin in cells in the same layer was occasionally noted. The zonation pattern of the markers is schematically illustrated in Figure 1-13.

Pepsinogen II, a marker of both pyloric and fundic glands, was less frequently expressed in signet ring cancer cells, but if positive, it showed a distinct zonation pattern at the lower layer of the mucosa. Sulfomucin in cancer cells occupying the bottom layer of the mucosa certainly reflects the fact that atrophic pyloric glands are occasionally positive for sulfomucin. Furthermore, by AB-PAS staining 39 of 50 tumors showed a predominance of neutral mucin in signet ring cancer cells. Acid mucin predominance was seen only in four tumors. Sialomucin-positive mature signet ring cells were fairly consistently scattered in the upper layer of the mucosa in all but three tumors, although the staining intensity

with alcian blue was mostly weak (Fig. 1-12c). The sialomucin-positive signet ring cancer cells are not necessarily a counterpart of goblet cells, since hyperplastic or regenerative foveolar cells without intestinal metaplasia often stain weakly positive for sialomucin.

When we observe intramucosal lesions of signet ring cell carcinoma, taking into account the above information, the multilamellar pattern formed by signet ring cancer cells is easily recognized even in H&E preparations (Figs. 1-12a and 1-14a). Typical signet ring cells occur in the upper and bottom layers of the mucosa, whereas immature-looking small cancer cells with scanty or finely vacuolated cytoplasm are distributed at the junctional zone between the above two layers, which correspond to the level of the generative zone of normal or inflamed antral mucosa. The immature-looking cancer cells in the junctional zone occasionally show mitoses. Signet ring cells in the upper layer are generally larger than those in the bottom layer. In many specimens with tumors arising from the fundic mucosa, the oxyntic glands especially adjacent to the tumors showed antralization, resulting in the formation of pseudopyloric glands with or without remaining parietal cells. Chief cells were absent from the antralized mucosa.

In a few cancers arising from the fundic mucosa with fairly intact oxyntic glands, the immature cancer cell layer occupied the level

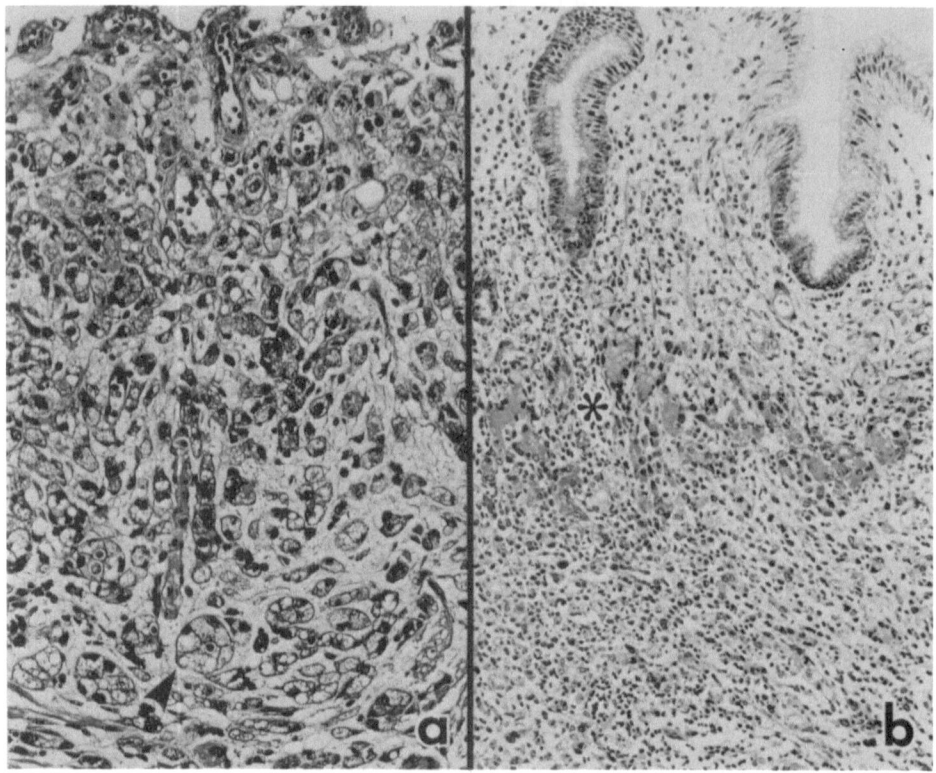

Fig. 1-14. Intramucosal lesion of signet ring cell carcinoma in the oxyntic mucosa. H&E; ×
200 (a) and ×120 (b).
    Signet ring cancer cells in the lower layer of the mucosa occasionally reveal an acinus-like
arrangement (arrowhead) simulating (pseudo) pyloric glands (a). In a few cases, the zone of immature-looking cancer cells lies at the level of the generative zone of normal oxyntic mucosa (b,
asterisk), and signet ring cells are scattered in the lamina propria mucosae above and below this
zone.

of the generative zone of normal fundic mucosa, but the differentiation toward parietal
cells or chief cells by cancer cells occupying
the lower half layer was hardly evident (Fig.
1-14b).[17,71] The cancer cells in the bottom
layer with histochemical characteristics of pyloric gland cells (pyloric gland-type signet ring
cells) varied in their morphological features
from case to case. In some tumors, (e.g., the
tumor in Figure 1-10), the pyloric gland-type
cancer cells looked so immature and small-
sized that we were unable to recognize the
junctional zone. In many such tumors, not
only lysozyme and CPS class III but also SC
reactivities were seen with a bottom-layered
pattern.

In other tumors, the pyloric gland-type cancer cells were so well developed as to form an
acinus-like arrangement (Fig. 1-14a). In the
latter case, pepsinogen II immunoreactive pyloric gland-type cancer cells were rather
frequently encountered, while immunoreactivity for SC was scarcely seen. In one tumor,
cancer cells in the lower half mucosal layer
showed quite a well organized arrangement
simulating normal pyloric glands, while cancer cells in the upper half layer were arranged
in abortive tubules consisting of columnar
atypical cells (Fig. 1-15). SC was exclusively
detected in the latter cancer cells, resulting in
a reversed distribution pattern of SC. The mature pyloric gland-like cancer cells were posi-

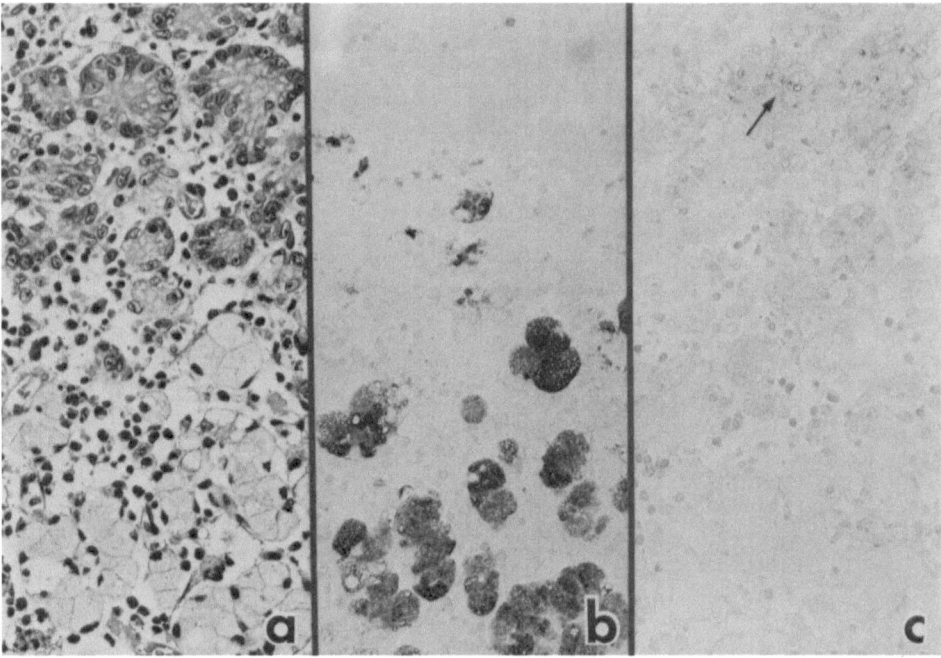

Fig. 1-15. Signet ring cell carcinoma with a reversed SC expression in the mucosa. H&E (a), CPS class III (b) and indirect immunoperoxidase method for SC (c). Methyl green counterstain (b & c), ×240.

This intramucosal cancer looks like mature pyloric glands (SC-negative) in the lower half of the mucosa, while cells in the upper layer display a tubular differentiation with SC immunoreactivity (arrow). The mode of marker expression corresponds to that in "incompletely" intestinalized mucosa.

tive for lysozyme, while the tubularly arranged part contained scattered goblet-like cells of small size and showed CEA immunoreactivity in cancer cells near the gastric lumen. Therefore, this cancer tissue resembled intestinalized mucosa with remaining pyloric glands at the bottom, not only morphologically, but also histochemically. The reversed pattern of SC staining was encountered in five tumors, three of which were focally associated with characteristics of adenoplastic carcinomas.

A varying number of signet ring cells with intracytoplasmic lumen (ICL) were seen in 29 of 50 early signet ring cell carcinomas examined. Four tumors showed many signet ring cells of the ICL type, 10 tumors showed a modest number, and 15 tumors contained a few. Ultrastructurally, the plasma membranes

of ICL have been described as comparable to the absorptive surface of intestinal-type epithelial cells.[30] ICL has been reported as a specific structure of various adenocarcinoma cells, especially of breast carcinoma.[72] In fact, signet ring cells with ICL were easily detected in tumors with admixed adenoplastic components. However, with AB-PAS staining the mucin in ICL was often neutral, but not acidic. Signet ring cells of the pyloric gland type also occasionally formed ICLs, as Figure 1-16 illustrates. Therefore, the detection of signet ring cells of the ICL type does not necessarily indicate their intestinal differentiation.

Discussion: It is worthy of note that gastric cancer cells in the mucosa often simulate the polarity of differentiation of their noncancer-

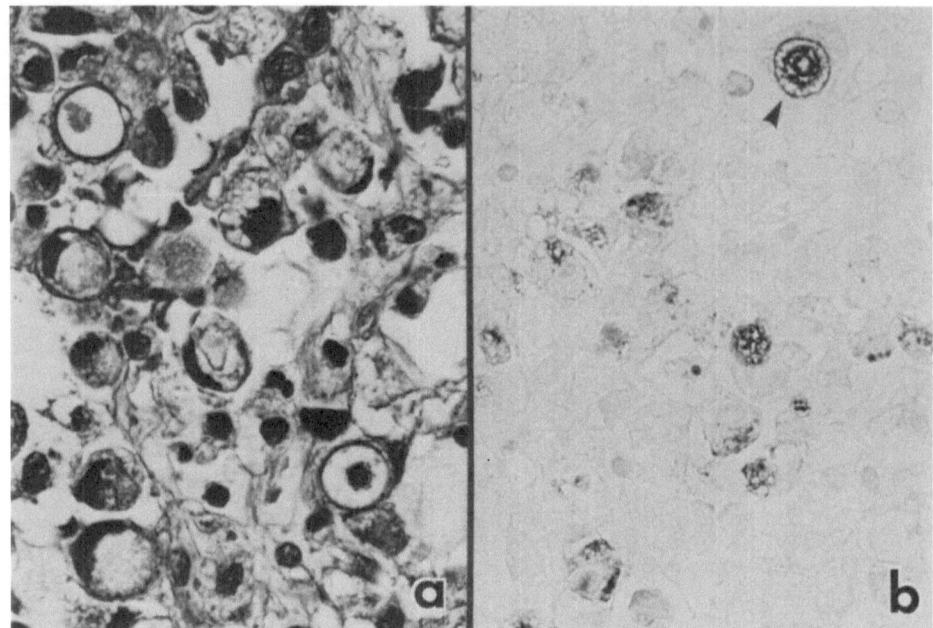

Fig. 1-16. Signet ring cells of the intracytoplasmic lumen (ICL) type. H&E (a) and CPS class III (b), ×600.

A varying number of signet ring cells with ICL are not infrequently intermingled with ordinary signet ring cells. They are often present in tumors focally showing a tubular component. Signet ring cells of the ICL type reactive to CPS class III are occasionally observed (b, arrowhead).

ous counterparts. The polarity is expressed as the zonal (lamellar or layered) distribution of the glycoprotein antigens and mucins of the pyloric gland and goblet cell types.[9,29,30,35,36] Such organized differentiation in the mucosa is more stable and more synchronized in signet ring cell carcinoma than in adenoplastic carcinoma.[35] Early cancer with rather intact noncancerous epithelial structures more clearly shows the zonation pattern than advanced cancer with severely distorted noncancerous epithelium. These findings suggest that the cancer cell differentiation is regulated by the microenvironment in the mucosa, as is shown in normal tissues.[73] In other words, stromal elements in the lamina propria mucosae are able to control the differentiation and growth of cancer cells, as has been described by Fujita.[8,9,74]

Tsuchihashi has clearly proved that mucosal microvascular networks in the stomach form a functional trilayered zonation corresponding to three such epithelial layers as glands, generative cells and surface lining cells.[75] Watanabe emphasized with experimental models of radiation pneumonia the importance of preceding changes of vascular and lymphatic microcirculation in pulmonary alveoli for the progression of interstitial inflammation and the formation of fibrosis.[76] Intact mucosal microcirculatory networks should, therefore, be greatly involved in establishing the cancer-regulating microenviroment. Meanwhile, certain degrees of the organoid differentiation were demonstrated at the site of invasion of some advanced carcinomas. This fact suggests a partial induction of cancer cell differentiation by the stromal elements even at extramucosal sites.

Quite interestingly, it has been clarified with [³H]-thymidine autoradiography that cancer cells with proliferation ability in the mucosal lesion of early signet ring cell carcinoma are solely distributed in the zone of the generative cells found in noncancerous mucosa.[9,77] These mitogenic cells are equivalent to immature cancer cells located between mature signet ring cells in the upper layer and pyloric gland-type signet ring cells in the bottom layer. With rare exceptions, typical signet ring cells filled with cytoplasmic mucin have been shown to lack mitotic activity.[9,77] Thus, the initial site of carcinogenesis in signet ring cell carcinoma must be logically in the zone of generative cells, as has been pointed out by Fujita.[9] CEA-positive mature signet ring cells in the upper layer of the mucosa react strongly to PAS, and weakly and inconsistently to alcian blue in most cases. Such histochemical reactions probably reflect the properties of hyperplastic or regenerative gastric foveolar epithelium. Katsuyama et al demonstrated the properties of gastric surface epithelial cell-type mucin in these mature signet ring cells with the galactose oxidase-Schiff (GOS) sequence.[30]

From our limited experience, MOS-positive and strongly alcianophilic signet ring cells (goblet cell-type), which are frequently present in mucinous adenocarcinoma, are also found in some early signet ring cell carcinomas. The presence of PA-SB-PH-PAS reactive goblet cell mucin in such signet ring cells has been described by Katsuyama et al.[30] It is concluded that neoplastic cells in the mucosa with signet ring cell carcinoma proliferate in the generative immature cell layer and differentiate upward to the surface to become surface epithelial-type cells or goblet-type cells, and downward to the deeper layer to become pyloric gland-type cells, as has been reported independently by groups of Katsuyama,[29,30] Fujita[9,74] and ourselves.[35,36] It is quite reasonable that the mitogenic and immature-looking cancer cells in the mucosa are a neoplastic counterpart of totipotent stem cells in the nonneoplastic mucosa. They, which may be called "malignant stem cells,"[78-81] are capable of mitosis and of differentiation under the appropriate influence of the mucosal microenvironment.

On the other hand, it has been shown by Fujita that adenoplastic cancer cells in the mucosa are able to incorporate [³H]-thymidine into DNA in any layer of the mucosa.[9] Namely, the proliferation site of adenoplastic carcinoma is not related to the generative zone of the noncancerous mucosa. This fact necessarily corresponds to our observation that the zonation pattern of histochemical markers is often focal and abortive in adenoplastic carcinomas.

Of great interest is the difference of CEA expression between lesions in the mucosa and lesions at the invading site of signet ring cell carcinoma. In noncancerous mucosa, CEA is localized in the uppermost surface lining cells with or without intestinalization, the cells without mitotic activity, as occurs in normal intestine.[49,82] Cells in the generative zone are negative for CEA. As discussed above, in the mucosal lesion of many signet ring cell carcinomas, CEA is expressed on mature signet ring cells without mitotic activity occupying the upper layer of the mucosa, while immature-looking proliferative cells are usually devoid of CEA immunoreactivity. On the other hand, the morphology of invading cancer cells in advanced signet ring cell carcinomas with scirrhous growth usually resembles that of immature-looking proliferative cells in the mucosa. It is quite different from the mucosal lesion, in that the immature-looking cancer cells at the invading site almost always display strong immunoreactivity for CEA or CEA/NCA in addition to occasional reactivities to lysozyme, SC and/or CPS class III.

Such a discrepancy of CEA expression between the mucosal and invading lesions is a genuine problem that must be solved. It is assumed that the expression of CEA in a given cell is time-dependent, but is not directly related to the cell cycle (i.e., CEA is a substance appearing on the cell membranes with a fixed time lag after the mitotic event, whether the cell has proliferative ability or not).

It has been described that both leukemia cells[83] and gastric cancer cells[9] show a decrease of the ratio of cells in the generative cycle and an elongation of cellular life span in comparison with their normal counterparts. It has further been disclosed that the [³H]-thymidine-labeling index is lower in invading cancer cells of scirrhous carcinomas than in mucosally located cancer cells.[84] The presence of postmitotic and nonproliferating tumor stem cells in G_0 phase has been described in invasive mammary adenocarcinoma of mice.[85] The maturation or differentiation of immature cancer cells should be quite reasonably restricted by the presence of thick fibrous tissue at the invading site. Consequently, the cancer cells with an elongated life span come to express CEA excessively with maturation in the upper layer of the mucosa, and with restricted maturation at the invading site.

5. DIFFERENTIATION TO ENDOCRINE CELLS IN SCIRRHOUS CARCINOMA

A wide variety of carcinomas, especially adenocarcinomas, are known to contain neoplastic cells with endocrine nature, even when they are not categorized as so-called neuroendocrine tumors.[31,86] Scirrhous carcinoma of the stomach is one of the representatives of such tumors, since plentiful endocrine-like cells with a positive argyrophil reaction have been detected among scirrhously invading cancer cells.[32,34,40] Such cancers are called as argyrophilic carcinoma.[32,34]

In this part, the differentiation to endocrine cells in scirrhous carcinoma is analyzed and characterized with the indirect immunoperoxidase method. First, the properties of endocrine cells in nontumorous mucosa are presented.[38,57,87] The specificity of the immunostaining was confirmed by absorption experiments using synthetic or purified antigens, as reported previously.[38,57]

In both antral and oxyntic mucosa, there are scattered argyrophil cells and argentaffin (enterochromaffin, EC) cells identified by Grimelius silver and Masson's silver, respectively. Argentaffin cells are argyrophilic, but argyrophil cells are not necessarily argentaffin. Argentaffin cells in nonmetaplastic gastric mucosa (gastric EC cells) are marked by their closed position (without direct contact to the gland lumen). These cells are fairly evenly distributed in the generative zone through the pyloric or oxyntic glands.

Gastrin cells and somatostatin cells are present mainly in the generative zone of antral mucosa and occasionally among the pyloric glands. Somatostatin cells are also scattered in the oxyntic glands where gastrin cells are absent. The occurrence of gastrin cells in pseudopyloric glands in fundic mucosa is exceptional. Glicentin (enteroglucagon or proglucagon) cells, in which pancreatic glucagon immunoreactivity is frequently, but not consistently detected, are distributed in fetal fundic mucosa, while adult oxyntic glands are devoid of glicentin immunoreactive cells.[38] Drastic changes of endocrine cells occur in the mucosa with intestinal metaplasia, as reported previously.[38,57] Selective and often hyperplastic increase of glicentin cells, argyrophil cells, and intestinal EC cells is quite characteristic of intestinal metaplasia. Intestinal EC cells with an open position (showing direct contact to the gland lumen) are easily recognized as basal granulated cells in H&E preparations.[57] The occurrence of pancreatic glucagon and PP immunoreactivities in the glicentin cells is infrequent.[38] Gastrin cells, somatostatin cells, and gastric EC cells are rarely present after the metaplastic change.[57]

Chromogranin is a substance present in cored granules of various endocrine cells including adrenomedullary cells and parathyroid cells,[40,88] and is known to be cosecreted with a variety of peptide hormones and amines.[89,90] In the gastrointestinal tract, chromogranin-positive endocrine cells correspond fairly well to the argyrophil and argentaffin cells.[40] Some of the gastrin cells and glicentin cells are chromogranin-positive, whereas most of the peptide-containing cells are argyrophobic.[40]

The occurrence of endocrine-like cells in the mucosal lesion of early signet ring cell carcinoma[33] is now commented on. Immunoperoxidase staining for chromogranin and Grimelius silver are used to detect such a

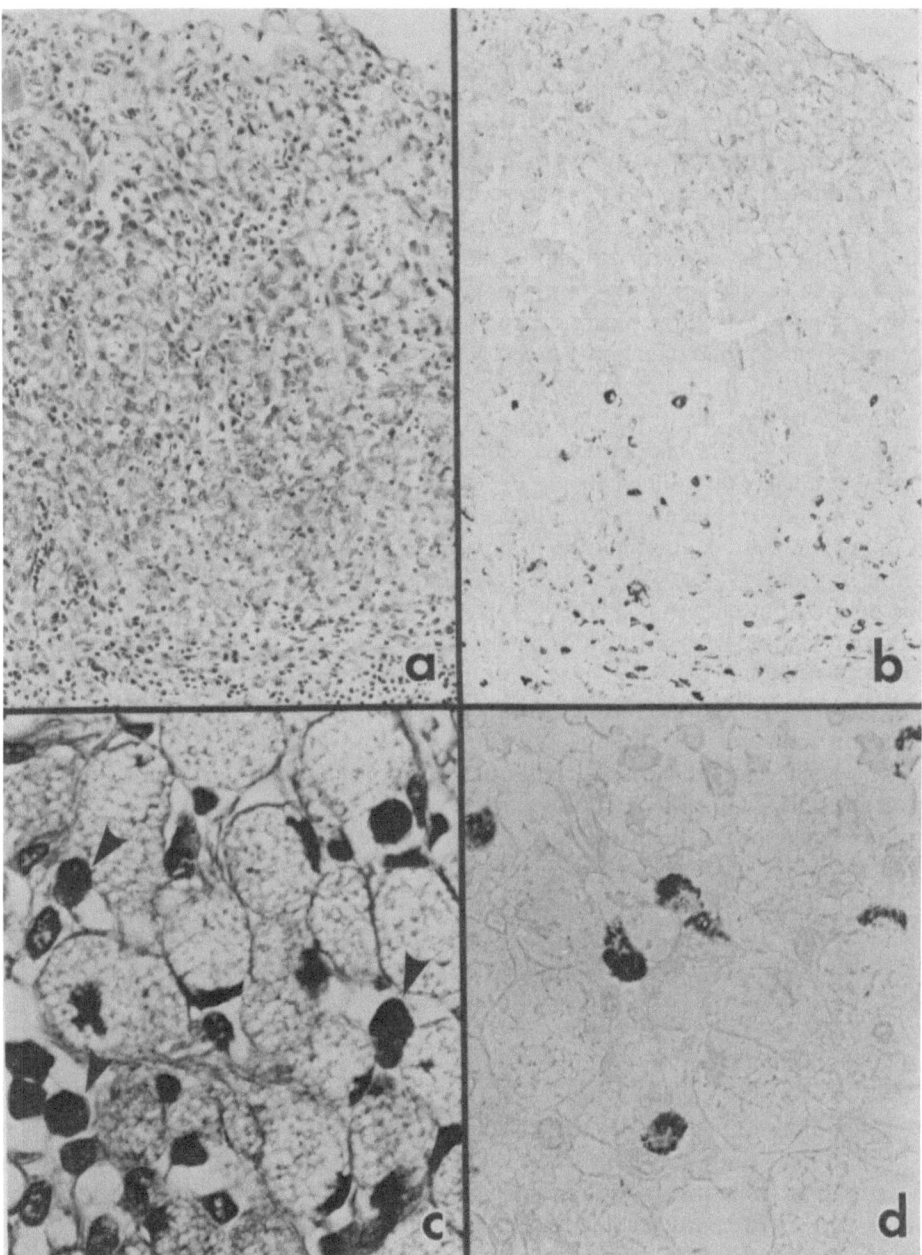

Fig. 1-17. Differentiation of intramucosal signet ring cell carcinoma to endocrine-like cells. H&E (a) and Grimelius silver (b), ×150. H&E (c) and indirect immunoperoxidase method for chromogranin (d), ×750.

Argyrophilic cancer cells are predominantly distributed in the bottom layer of the mucosa. High power view reveals that the endocrine-like cells with granular cytoplasmic reaction to chromogranin are small in size and correspond to small non-signet ring cells with eosinophilic granularity in the cytoplasm (arrowheads).

component. Both methods gave almost the same results for the detection of endocrine-like cells. Keen attention was paid to evaluation of whether the positive cells were neoplastic or not, since (1) atrophic pyloric glands commonly persist in the cancerous mucosa and (2) isolated micronodules of endocrine cells are frequently distributed in the lamina propria of the mucosa with atrophic gastritis.[33,57,87] Of 59 lesions examined, 14 showed many endocrine-like cancer cells, 20 showed scattered cells, nine showed only a few cells, and 16 were devoid of such cells. It is noteworthy that the endocrine-like cells were almost always distributed in the lower half layer or, more frequently, at the bottom of the mucosa, as are endocrine cells in noncancerous mucosa.

This distribution pattern of endocrine-like cells should be another example of the zonal differentiation shown by signet ring cancer cells in the mucosa. Figure 1-17(a,b) shows a representative picture of intramucosally located cancer differentiating to argyrophilic endocrine-like cells. Figure 1-17(c,d) illustrates a high power view of the bottom layer of the mucosa of another case, where numbers of chromogranin-positive cells are intermingled with signet ring cells of the pyloric gland-type. Characteristically, the endocrine-like cells have small amounts of granular cytoplasm without mucin in H&E preparations.

Table 1-9 summarizes results of histochemical analysis of endocrine-like cells in 26 scirrhous carcinomas of the stomach. Seven scirrhous carcinomas contained numbers of cells with a positive Grimelius reaction in the gastric wall, and could be categorized as argyrophilic carcinoma (Fig. 1-18). Varying numbers of argyrophilic neoplastic cells were seen at the invading site of 15 of 26 tumors. An additional five tumors exhibited argyrophilic cancer cells only in the mucosa. Thus, the occurrence of argyrophilic cancer cells in scirrhous carcinoma is quite frequent.[32,34,38]

On the contrary, Masson's silver-positive argentaffin tumor cells were infrequently noted in those specimens. Of five peptide hormones examined, glicentin immunoreactive

TABLE 1-9

Endocrine-like Cells at Invading Site of 26 Scirrhous Carcinomas of the Stomach

	++	+	(+)	−	ND
Argyrophil	7	4	4	11[5]	0
Argentaffin	0	0	2	20	4
Glicentin					
49– 69	2	2	4	18[1]	0
Glucagon					
19– 29	0	2	0	21	3
PP	0	0	0	13	13
Somatostatin	0	3	3	10	10
Gastrin	0	0	1	15	10

++: plentiful positive cells seen

+: positive cells scattered

(+): only a few cells positive

−: negative

ND: not done

Glicentin 49–69: enteroglucagon or proglucagon

Glucagon 19–29: pancreatic-type glucagon

PP: pancreatic polypeptide

[ ]: the number of tumors with positive cells only in the mucosa

cells were most frequently demonstrated (Fig. 1-18c). Cancers with two-plus or one-plus glicentin cells in Table 1-9 were all argyrophilic carcinomas, although most, if not all, glicentin cells have been shown to be argyrophobic.[38] Pancreatic glucagon immunoreactivity was detected in the glicentin-containing cells in two tumors, while no PP immunoreactive cells were noted. A small to modest number of somatostatin-containing cells were present in six of 16 tumors (Fig. 1-18d).[34] The infrequency of gastrin-positive scirrhous cancer cells possibly reflects the fact that most tumors originated from the oxyntic mucosa. However, Tahara et al described the rather frequent occurrence of gastrin-positive cells in scirrhous carcinomas.[34]

The occurrence of glicentin immunoreactive cells in scirrhous carcinoma is preferably interpreted to be an expression of fetalism in cancer cells, since glicentin is present in endocrine cells of fetal oxyntic mucosa, but it is absent from those of adult oxyntic mucosa.[38]

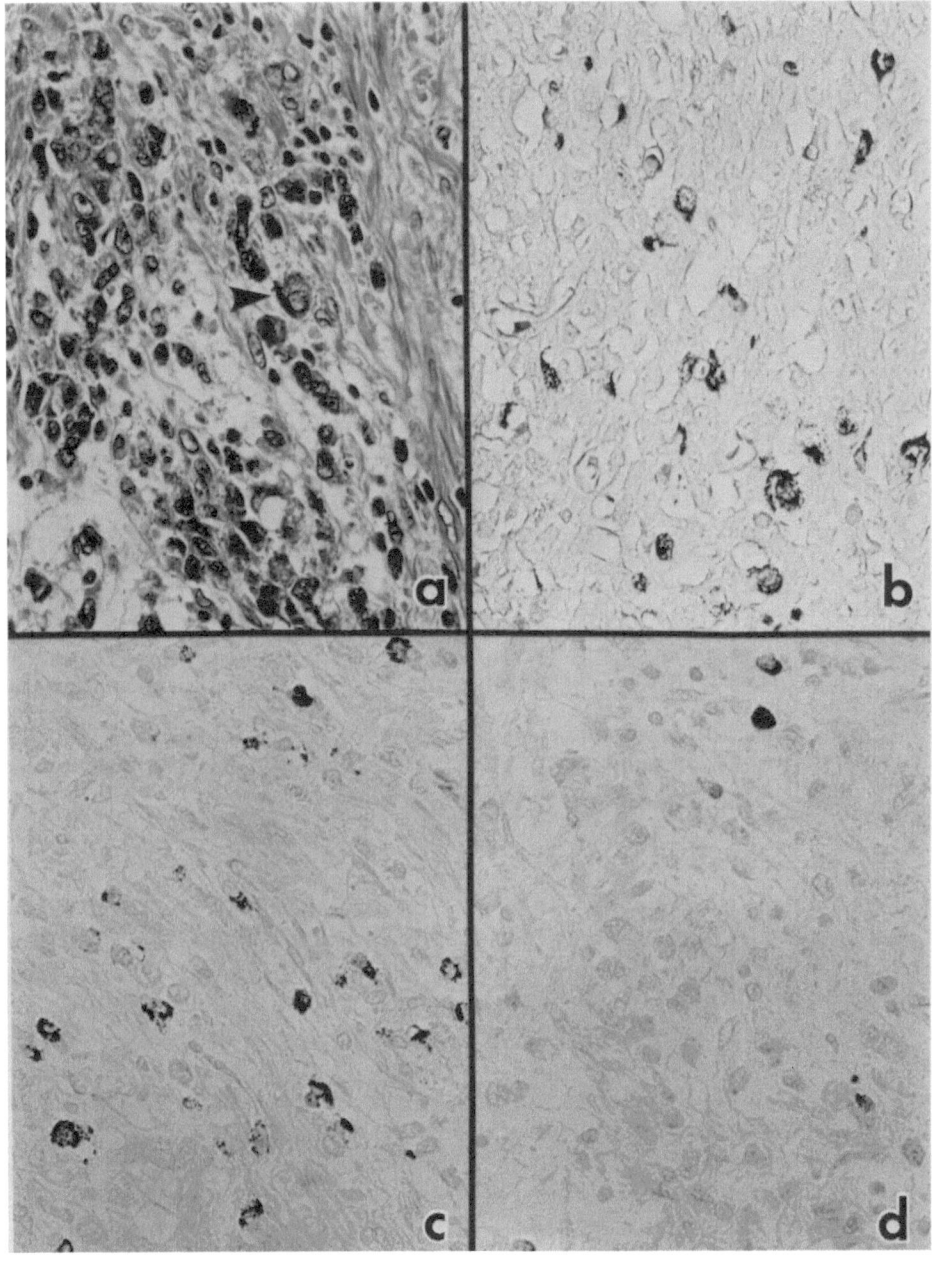

Fig. 1-18. Scirrhous argyrophil carcinoma of the stomach. H&E (a), Grimelius silver (b) and immunoperoxidase method for glicentin (c) and somatostatin (d). Methyl green counterstain (c & d), ×400.

Scirrhously infiltrating cancer cells usually look immature and occasionally show a cytoplasmic granularity (arrowhead). Argyrophil reaction and peptide hormone immunoreactivity (especially of glicentin) are often positive in such cancer cells.

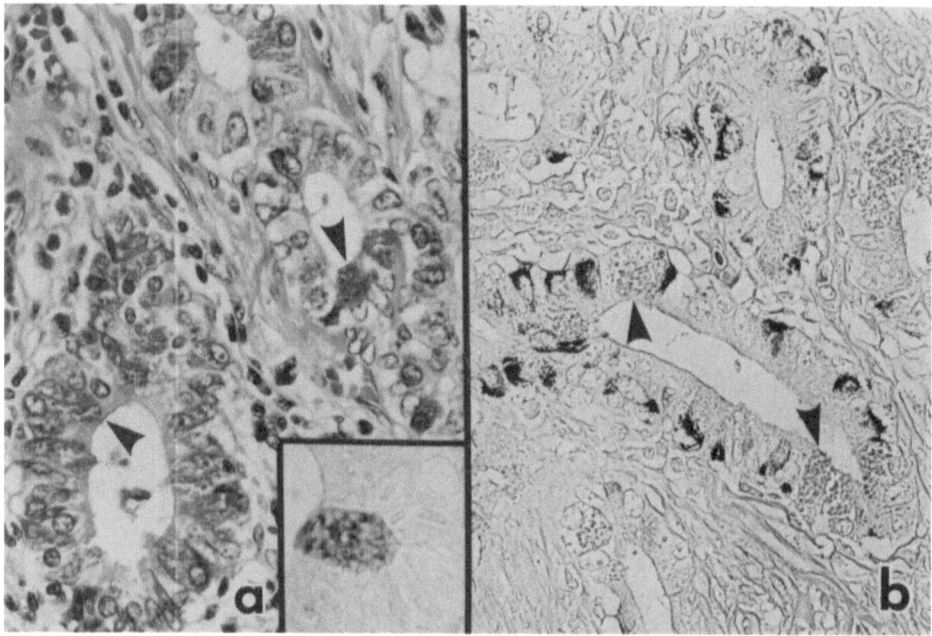

Fig. 1-19. Advanced adenoplastic carcinoma (tub$_1$) partially differentiating toward Paneth cells and endocrine-like cells. H&E (a) and Grimelius silver (b), ×400. Indirect immunoperoxidase method for lysozyme (inset), ×750.

Infiltrating tubular adenocarcinoma contains numbers of Paneth cells (arrowheads) with immunoreactive lysozyme. In addition, the existence of plentiful argyrophil cells is characteristic of this tumor.

Intestinalized mucosa has been proved to exhibit a number of glicentin-containing endocrine cells,[38,57] but the above phenomenon is unlikely to represent an intestinal phenotype, because most scirrhous carcinomas have their origin in nonintestinalized oxyntic mucosa. The frequent association of endocrine differentiation in diffuse carcinoma of the stomach is closely related to the facts that (1) from the standpoint of cell kinetics, the endocrine cell in the gastric mucosa belongs to a dissociative cell group,[91] and the tumor cell of diffuse carcinoma is literally an extreme expression of a dissociative cell;[8,9] and that (2) nontumorous endocrine cells under fibrotic conditions frequently show hyperplastic proliferations, including islet cells in chronic pancreatitis,[92] endocrine cell micronodules in chronic gastritis,[33,57,87] and pulmonary tumorlets with fibrotic derangement of peribronchial tissue.[93,94]

On the other hand, the detection of endocrine-like cells in adenoplastic carcinomas is a rare occasion. In fact, of 23 adenoplastic carcinomas invading into the submucosa or deeper areas, only three tumors exhibited a few or scattered Grimelius-positive cancer cells at the invading site, whereas four of seven intramucosally located adenoplastic carcinomas contained scattered endocrine-like cells in the cancerous glands. Adenoplastic carcinomas with plentiful endocrine-like cells as a neoplastic component are very limited in our experience so far. In a few adenoplastic carcinomas, such cells were easily recognized in H&E preparations as basal granulated cells, which clearly revealed both argyrophil and argentaffin reactions. Interestingly enough, many of such tumors also contained typical Paneth cells with strong immunoreactivity for lysozyme as shown in

Figure 1-19.[95] Immunohistochemically, most argyrophilic tumor cells stained positive for chromogranin, while a number of cells immunoreactive to glicentin were also commonly distributed in the cancerous glands.[40] Cells immunoreactive to pancreatic glucagon, PP, somatostatin, or gastrin were less or a few in number. The expression pattern is intimately related to that of intestinal metaplasia.

Comment: When we note the occurrence of endocrine-like cells in nonneuroendocrine carcinoma, it is quite fascinating to suppose there is a totipotent neoplastic stem cell, as has been vigorously investigated in hematopoietic malignancies.[96] The carcinogenesis occurs at the level of the tumor stem cell or differentiation-committed immature cell,[78–81] and it then differentiates, under the influence of mucosal microenvironment, into various epithelial cell types such as surface epithelial cell, absorptive cell, goblet cell, pyloric gland cell, Paneth cell, and endocrine cell. The same assumption has been proposed in teratocarcinoma[97] and in other nonhematopoietic malignancies[78,79] including lung cancer.[80,81]

In fact, the endodermal origin of dispersed endocrine cells in the alimentary and respiratory tracts has been clarified,[79,98] denying the original Pearse hypothesis of their neural crest (neuroectodermal) origin. He proposed the concept of the APUD (amine precursor uptake and decarboxylation) system.[99] With the assumption of the totipotent tumor stem cell,[78–81] we as pathologists can reasonably understand our frequent experiences of such mixed forms of endocrine and nonendocrine tumors as goblet cell carcinoid of the vermiform appendix,[100] an intermediate form of papillary and medullary carcinoma of the thyroid gland,[101] small cell lung carcinoma with glandular and squamous cells,[102] and a variety of adenocarcinomas with endocrine-like cells.[31,86] We have further disclosed that SC-immunoreactive nonneuroendocrine neoplastic cells are occasionally present in ordinary gastrointestinal carcinoid tumors and in pancreatic islet cell tumors.[94]

6. PRODUCTION OF ALPHA-FETOPROTEIN AND HUMAN CHORIONIC GONADOTROPIN BY GASTRIC CANCER: EXPRESSION OF "RETRODIFFERENTIATION"

Production of α-fetoprotein (AFP) is characteristic of hepatocellular carcinoma, hepatoblastoma, and teratocarcinoma.[103] Increased levels of serum AFP have been described repeatedly, however, in patients with neoplasms of foregut origin.[21–23,104] Especially in Japan, many of these patients suffer from gastric cancer.[104] About 15% of patients with gastric cancer are known to show elevated serum AFP levels.[105] AFP has been directly demonstrated in gastric cancer tissue by both immunoassay[106] and immunohistochemistry.[21–23,39]

Our immunohistochemical analyses to characterize AFP-producing gastric cancer are presented below, in which 20 surgical specimens of gastric cancer with elevated serum AFP levels and 10 control surgical specimens of gastric cancer with negative serum AFP were studied.[39] Samples from metastatic sites (lymph nodes, livers or pancreas) including autopsy materials were also examined. Serum AFP was measured by the enzyme immunoassay, and 20 ng/ml or more were judged as positive.

Group A included 11 cases with preoperatively elevated levels of serum AFP. Group B included nine cases whose preoperative sera failed to show the elevation of AFP, but AFP levels were elevated after surgery. Group C included 10 unselected serial cases with negative serum AFP levels throughout the clinical course. The indirect immunoperoxidase staining was performed to detect CEA, human chorionic gonadotropin (HCG), placental alkaline phosphatase (PALP), SC and lysozyme as well as AFP. AntiCEA was prepared to be unreactive to NCA by previous absorption. AntiHCG is reactive to both alpha and beta subunits of HCG. AntiPALP partially cross-reacts to alkaline phosphatase of the intestinal type,[107] since the brush border of normal duodenal lining cells and of some, but not all, intestinalized epithelia stains positive in addition to plasma membranes of normal placental syncytiotrophoblasts and seminoma cells.[108] To demonstrate glycogen and mucin, PAS reactions with or without diastase treatment and the AB-PAS sequence were employed.

Clinical and histochemical data are summarized in Table 1-10. With regard to immunostaining of AFP, nine of 11 tumors in group A, five of nine tumors in group B, and none of 10 in group C were positive. Noncancerous gastric tissue was uniformly negative for AFP. Serum AFP levels of AFP stain-negative cases in groups A and B were relatively low (211 ng/ml maximum). In contrast with the observation by Kodama et al,[23] a rough correlation between serum AFP levels and staining tendency for AFP was noted. Namely, all four tumors accompanying extremely high levels of serum AFP (more than 10,000 ng/ml) immunohistochemically revealed a number of AFP-positive tumor cells (++ or +++). A case with relatively low serum AFP (141 ng/ml) but with two-plus AFP stain (case 4 in Table 1-10) suffered from early gastric cancer invading into the submucosa. Positive AFP staining was demonstrated in all nine cases with serum AFP levels of more than 1,000 ng/ml, in four of six cases with serum AFP levels between 100–1,000 ng/ml, and in only one of five cases with serum AFP levels between 20–100 ng/ml. In group B, there were two cases whose AFP staining was positive in the metastatic site but negative in the primary. This possibly reflects the postoperative elevation of serum AFP. All tumors with positive AFP staining in the primary site showed AFP-positive cells also in the metastatic site.

High incidence of liver metastasis in AFP producing gastric cancer has been pointed out.[26,104] Since mild to moderate elevation of serum AFP in patients with chronic hepatitis or liver cirrhosis has been described,[109] the production of AFP by nonneoplastic hepatocytes should also be considered,[104] especially in AFP stain-negative cases. In five liver tissues immunohistochemically examined, however, AFP was localized only in the metastatic tumors, and no hepatocytes were stained.

AFP immunoreactivity was mainly observed as vesicular or granular structures in the cytoplasm, which probably correspond to rough endoplasmic reticula and Golgi apparati as its localization sites. This intracytoplasmic pattern of positivity is totally identical to that in fetal hepatocytes and yolk sac tumor cells.[110]

It has been noted that histologically, AFP-producing gastric cancer tends to show a poorly differentiated medullary or well-differentiated papillary growth pattern.[23] In the present series, medullary carcinomas with paucity of mucin were often strongly positive for AFP (Fig. 1-20a,b). Four tumors were at least focally papillary adenocarcinomas, three of which were positive for AFP staining (Fig. 1-20c). Six tumors were signet ring cell (scirrhous) carcinomas including three with positive AFP staining (Fig. 1-20d). It is noteworthy that four neoplasms focally or diffusely showed histological features of embryonal carcinoma with positive AFP staining, as is shown and discussed later.

The common cytological feature of AFP-positive cancer cells was a clear and finely granular appearance of the cytoplasm, and the cells possessed abundant glycogen (Fig. 1-20a). The abundance of glycogen was also true for the AFP-positive tumor cells in signet ring cell carcinoma. On the basis of such a cytological feature, we can anticipate the occurrence of immunoreactive AFP in a given gastric cancer. Gitlin et al disclosed a small amount of AFP in gastrointestinal tissue extracts of human fetus.[111] Lee et al[22] and Miyayama and Miyayama[21] observed AFP immunoreactivity in fetal gastrointestinal epithelium of 9 to 16 or 21 gestational weeks. The gastrointestinal epithelium of the fetus is known to be rich in glycogen. Namely, fetal cells are shown to be relatively resistant to hypoxia and to have a well-developed anaerobic glycolysis system.[112] Accordingly, it is appro-

TABLE 1-10

Immunohistochemical Analysis of AFP-Producing Gastric Cancer

Case Age/Sex	Site	Histology	Serum AFP Level (ng/ml) Pre-op.	Post-op.	Mucin/Glycogen	AFP	CEA	HCG	PALP	SC	Lysozyme
group A											
1. 62M	St(sm)	por(med)	1000<	1000<	-**	+++	+	-	-	(+)	-
	Liver	por(med)			-**	+++	++	-	+	-	-
	Liver#	por(med)			-**	+++	-	-	-	-	-
2. 68M	St(se)	emb	99.3	20.4–28200	-**	++	+	(+)	(+)	-	-
	LN	emb			-**	++	+	(+)	(+)	-	-
	LN	tub₂			++(c)	-	+++	-	-	+++	++
	Liver#	emb			-**	++	+	-	-	-	-
3. 52M	St(se)	por(med)	3500	54–15100	+(s)*	+	+++	+	+	(+)	(+)
	LN	por(med)			+(s)**	+	+++	(+)	-	(+)	-
	Liver#	por(med)			+(s)**	(+)	+++	-	-	-	(+)
4. 67M@	St(sm)	por(med)	141	67–3.2	(+)(s/c)**	++	+	(+)	-	+	+
		emb			-**	+	+	-	-	-	-
5. 54F	St(se)	por(med)	430	4300	+(s/c)**	+	++	-	-	+	(+)
	LN	por(med)			-**	(+)	(+)	-	-	-	(+)
6. 72F@	St(se)	pap	160	13.5–49	+++(s)	(+)	+++	-	-	+	-
		por(med)			+(s)	-	(+)	-	-	-	-
	LN	por(med)			+(s)**	+	+	-	-	-	(+)
7. 72M	St(se)	tub₁	36.4	168–1800	+(s/c)	-	+++	(+)	++	(+)	(+)
		emb			-**	(+)	++	(+)	+	+++	(+)
8. 73M	St(pm)	tub₁/pap	161	51.5–2.8	(+)(s/c)**	+	+	(+)	+++	+	-
	LN	pap			-**	++	+++	(+)	+++	+	-
	LN	por(med)			++(c)**	++	+++	-	-	-	+++
9. 69F	St(se)	pap	38.0	21.1–1.0	+++(s)*	-	+++	(+)	(+)	++	+
	LN	pap			+++(s)*	-	+++	(+)	(+)	++	(+)
	Liver	pap			+++(s)*	-	+++	(+)	(+)	(+)	+++
10. 42F	St(se)	sig(sci)	46.0	3.3–2300	++(s/c)**	+	+++	(+)	+++	++	(+)
	LN	sig			++(s/c)**	(+)	+++	-	+++	+++	(+)
11. 29F	St(se)	sig(sci)	211	27.7	+++(s/c)*	-	+++	+	++	+++	+
	LN	sig			+++(s/c)	-	++	+	+++	+++	++

Case Age/Sex	Site	Histology	Serum AFP Level (ng/ml)		Mucin/Glycogen*,**	Immunohistochemistry					
			Pre-op.	Post-op.		AFP	CEA	HCG	PALP	SC	Lysozyme
group B											
12. 78M	St(ss)	emb	negative	10000<	-**	++	+	-	-	(+)	-
	LN	emb			-**	+++	+	-	+	(+)	-
	Panc#	emb			-**	+	-	-	-	-	(+)
13. 58F	St(se)	por(med)	13.0	108	(+)(s)	-	(+)	-	-	(+)	-
	LN	por(med)			(+)(s)*	(+)	-	-	-	-	-
14. 60F@	St(sm)	tub₁	1.0	91–14.0	+++(s)	-	+++	-	(+)	+++	(+)
		por(med)			(+)(s)	-	+++	-	(+)	+	-
	LN	por(med)			++(s)	-	+++	-	+	++	(+)
15. 68F	St(se)	tub₁/pap	6.0	1600–3550	+(s/c)**	+	+++	(+)	+	++	-
	LN	pap			+++(s/c)**	+	+++	-	-	+	-
	Liver#	tub₁/pap			+(s/c)**	(+)	+++	(+)	-	-	(+)
16. 39F	St(se)	sig(sci)	3.8	168–1200	++(s/c)**	(+)	+++	(+)	+++	+	+
	LN	sig			+++(s/c)**	+	+++	-	+++	++	++
17. 32F	St(se)	sig(sci)	9.0	78	+++(c)	-	+++	+	++++	++	(+)
	LN	sig			++(c)**	+	+++	+	++++	(+)	(+)
18. 32F	St(se)	sig(sci)	2.0	2.8–48	++(c)**	-	+++	-	++++	++	(+)
	LN	sig			++(c)	-	+++	-	-	+	-
19. 62F	St(ss)	sig(sci)	negative	22–2.0	+++(c)	-	++	-	-	++	++
	Panc#	sig			+++(c)	-	+++	-	-	++	(+)
20. 48M	St(ss)	sig(sci)	negative	41–122	++(s/c)	-	++	(+)	+	++	+
	LN	sig			++(c)	-	+++	-	-	+++	+
	LN#	tub₁			++(s)	-	+++	-	-	++	-

group C

21. 68M	St(se)	pap	3.4	15.5	++(c)*	−	+++	−	+	+++	(+)
22. 59M@	St(m)	tub$_1$	2.1	2.3	+++(s)	−	++	−	−	+++	(+)
23. 42M	St(se)	tub$_1$	2.8	1.9	+++(s)	−	++	(+)	(+)	+++	+
24. 64M@	St(ss)	tub$_2$	1.1	5.9	+++(s)	−	+	(+)	+	+	(+)
	LN	tub$_1$			+++(s)	−	+++	−	+++	++	(+)
25. 61F	St(se)	tub$_2$	1.1	2.0	++(s)	−	+++	−	++	+++	+++
	LN	tub$_2$			++(s)	−	++	−	(+)	−	++
26. 62M@	St(m)	sig	1.0	1.5	+++(c)	−	+++	(+)	(+)	+	+
27. 48M@	St(sm)	sig	negative	1.4	+++(c)	−	++	(+)	−	+++	++
28. 47M	St(se)	por(med)	1.0	1.8	+(s/c)*	−	+++	+	+++	+	−
	LN	sig			+++(c)	−	+++	−	+	+	(+)
29. 48M@	St(se)	sig	negative	1.0	++(s/c)*	−	+++	−	(+)	−	(+)
30. 56F	St(se)	sig(sci)	2.2	7.6	+++(s/c)	−	+++	−	+	+	(+)

+ + +: Many cancer cell are positive (>%).

+ +: A moderate number of cancer cells are positive (% ~ %).

+: A small number of cancer cells are positive (<%).

(+): Only a few cancer cells are positive.

−: No cancer cells are positive.

@: Patient alive

#: Autopsy material

med: medullary; sci: scirrhous; emb; embryonal carcinoma

(s): surface coat-type mucin

(c): intracytoplasmic mucin

**: Many cancer cells are glycogen-rich.

* Glycogen-rich cancer cells are focally seen.

St: stomach; LN: lymph node; Panc: pancreas; m, sm, pm, ss, se: indicate the depth of invasion: m: mucosa, sm: submucosa, pm: proper muscle layer, ss: subserosa, and se: exposure onto the serosa

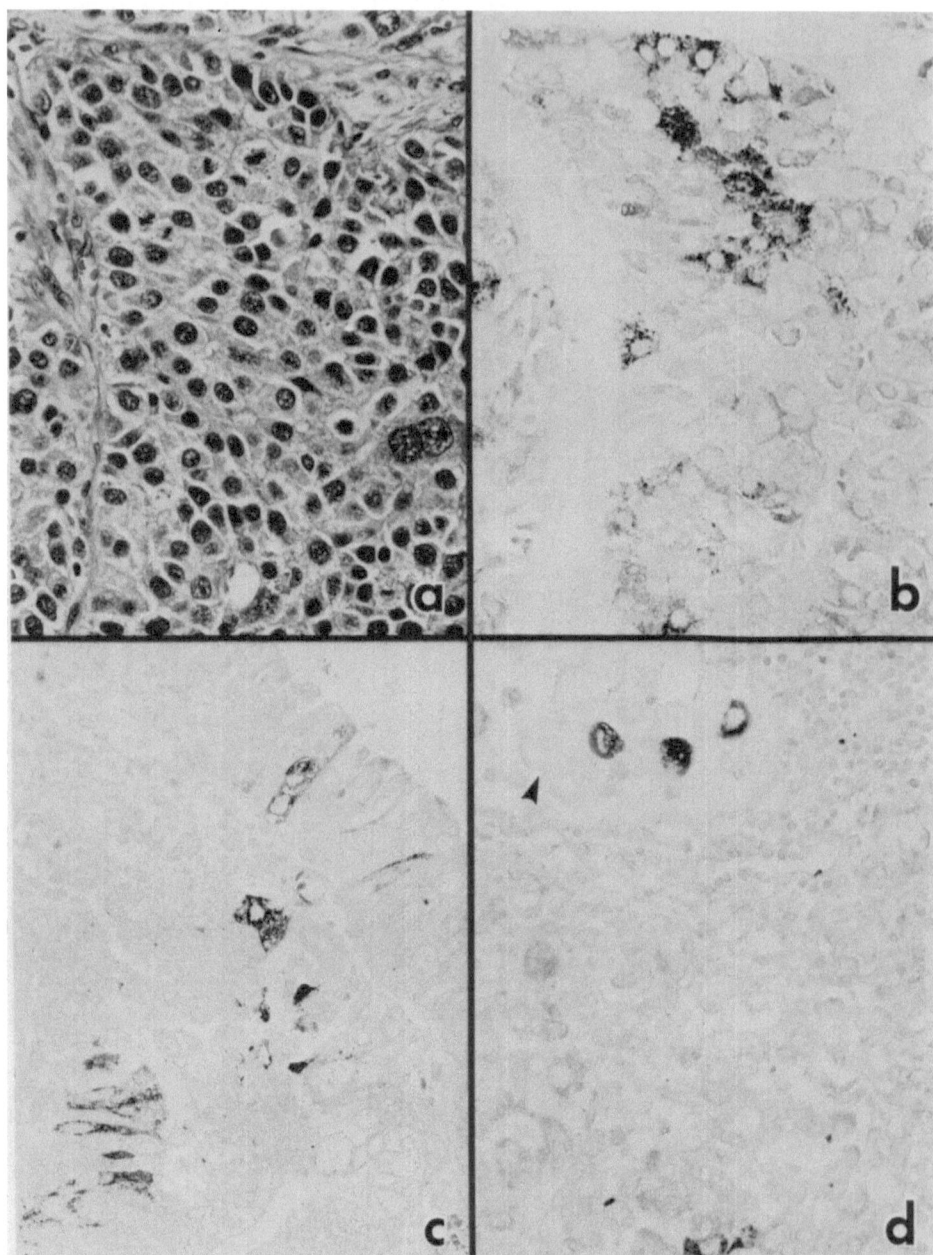

Fig. 1-20. Morphological variation of AFP-producing gastric carcinoma. Medullary carcinoma (case 1), a: H&E, b: AFP, ×300; papillary adenocarcinoma (case 15), c: AFP, ×240; and signet ring cell carcinoma (case 17, lymph node metastasis), d: AFP, ×300. Indirect immunoperoxidase method with methyl green counterstain.

Poorly differentiated medullary carcinoma consisting of cells with clear and finely granular cytoplasm frequently is accompanied by high serum AFP levels and numbers of AFP-positive cancer cells. Well-differentiated papillary adenocarcinoma and signet ring cell carcinoma occasionally show scattered AFP-positive cells. Mature signet ring cells (arrowhead) are usually devoid of AFP.

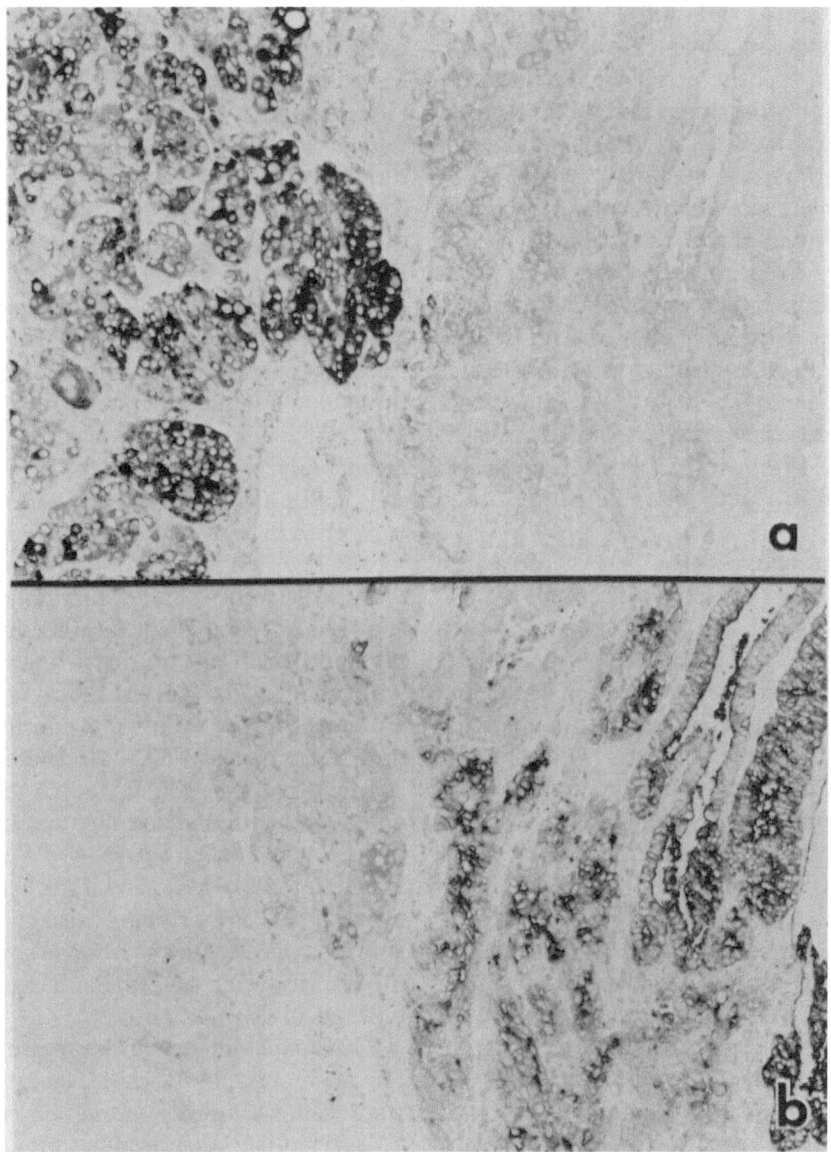

Fig. 1-21. Reciprocal localization of AFP (a) and CEA (b) in the mucosal lesion of case 4. Indirect immunoperoxidase method with methyl green counterstain, ✕ 120.
AFP-positive area shows a medullary growth pattern whereas CEA-positive cancer cells proliferate in a papillotubular fashion.

priate to assume that AFP-producing gastric cancer has regained the properties of fetal gastrointestinal epithelium.

The intriguing contrast of the staining pattern between AFP and CEA[39] is presented next. CEA was again positive in all tumors examined. In tumors with a number of AFP-positive cells, however, CEA showed a tendency to be only focally positive (Table 1-10). Figure 1-21 demonstrates a reciprocal localization pattern of AFP and CEA in a poorly differentiated carcinoma (case 4 in Table 10). Namely, AFP-positive cells proliferate in a medullary growth pattern and are CEA-negative, whereas the CEA-positive area shows a papillotubular growth pattern and is AFP-negative. The latter area seems to represent an ordinary type of adenocarcinoma. The specialities of AFP-positive gastric cancer cells as cells retrodifferentiating toward fetal gastrointestinal cells become herein evident. SC and lysozyme are also regarded as strict markers of the ordinary type of gastric carcinoma, although their expression was less consistent than CEA. AFP-positive cells hardly revealed any immunoreactivities with SC and lysozyme.

Immunoreactive PALP was detected in a varying number of gastric cancer cells in 23 of 30 tumors (Fig. 1-22a, b), as has already been pointed out.[21,25,26] The plasma membranes were the main site of staining for PALP, but some signet ring cancer cells showed positivity in Golgi areas. Cancers with plentiful PALP-positive cells were often diffuse carcinomas strongly positive for CEA. A reciprocal staining pattern was noted between PALP and lysozyme (Table 1-10). PALP staining in cancer with a pronounced AFP reactivity was often focal.

Regarding immunoreactive HCG, a few cancer cells were positive in 17 of 30 cases without evidence of a correlation with the staining for AFP, CEA, and PALP. HCG-positive cancer cells in the series of Table 1-10 never showed syncytiotrophoblastic morphology, as seen in Figure 1-22(c,d). Similar results have been reported by other investigators.[21,23,24,34] In a separate study, we have observed that the HCG-like substance in some gastric carcinomas is predominantly an alpha-subunit of HCG. The Alpha-subunit of HCG is further demonstrated in some endocrine-like cells of noncancerous antral mucosa. Unbalanced synthesis and secretion of HCG subunits are well known characteristics of cultured tumor cell lines[113,114] and various endocrine neoplasms.[40,115] Therefore, the detection of HCG immunoreactivity with antiHCG conventional antibody by itself does not necessarily indicate the retrodifferentiation toward trophoblastic cells.

In the next condition, embryonal carcinoma arising from the stomach as a AFP-producing tumor is shown and discussed.[39] As Figure 1-23 illustrates, the tumor cells (case 2 in Table 1-10) possess clear and finely granular cytoplasm. They proliferate with a sheet-like solid arrangement, and the formation of glandular structures with papillary projections is characteristic. Other areas reveal those glomeruloid structures with a few hyaline globules that are typical of yolk sac tumor. Glycogen is abundant in the tumor cells, and mucin is completely negative. AFP is positive in many tumor cells, while CEA is focally detected along the surface of the papillary projections. This peculiar tumor further shows foci of tubular adenocarcinoma both in the mucosa of the primary tumor and in lymph node metastasis. As shown in Figure 1-24, these foci are positive for mucin and immunoreactive for CEA, SC, and lysozyme, but negative for AFP. In the present series, another three tumors focally (two cases) or almost totally (one case) showed features resembling embryonal carcinoma, an admixture of solid and papillary areas without the glomeruloid structures. The cells were uniformly glycogen-rich, mucin-negative, and AFP-positive.

These phenomena can be regarded as the retrodifferentiation of gastric cancer cells toward yolk sac or very immature embryonal cells. A similar hypothesis has been proposed for the histogenesis of choriocarcinoma of the stomach,[116] which is presented below. Endo et al found with the Concanavalin A binding analysis that the sugar moiety of serum AFP in patients with gastrointestinal cancer is very similar to that of yolk sac tumor, but is different from that of fetal liver and hepatocellular carcinoma.[117] Therefore, it may be relevant that while the degree of retrodifferentiation in AFP-producing nonembryonal carcinoma of the stomach comes toward fetal gastrointestinal cells (fetalism), the degree of retrodifferentiation in AFP-producing embryonal carci-

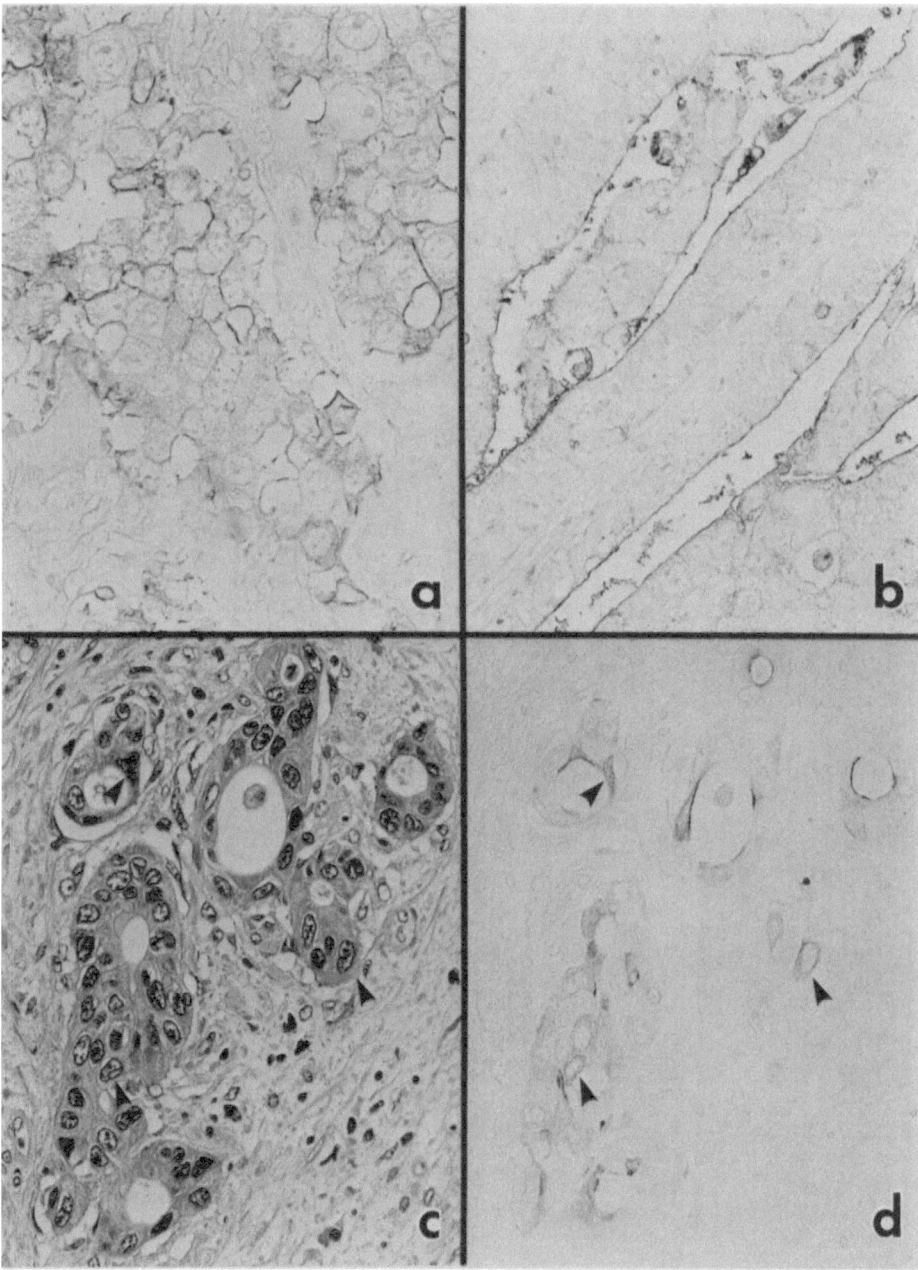

Fig. 1-22. Immunohistochemical localization of PALP and HCG in gastric cancer. Signet ring cell carcinoma (case 11, a: PALP), ×400; papillary adenocarcinoma (case 8, b: PALP), ×300; papillary adenocarcinoma (case 9, c: H&E, d: HCG), ×300. Indirect immunoperoxidase method with methyl green counterstain.

PALP is often strongly positive on the plasma membranes of scirrhous cancer cells. PALP is also demonstrated on the apical surface of some adenoplastic carcinoma cells. HCG-positive gastric cancer cells are not necessarily syncytiotrophoblastic (arrowheads).

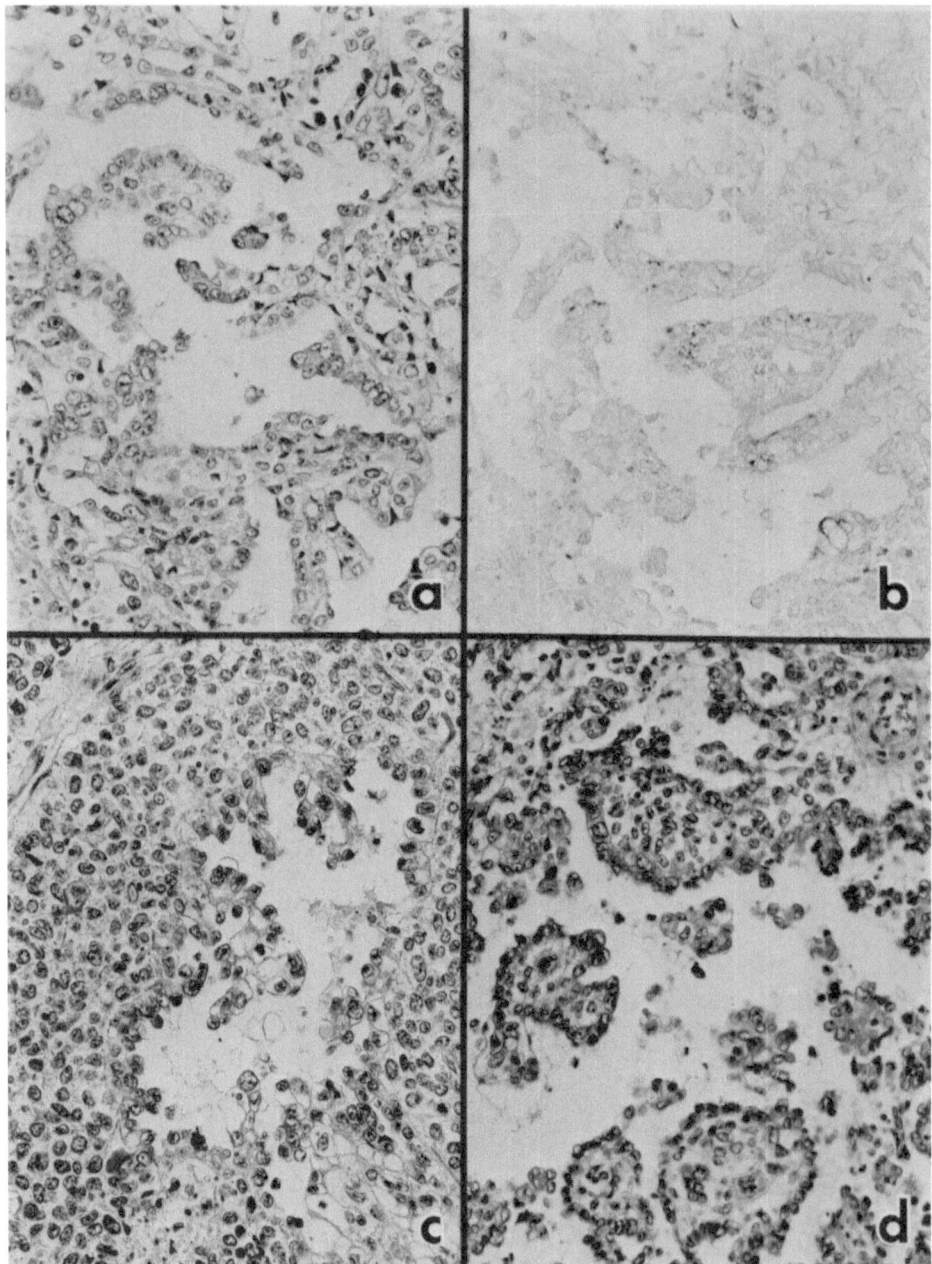

Fig. 1-23. Primary embryonal carcinoma of the stomach (case 2). H&E (a, c and d) and indirect immunoperoxidase method for AFP (b), ×200.

The tumor is composed of an admixture of solid and papillary areas. Glomeruloid structure is focally noted (d). Granular or vesicular positivity of AFP is easily seen in the papillary area (a and b). CEA is focally positive along the apical surface of a lumen in (c). Mucin, SC and lysozyme are negative in these areas.

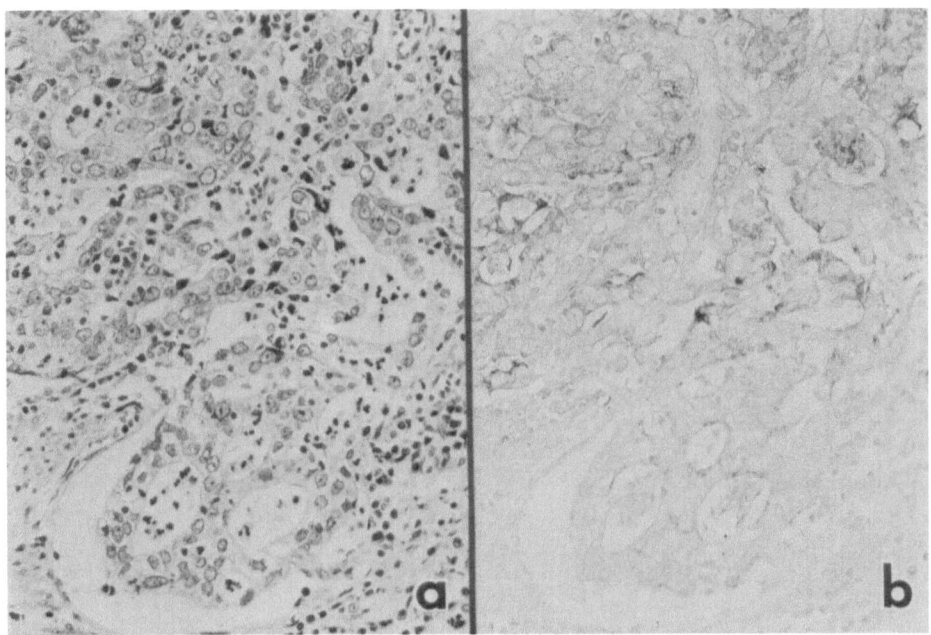

Fig. 1-24. Component of adenoplastic carcinoma in a case of primary gastric embryonal carcinoma. Intramucosal lesion of case 2. H&E (a) and indirect immunoperoxidase method for SC (b), ×200.

Not only in the mucosa but also in lymph node metastasis, foci of adenoplastic carcinoma with SC immunoreactivity are found, although the predominant histology is embryonal carcinoma. Note lymphatic invasion.

noma of the stomach comes back to yolk sac cells or very immature embryonal cells (embryonism).

Meanwhile, primary gastric choriocarcinoma has been described, whose histological pictures are identical to those of ordinary choriocarcinoma.[116,118] So far, we have experienced one surgical and two autopsy specimens of primary gastric choriocarcinoma with clinical and laboratory manifestations of HCG overproduction. All patients died within a short clinical period of generalized metastases including to the liver. Large volumes of the tumors showed massive hemorrhagic necrosis intermingled with syncytiotrophoblastic and cytotrophoblastic tumor cells. Immunohistochemically, the syncytiotrophoblastic cells were strongly positive for HCG (and its alpha and beta subunits), but were negative for CEA, AFP, PALP, SC, and lysozyme (Fig. 1-25). The cytotrophoblastic cells were devoid of such markers (keratin is

clearly positive). In metastatic lesions, two cases further showed a component of yolk sac tumor with typical histological and immunohistochemical features (AFP and CEA positive but PALP, HCG, SC, and lysozyme negative).

A similar case has recently been presented by Yonemura et al.[119] The components of choriocarcinoma and yolk sac tumor were detected as separate metastatic nodules in the lymph node and/or liver. The co-occurrence of choriocarcinoma and yolk sac tumor from a single primary is very common phenomenon in gonadal and extragonadal malignant germ cell tumors.[120] Quite distinct from the ordinary malignant germ cell tumors is the consistent existence of a component of adenocarcinoma in the gastric tumor,[116,118,119] as was mentioned above for embryonal carcinoma of the stomach. All three cases of gastric choriocarcinoma disclosed foci of adenoplastic (tubular or papillary) carcinoma with pos-

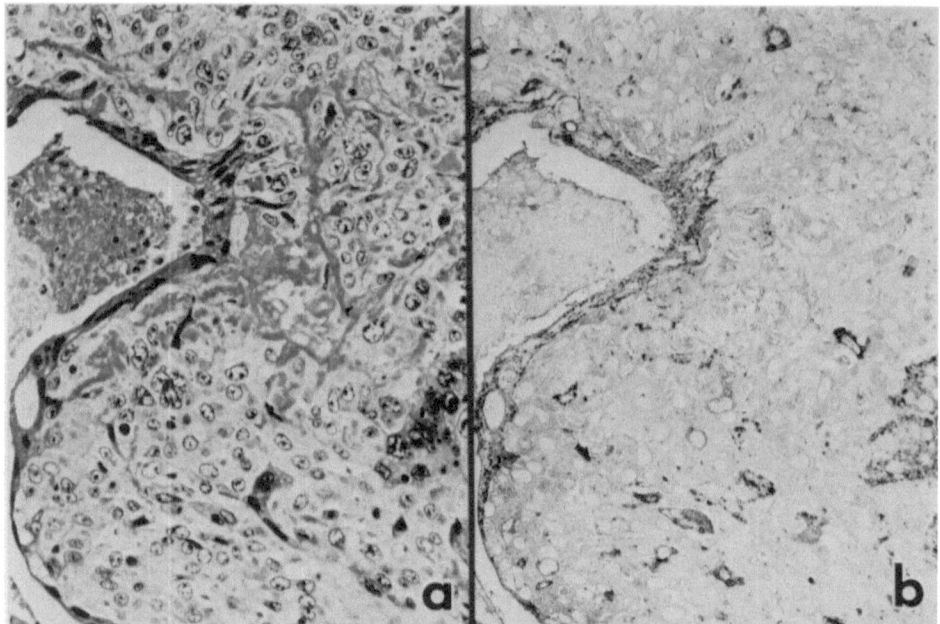

Fig. 1-25. Primary gastric choriocarcinoma. H&E (a) and indirect immunoperoxidase method for HCG (b), ×200.

Syncytiotrophoblastic tumor cells are clearly positive for HCG. Foci of yolk sac tumor and adenoplastic carcinoma are also seen in both the primary and metastatic sites.

itive reactions to mucin, CEA, SC, and/or lysozyme within the gastric wall, including the mucosa. Lymph node metastasis of adenoplastic carcinoma was also noted in one case.

The clinical and morphological transformation of papillary thyroid cancer into anaplastic cancer is regarded as "malignant transformation of less malignant cancer cells."[121] Similarly, the occurrence of malignant germ cell tumors from the stomach may be understood when such a concept is extended to the gastric cancer (i.e., the transformation occurs at the stem cell level of ordinary adenoplastic cancer), resulting in retrodifferentiation into highly malignant cancer of embryonal, yolk sac, or trophoblastic nature.

OVERALL SUMMARY AND CONCLUSIONS

In this chapter, highly variegated but harmonized differentiations of gastric cancer cells were presented and analyzed with the aid of immunohistochemistry and mucin histochemistry. The demonstration of dual differentiation toward gastric and intestinal epithelial cells in both diffuse and adenoplastic carcinomas supports questioning the view of histogenesis that diffuse carcinoma arises from almost intact gastric mucosa, while adenoplastic carcinoma arises from intestinalized mucosa. In fact, not only carcinomas predominantly composed of signet ring cells with an intestinal phenotype, but also tubular adenocarcinomas predominantly with a gastric phenotype (e.g., adenocarcinoma with lymphoid stroma) were identified.

It is very surprising that many signet ring cell carcinomas in the mucosa reveal well organized zonal (lamellar or layered) differentiations, especially when the destruction of preexisting mucosal structures is minimal. The marker substances are expressed in the intramucosal cancer cells with a consistent localization pattern similar to that of nonneoplastic epithelial cells.

These observations are very important in a

sense that the differentiation of cancer cells is possibly controlled by the appropriate mucosal microenvironment that contains well developed microcirculatory networks. Such a notion becomes most understandable when we take the cell kinetics in the lesion carefully into account. The proliferative cells of intramucosal signet ring cell carcinoma occupy solely the layer that corresponds to the generative zone of noncancerous mucosa, and mature signet ring cells, which occupy the upper and bottom layers of the mucosa are no longer mitogenic. Consequently, immature-looking proliferative cancer cells, "neoplastic stem cells," in the mucosa differentiate upward to signet ring cells of the surface epithelial cell-type or goblet cell-type and downward to those of the pyloric gland-type. The incompletion of the zonal differentiation in adenoplastic carcinoma in the mucosa may reflect the random distribution of mitogenic cancer cells.

The differentiation toward endocrine-like cells is another characteristic of diffuse (scirrhous) carcinoma, in which argyrophilic and chromogranin-immunoreactive cells are frequently encountered. Some argyrophilic carcinomas exhibited a number of glicentin-immunoreactive cells. This probably represents a fetal-type expression (fetalism), since most scirrhous carcinomas occur in scarcely intestinalized oxyntic mucosa, and the demonstration of glicentin cells in the oxyntic mucosa is peculiar to fetal stomach. The presence of multipotent tumor stem cells that differentiate into various cell components including endocrine cells should be speculated upon again.

Finally, the notion of "retrodifferentiation" of gastric cancer cells was insistently favored. Tumors with extremely high levels of serum AFP or a number of AFP stain-positive cells mostly belonged to poorly differentiated medullary carcinoma or embryonal carcinoma arising from the stomach, while papillary adenocarcinoma or signet ring cell carcinoma was also occasionally AFP-positive. A component of yolk sac tumor was seen in two of three primary gastric choriocarcinomas. Clear cytoplasm with abundance of glycogen was a common cytological feature of AFP-positive cancer cells. For these tumors, the acquisition of the properties of fetal gastrointestinal epithelium, which has been reported to be AFP-positive, or of more immature retrodifferentiated embryonal cells would be a relevant explanation. The common existence of a component of ordinary adenoplastic carcinoma in tumor tissues of embryonal carcinoma and choriocarcinoma of the stomach may lead to the concept of "malignant transformation" of ordinary gastric cancer cells into highly retrodifferentiated embryonal, yolk sac or trophoblastic tumor cells.

ACKNOWLEDGEMENTS

The author expresses gratitude to Professor Keiichi Watanabe, Department of Pathology, Tokai University School of Medicine, Isehara, for his efforts in reviewing and criticizing the manuscript. The author is also deeply indebted to Professor Hiroshi Nagura, Laboratory of Germfree Life Research, Institute for Disease Mechanism and Control, Nagoya University School of Medicine, Nagoya, and to Associate Professor Tsutomu Katsuyama, Pathology Division of Central Clinical Laboratories, Shinshu University Hospital, Matsumoto, for their valuable advice and suggestions. The skillful technical assistance of Mr. Johbu Ito, Cell Biology Research Laboratory, Tokai University School of Medicine, Isehara, for taking photographs is also gratefully acknowledged. This work was in part supported by the Grant-in-Aid from the Ministry of Education, Japan #61010035.

REFERENCES

1. Markert C.L.: Cell differentiation in neoplasia, in: Tumor Cell Heterogeneity. Origins and Implications (eds. Owens A.H. Jr, Coffey D.S., Baylin S.B.), New York, London, Academic Press, 1982, pp 237–247
2. Sugano H., Nakamura K., Kato Y.: Pathological studies of human gastric cancer. Acta Pathol Jpn 32 (Suppl 2):329–347, 1982
3. Osamura R.Y.: Review: gastric carcinoma in Japan. Tokai J. Exp Clin Med 8:405–410, 1983
4. Lauren P.: The two histologic main types of gastric carcinoma; diffuse and so-called intestinal-type car-

cinoma. An attempt at a histoclinical classification. Acta Pathol Microbiol Scand **64**:31–49, 1965

5. Nakamura K.: Structure of the gastric cancer. Igaku-Shoin, Tokyo, 1982 (in Japanese)

6. Hattori T., Fujita S.: Tritiated thymidine autoradiographic study on cellular migration in the gastric gland of the golden hamster. Cell Tiss Res **172**:171–184, 1976

7. Hattori T., Fujita S.: Tritiated thymidine autoradiographic study of cellular migration and renewal in the pyloric mucosa of golden hamsters. Cell Tiss Res **175**:49–57, 1976

8. Fujita S., Hattori T.: Cell proliferation, differentiation, and migration in the gastric mucosa: a study on the background of carcinogenesis, in: Pathophysiology of Carcinogenesis in Digestive Organs (eds. Farber F., Kawachi T., Nagayo T., Sugano H., Sugimura T., Weisburger J.H.), Tokyo University/Park Press, 1977, pp 21–36

9. Fujita S.: Histogenesis and progression of gastric cancer from a viewpoint of cell kinetics. Tr Soc Pathol Jpn **70**:23–54, 1981 (in Japanese)

10. Imai T., Kubo T., Watanabe H.: Chronic gastritis in Japanese with reference to high incidence of gastric carcinoma. J Natl Cancer Inst **47**:179–195, 1971

11. Nakamura K., Sugano H., Takagi K.: Carcinoma of the stomach in incipient phase. Its histogenesis and histological appearances. Gann **59**:251–258, 1968

12. Matsukura N., Suzuki K., Kawachi T., Aoyagi M., Sugimura T., Kitaoka H., Numajiri H., Shirota A., Itabashi M., Hirota T.: Distribution of marker enzymes and mucin in intestinal metaplasia in human stomach and relation of complete and incomplete types of intestinal metaplasia to minute gastric carcinomas. J Natl Cancer Inst **65**:231–240, 1980

13. Isaacson P.: Immunoperoxidase study of the secretory immunoglobulin system and lysozyme in normal and diseased gastric mucosa. Gut **23**:578–588, 1982

14. Kittas C., Aroni K., Kotsis L., Papadimitriou C.S.: Distribution of lysozyme, α_1-antichymotrypsin and α_1-antitrypsin in adenocarcinomas of the stomach and large intestine. An immunohistochemical study. Virchows Arch [Pathol Anat] **398**:139–147, 1982

15. Tahara E., Ito H., Shimamoto F., Iwamoto T., Nakagami K., Niimoto H.: Lysozyme in human gastric carcinoma: a retrospective immunohistochemical study. Histopathology **6**:409–421, 1982

16. Ejeckam G.C., Huang S.N., McCaughey W.T.E., Gold P.: Immunohistopathologic study on carcinoembryonic antigen (CEA)-like material and immunoglobulin A in gastric malignancies. Cancer **44**:1606–1614, 1979

17. Tome Y., Hirohashi S., Sekine T., Itabashi M., Hirota T., Shimosato Y.: Production of pepsinogen by gastric carcinoma. Igaku-no-ayumi **123**:999–1000, 1982 (in Japanese)

18. Reis W.A., Thompson W.D., Kay J.: Pepsinogen in gastric carcinoma cells. J Clin Pathol **36**:137–139, 1983

19. Denk H., Tappeiner G., Davidovits A., Eckerstorfer R., Holzner J.H.: Carcinoembryonic antigen and blood group substances in carcinomas of the stomach and colon. J Natl Cancer Inst **53**:933–942, 1974

20. Mori T., Lee P.-K., Nakajo Y., Awata K., Kosaki G.: Biological features of CEA-positive cells in gastric cancer and fetal tissues, in: Carcino-Embryonic Proteins: Chemistry, Biology, Clinical Applications, vol II (ed. Lehmann F.G.), Elsevier/North Holland Biomedical Press, New York, 1979, pp 23–28

21. Miyayama H., Miyayama Y.: Immunohistochemical study of αFP, CEA, hCG, and placental A1-P expressed in human gastrointestinal cancers in comparison to embryo-fetal gastrointestinal mucosa. Pathol Clin Med **3**:905–915, 1985 (in Japanese with English abstr)

22. Lee P.-K., Mori T., Fujimoto N., Nakamura T., Kosaki G.: Relationships of AFP-producing cells in gastric cancer, hepatocellular cancer and fetal tissues, in: Carcino-Embryonic Proteins: Chemistry, Biology, and Clinical Applications (ed. Lehmann FG), vol II, Elsevier/North Holland Biomedical Press, New York, 1979, pp 373–378

23. Kodama T., Kameya T., Hirota T., Shomosato Y., Ohkura H., Mukojima T., Kitaoka H.: Production of alpha-fetoprotein, normal serum protein, and human chorionic gonadotropin in stomach cancer: histologic and immunohistochemical analyses of 35 cases. Cancer **48**:1647–1655, 1981

24. Ito T., Tahara E.: Human chorionic gonadotropin in human gastric carcinoma. A retrospective immunohistochemical study. Acta Pathol Jpn **33**:287–296, 1983

25. Kawasaki H., Takeuchi M., Kimoto E.: Immunofluorescent staining of placental alkaline phosphatase in gastric and rectal carcinoma. Gann **65**:473–479, 1974

26. Kojima J., Kanatani M., Yamamoto T., Tateishi R., Nakamura N.: Carcinoembryonic proteins in gastric carcinoma metastatic to the liver. Gastroenterol Jpn **14**:596–603, 1979

27. Rapp W., Windisch M., Peschke P., Wurster K.: Purification of human intestinal goblet cell antigen (GOA): its immunohistological demonstration in the intestine and in mucus producing gastrointestinal adenocarcinomas. Virchows Arch [Pathol Anat] **382**:163–177, 1979

28. Furihata C., Tatematsu M., Miki K., Katsuyama T., Sudo K., Miyagi N., Kubota T., Jin S.-S., Kodama K., Ito N., Konishi Y., Suzuki K., Matsushima T.: Gastric-and intestinal-type properties of human gastric cancers transplanted into nude mice. Cancer Res **44**:727–733, 1984

29. Katsuyama T., Tsukahara M., Nasu T.: Application of paradoxical Concanavalin A staining to gastrointestinal pathology. II. Mucosubstance histochemistry of human gastric carcinoma. Igaku-no-ayumi **111**:156–158, 1979 (in Japanese)

30. Katsuyama T., Ono K., Nakayama J., Kanai M.: Recent advances in mucosubstance histochemistry, in: Gastric Mucus and Mucus Secreting Cells (ed. Kawai K), Excerpta Medica, Tokyo, 1985, pp 3–18

31. Azzopardi J.G., Pollock D.J.: Argentaffin cells and argyrophil cells in gastric carcinoma. J Pathol Bacteriol **86**:443–452, 1963

32. Kubo T., Watanabe H.: Neoplastic argentaffin cells in gastric and intestinal carcinomas. Cancer **27**:447–454, 1971

33. Tahara E., Ito H., Shimamoto F., Taniyama K., Iwamoto T., Sumiyoshi H., Kajihara H., Yamamoto M.: Argyrophil cells in early gastric carcinoma: an immunohistochemical and ultrastructural study. J Cancer Res Clin Oncol **103**:187–202, 1982

34. Tahara E., Ito H., Nakagami K., Shimamoto F., Yamamoto M., Sumii K.: Scirrhous argyrophil cell carcinoma of the stomach with multiple production of polypeptide hormone, amine, CEA, lysozyme and HCG. Cancer **49**:1904–1915, 1982

35. Tsutsumi Y., Nagura H., Kamoshida E., Ishii M., Mikata A.: Immunohistochemical studies on secre-

tory glycoproteins produced by gastric cancer. Digest Org Immunol 7:168–174, 1981 (in Japanese)

36. Tsutsumi Y., Mikata A., Nagura H.: Histochemical studies on mucins and secretory glycoproteins in early gastric carcinoma. Acta Histochem Cytochem 14:82, 1981 (Abstract)

37. Nagura H., Tsutsumi Y., Shioda Y., Watanabe K.: Immunohistochemistry of gastric carcinomas and associated diseases: novel distribution of carcinoembryonic antigen and secretory component on the surface of gastric cancer cells. J Histochem Cytochem 31:193–198, 1983

38. Tsutsumi Y.: Immunohistochemical studies on glucagon, glicentin and pancreatic polypeptide in human stomach: normal and pathological conditions. Histochem J 16:869–883, 1984

39. Tsutsumi Y., Sato T., Kondo Y., Ogoshi K.: Immunohistochemical analysis of alpha-fetoprotein producing gastric carcinomas. Digest Org Immunol 13:31–39, 1984 (in Japanese)

40. Tsutsumi Y.: Immunohistochemistry of hormone (4). Neuroendocrine-related substances. Pathol Clin Med 2:1610–1623, 1984 (in Japanese)

41. Grimelius L.: A silver nitrate stain for α_2 cells in human pancreatic islets. Acta Soc Med Upsal 73:243–270, 1968

42. Masson P.: Carcinoids (argentaffin cell tumors) and nerve hyperplasia of the appendicular mucosa. Am J Pathol 4:181–212, 1928

43. Japanese Research Society of Gastric Cancer: The general rules for the gastric cancer study in surgery and pathology (11th ed), Kanehara-Shuppan, Tokyo, 1985 (in Japanese)

44. Spicer S.S.: Diamine methods for differentiating mucosubstances histochemically. J Histochem Cytochem 13:211–234, 1965

45. Katsuyama T., Spicer S.S.: Histochemical differentiation of complex carbohydrates with variants of the Concanavalin A-horseradish peroxidase method. J Histochem Cytochem 26:233–250, 1978

46. Culling C.F.A., Reis P.E., Dunn W.L.: A new histochemical method for the identification and visualization of both side chain acylated and nonacylated sialic acids. J Histochem Cytochem 24:1225–1230, 1976

47. Nakane P.K.: Recent progress in peroxidase-labeled antibody method. Ann NY Acad Sci 254:203–211, 1975

48. Sternberger L.A. Hardy P.H. Jr, Cuculis J.J., Meyer H.G.: The unlabeled antibody enzyme method of immunohistochemistry. Preparation and properties of soluble antigen-antibody complex (horseradish peroxidase-antihorseradish peroxidase) and its use in identification of spirochetes. J Histochem Cytochem 18:315–333, 1970

49. Tsutsumi Y., Nagura H., Watanabe K.: Immunohistochemical observations of carcinoembryonic antigen (CEA) and CEA-related substances in normal and neoplastic pancreas. Pitfalls and caveats in CEA immunohistochemistry. Am J Clin Pathol 82:535–542, 1984

50. Wagener C., Csaszar H., Totović V., Breuer H.: A highly sensitive method for the demonstration of carcinoembryonic antigen in normal and neoplastic colonic tissue. Histochemistry 58:1–11, 1978

51. Tourville D.R., Adler R.H., Bienenstock J., Tomasi T.B. Jr: The human secretory immunoglobulin of γA, secretory "piece", and lactoferrin in normal human tissue. J Exp Med 129:411–429, 1969

52. Brandzaeg P., Bahlien K.: Immunohistochemical studies of the formation and epithelial transport of immunoglobulins in normal and diseased human intestinal mucosa. Scand J Gastroenterol 11 (Suppl 36):1–45, 1976

53. Brown W.R., Isobe Y., Nakane P.K.: Studies on translocation of immunoglobulins across intestinal epithelium. II. Immunoelectronmicroscopic localization of immunoglobulins and secretory component in human intestinal mucosa. Gastroenterology 71:985–995, 1976

54. Tsutsumi Y., Nagura H., Watanabe K.: Immune aspects of intestinal metaplasia of the stomach: an immunohistochemical study. Virchows Arch [Pathol Anat] 403:345–359, 1984

55. Mason D.Y., Taylor C.R.: The distribution of muramidase (lysozyme) in human tissues. J Clin Pathol 28:124–132, 1975

56. Adinolfi M., Glynn A.A., Lindsay M., Milne C.M.: Serological properties of γ-A antibodies to *Escherichia coli* present in human colostrum. Immunology 10:517–526, 1966

57. Tsutsumi Y., Nagura H., Watanabe K., Yanaihara N.: A novel subtyping of intestinal metaplasia of the stomach, with special reference to the histochemical characterizations of endocrine cells. Virchows Arch [Pathol Anat] 401:73–88, 1983

58. Mason D.Y., Taylor C.R.: Distribution of transferrin, ferritin, and lactoferrin in human tissues. J Clin Pathol 31:316–327, 1978

59. Parmley R.T., Takagi M., Barton J.C., Boxer L.A., Austin R.L.: Ultrastructural localization of lactoferrin and iron-binding protein in human neutrophils and rabbit heterophils. Am J Pathol 109:343–358, 1982

60. Nishida O., Kano T., Tsukada H., Yasuda N., Kobayashi Y., Sakai M., Uchino H., Miyake T.: Localization of lactoferrin in gastric mucosa. Jap J Gastroenterol 82:1–8, 1985 (in Japanese with English abstr)

61. Samloff I.M., Liebman W.M.: Cellular localization of the group II pepsinogens in human stomach and duodenum by immunofluorescence. Gastroenterology 65:36–42, 1973

62. Gold P., Freedman S.O.: Specific carcinoembryonic antigens in human digestive system. J Exp Med 122:467–481, 1965

63. Klockars M., Reitamo S., Reitamo J.J., Möller C.: Immunohistochemical identification of lysozyme in intestinal lesions in ulcerative colitis and Crohn's disease. Gut:18:377–381, 1977

64. Watanabe H., Enjoji M., Imai T.: Gastric carcinoma with lymphoid stroma. Cancer 38:232–243, 1976

65. Ridolfi R.L., Rosen P.P., Port A., Kinne D., Miké V.: Medullary carcinoma of the breast. A clinicopathologic study with 10 years follow-up. Cancer 40:1365–1385, 1977

66. Higuchi Y., Ishida M., Hayashi H.: A lymphocyte chemotactic peptide released from immunoglobulin G by neutrophil neutral thiol protease. Cell Immunol 46:297–308, 1979

67. Selby W.S., Janossy G., Jewell D.P.: Immunohistochemical characterization of intraepithelial lymphocytes of human gastrointestinal tract. Gut 22:169–176, 1981

68. Sato T., Yamazaki H., Tsutsumi Y., Mori I., Hata J., Tamaoki N., Noto T., Nagura H.: Quantitative analysis of subsets of intraepithelial T lymphocytes in carcinoma of the colon. Digest Org Immunol 13:61–65, 1984 (in Japanese)

69. Asano S., Sato N., Mori M., Ohsawa N., Kosaka K.,

Ueyama Y.: Detection and assessment of human tumors producing granulocyte-macrophage colony-stimulating factor (GM-CSF) by heterotransplantation into nude mice. Br J Cancer 41:689–694, 1980

70. Tamaoki N.: Pathology of human cancer transplanted into nude mice. Experimental approach to the pathology of tumor-bearing individuals. Tr Soc Pathol Jpn 93:93–125, 1985 (in Japanese)

71. Tsutsumi Y.: Application of parietal cell autoantibody to histopathological studies. Acta Pathol Jpn 35:823–829, 1985

72. Fisher E.R.: Ultrastructure of the human breast and its disorders. Am J Clin Pathol 66:291–305, 1976

73. Ruoslahti E.: Cell-matrix interactions as determinants of differentiation and tumor invasion, in: Oncodevelopmental Markers. Biologic, Diagnostic, and Monitoring Aspects (ed. Fishman W.H.), Academic Press, New York, London, 1983, pp 21–35

74. Fujita S.: Stroma as a rate limiting factor for growth of tumors *in vivo*. Gann Monogr Cancer Res 25:57–66, 1980

75. Tsuchihashi Y.: Studies on structure and function of the mucosal microvascular system of the gastrointestinal tract with special references to their relations to epithelial functions. J Kyoto Pref Univ Med 92:59–81, 1983 (in Japanese with English abstr)

76. Watanabe K.: Microcirculation in lung, in: Microcirculation (eds. Azuma T., Tsuchiya M., Mishima Y.), Lifetime Education Series 6, Nakayama Books, Tokyo, 1979, pp 186–196 (in Japanese)

77. Sugihara H.: Proliferation and differentiation of human signet ring cell carcinoma in gastric mucosa. Fine structural basis of the morphogenesis of "layered structure." J Kyoto Pref Univ Med 93:591–605, 1984 (in Japanese with English abstr)

78. Pierce G.B., Nakane P.K., Mazurkiewicz J.E.: Natural history of malignant stem cells, in: Differentiation and Control of Malignancy of Tumor Cells. Proceedings of the 4th International Symposium of the Prince Takamatsu Cancer Research Fund, Tokyo, 1973, University of Tokyo Press, Tokyo, 1974, pp 453–469

79. Pierce G.B., Nakane P.K. Martinez-Hernandez A., Ward J.M.: Ultrastructural comparison of differentiation of stem cells of murine adenocarcinomas of colon and breast with their normal counterparts. J Natl Cancer Inst 58:1329–1345, 1977

80. Yesner R.: Spectrum of lung cancer and ectopic hormones. Pathol Annu 13:(Part 1)217–240, 1978

81. Gazdar A.F., Carney D.N., Guccioni J.G., Baylin S.B.: Small cell carcinoma of the lung: cellular origin and relationship to other pulmonary tumors, in: Small Cell Lung Cancer (eds. Greco F.A., Oldham R.K., Bunn P.A. Jr), Grune & Stratton, New York, 1981, pp 145–175

82. Ahnen D.J., Nakane P.K., Brown W.R.: Ultrastructural localization of carcinoembryonic antigen in normal intestine and colon cancer. Abnormal distribution of CEA on the surface of colon cancer cells. Cancer 49:2077–2090, 1982

83. Schumacher H.R., McFeely A.E., Davis K.D., Maugel T.K.: The acute leukemia cell. IV. DNA synthesis in peripheral blood and bone. Am J Clin Pathol 56:508–514, 1971

84. Nakamura S., Kino I., Baba S.: *Ex vivo* autoradiographic study on the labeling index of gastric cancers. Proc Jap Cancer Assoc, the 44th Annual Meeting, 1985, p 379 (Abstr)

85. Wylie C.V., Nakane P.K., Pierce G.B.: Degree of differentiation in nonproliferating cells in mammary carcinoma. Differentiation 1:11–20, 1973

86. Hamperl H.: Über die "gelben" (chromaffinen) Zellen in gesunden und kranken Magendarmschlauch. Virchows Arch [Pathol Anat] 266:509–548, 1927

87. Solcia E., Cappela C., Buffa R., Usellini L., Frigerio B., Fontana P.: Endocrine cells of the gastrointestinal tract and related tumors. Pathobiol Annu 9:163–204, 1979

88. O'Connor D.T., Burton D., Deftos L.J.: Immunoreactive human chromogranin A in diverse polypeptide hormone producing human tumors and normal endocrine tissues. J Clin Endocrinol Metab 57:1084–1086, 1983

89. Cohen D.V., Elting J.: Biosynthesis, processing, and secretion of parathormone and secretory protein-I. Recent Prog Horm Res 39:181–209, 1983

90. O'Connor D.T., Frigon R.P., Sokoloff R.L.: Human chromogranin A. Purification and characterization from catecholamine storage vesicles of human pheochromocytoma. Hypertension 6:2–12, 1984

91. Fujimoto S., Hattori T., Kimoto K., Yamashita S., Fujita S., Kawai K.: Tritiated thymidine autoradiographic study on origin and renewal of gastrin cells in antral area of hamsters. Gastroenterology 79:785–791, 1980

92. Bartow S.A., Mukai K., Rosai J.: Pseudoneoplastic proliferation of endocrine cells in pancreatic fibrosis. Cancer 47:2627–2633, 1981

93. Torikata C., Kawai T., Yakumaru K., Kageyama K.: Histopathological studies on the tumorlet of the lung with special reference to the cytogenesis of proliferating cells. Acta Pathol Jpn 25:539–553, 1975

94. Tsutsumi Y., Osamura R.Y., Watanabe K., Yanaihara N.: Cytogenesis and pathological alterations of human bronchial neuroendocrine cells: an immunohistochemical study. Pathol Clin Med 1:298–319, 1983 (in Japanese with English abstr)

95. Heitz P.U., Wegmann W.: Identification of neoplastic Paneth cells in an adenocarcinoma of the stomach using lysozyme as a marker, and electron microscopy. Virchows Arch [Pathol Anat] 386:107–116, 1980

96. Clarkson B., Marks P.A., Till J.E. (eds): Differentiation of Normal and Neoplastic Hematopoietic Cells. Cold Spring Harbor Laboratory, 1978

97. Pierce G.B., Wills R.S.: Embryonic microenvironment in the regulation of cancer cells, in: Tumor Cell Heterogeneity. Origins and Implications (eds. Owens A.H. Jr, Coffey D.S., Baylin S.B.), Academic Press, New York, London, 1982, pp 249–258

98. Sidhu G.S.: The endodermal origin of digestive and respiratory tract APUD cells. Histopathologic evidence and a review of the literature. Am J Pathol 96:5–20, 1979

99. Pearse A.G.E.: the cytochemistry and ultrastructure of polypeptide hormone-producing cells of the APUD series and the embryologic, physiologic, and pathologic implications of the concept. J Histochem Cytochem 17:303–313, 1969

100. Subuswamy S.G., Gibbs N.M., Ross C.F., Morson B.C.: Goblet cell carcinoid of the appendix. Cancer 34:338–344, 1974

101. Ljungberg O., Bondeson L., Bondeson A-G: Differentiated thyroid carcinoma, intermediate type: a new tumor entity with features of follicular and parafollicular cell carcinoma. Hum Pathol 15:218–228, 1984

102. Matthews M.J., Hirsch F.R.: Problems in the diag-

nosis of small cell carcinoma of the lung. In: Small Cell Lung Cancer (eds. Greco F.A., Oldham R.K., Bunn P.A. Jr), Grune & Stratton, New York, 1981, pp 35–50

103. Masopust J., Kithier K., Rádl J., Koutecký J., Kotal L.: Occurrence of fetoprotein in patients with neoplasms and non-neoplastic diseases. Int J Cancer 3:364–373, 1968

104. Mori H., Onji M., Yoshida A., Fukunishi R.: Serum alpha-fetoprotein-positive gastric carcinoid with liver metastasis. Virchows Arch [Pathol Anat] 387:107–116, 1980

105. McIntire K.R., Walsmann T.A., Moertel C.G., Co V.L.W.: Serum α-fetoprotein in patients with neoplasms of the gastrointestinal tract. Cancer Res 35:991–996, 1975

106. Kitaoka Y., Hattori N., Mukojima T., Ohkura H., Nakayama N., Okada H.: Alpha-fetoprotein content in tissues from patients with gastric cancer. Tumor Res 8:171–177, 1973

107. Lehmann F.G.: Immunological relationship between human placental and intestinal alkaline phosphatase. Clin Chim Acta 65:257–269, 1975

108. Uchida T., Shjimoda T., Miyata H., Shikata T., Iino S., Suzuki H., Oda T., Hirano K., Sugiura M.: Immunoperoxidase study of alkaline phosphatase in testicular tumor. Cancer 48:1455–1462, 1981

109. Ishii M.: Radioimmunoassay of α-fetoprotein. Gann Monogr Cancer Res 14:89–98, 1973

110. Hata J., Ueyama Y., Tamaoki N., Akatsuka A., Yoshimura S., Shimizu K., Morikawa Y., Furukawa T.: Human yolk sac tumor serially transplanted in nude mice: its morphologic and functional properties. Cancer 46:2446–2455, 1980

111. Gitlin D., Perricelli A., Gitlin G.M.: Synthesis of α-fetoprotein by liver, yolk sac, and gastrointestinal tract of the human conceptus. Cancer Res 32:979–982, 1972

112. Villee C.A., Hagerman D.D., Holmberg N., Lind J., Villee D.B.: The effects of anoxia on the metabolism of human fetal tissues. Pediatrics 22:953–971, 1958

113. Tashjian A.H. Jr, Weintraub B.D., Barowsky N.J., Rabson A.S, Rosen S.W.: Subunits of human chorionic gonadotropin: unbalanced synthesis and secretion by clonal cell strains derived from a bronchogenic carcinoma. Proc Natl Acad Sci USA 70:1419–1422, 1973

114. Stanbridge E.J., Rosen S.W., Sussman H.H.: Expression of the α-subunit of human chorionic gonadotropin is specifically correlated with tumorigenic expression in human cell hybrids. Proc Natl Acad Sci USA 79:6242–6245, 1982

115. Heitz P.V., Kasper M., Klöppel G., Polak J.M., Vaitukaitis J.L.: Glycoprotein-hormone alpha-chain production by pancreatic endocrine tumors: a specific marker for malignancy. Immunocytochemical analysis of tumors of 155 patients, Cancer 51:277–282, 1983

116. Kameya T., Shimosato Y., Tsumuraya M., Ohsawa N., Nomura T.: Human gastric choriocarcinoma serially transplanted in nude mice. J Natl Cancer Inst 56:325–332, 1976

117. Endo Y., Tsuchida Y., Miyazaki J., Kaneko M.: Analysis of lectin affinity of alpha-fetoprotein. Application to diagnosis. Jap J Cancer Chemother 10:636–641, 1983 (in Japanese)

118. Mori H., Soeda O., Kamano T., Tsunekawa K., Ueda N., Yoshida A., Fukunishi R.: Choriocarcinomatous change with immunohistochemically HCG-positive cells in the gastric carcinoma of the males. Virchows Arch [Pathol Anat] 396:141–153, 1982

119. Yonemura Y., Hashimoto T., Sawa T., Shimizu K., Miyazaki I.: A case of gastric carcinoma producing chorionic gonadotropin and alpha fetoprotein. Pathol Clin Med 3:541–545, 1985 (in Japanese with English abstr).

120. Teilum G.: Special Tumors of Ovary and Testis. Comparative Pathology and Histologic Identification (2nd ed), Philadelphia, J.B., Lippincott, 1976

121. Hutter R.V.P., Tollefsen H.R., De Cosse J.J., Foote F.W., Frazell E.L.: Spindle and giant cell metaplasia in papillary carcinoma of the thyroid. Am J Surg 110:660–668, 1965

2

Prognosis in Gastric Carcinoma
The preeminence of staging and futility
of histological classification.

Manuel Moutinho Ribeiro
Mário Seoxas
Manuel Sobrinho-Simões

Numerous studies dealing with the predictive value of epidemiological and morphological factors in gastric carcinoma are on record.[1-53] Excluding a few of the earliest published papers,[2,11,25,35] all of the aforementioned studies stress the major prognostic significance of the extent of the neoplastic disease. From this agreement on, however, controversy is the rule.

Some authors claim that the finding of lymphatic and/or venous invasion carries a worse prognosis[18,27,32,38,56] while others stress the lack of influence of this finding,[3] and most do not mention it at all.

Sex and age of patients have been considered either as meaningful[6,8,14] or as meaningless prognostic factors.[4,11,23,38]

Most authors stress that patients with tumors located in the cardia and/or fundus do worse than those with tumors located elsewhere.[7,10,12,13,17,23,31,33] Discrepant results are reported, however, in the comparison of the relative survival of patients with tumors located in the antrum and in body of the stomach.[11-13,23,33,51]

Size and/or shape of tumors are regarded as major prognostic factors in some papers,[2,13,15,18,23,25,31,38] as minor in others,[27,35] and as nonsignificant in a few.[17,19]

The prognostic significance of some quite specific features such as the "breach of the capsule of metastatic lymph nodes" and "tumor necrosis" has been emphasized by a few authors[3,30,53] and ignored by the majority.

The predictive value of the analysis of the so-called host immunologic response (lymphoid infiltration of the primary tumor, predominant pattern of regional lymph nodes and degree of nodal histiocytosis) has been found either as (very) rewarding[3,4,17,30,35,36,47,49] or as relatively useless.[5,12]

The controversy attains its maximum in the discussion of the prognostic significance of several microscopical features of the tumors.

Some authors claim that the histological grading provides valuable prognostic information,[11,17,22,25] while others deny it.[8]

The prognostic significance of nuclear grading has only been reported once[4] and the influence on survival of the morphological pattern of tumoral growth is not equally estimated in different studies.[35,37,41,49]

The predictive value of most (if not all) the

histological classifications still is an open question, [8,12,15,19,31,41,42,46] despite the general agreement on the dreadful prognosis carried by the so-called scirrhous carcinoma. [15,18,21,30,36,44]

Several reasons contribute to these discrepancies. First, there is too large a variation of factors, as well as of the criteria employed in their definition, from series to series. Second, the evaluation of the prognostic significance of the different factors is frequently performed without controlling the influence of the interrelated variables. Third, many authors concentrate on a single surgical, pathological, or clinico-pathologic entity and are, therefore, prone to overemphasize the significance of their findings. Finally, the misuse of statistics, namely in what concerns the utilization of linear multivariable regression analysis without checking the adequacy of the models, has frequently contributed to increase the confusion.

We undertook the present study of prognostic factors in gastric carcinoma using several methods of analysis in an attempt to settle the aforementioned controversies. In addition, we intended to see if the accuracy of the TNM method might be improved and if histology kept any predictive value when survival was adjusted for the extent of neoplastic disease. Finally, we also intended to find which of the available histological classifications should be considered the best for prognostic purposes.

MATERIAL AND METHODS

From 1960 to 1983, 610 patients were operated on for gastric carcinoma in the Serviço de Cirurgia—4 of Hospital S. João in Portugal. Two-hundred and fifty eight patients were submitted to "curative" resection, 29 to "palliative" resection, 174 to bypass procedures and 149 patients to laparotomy. The diagnosis of gastric carcinoma was histologically confirmed in every case. The procedure was considered as "palliative" whenever there were distant metastases to lymph nodes, peritoneal surface or liver, and/or neoplastic invasion of neighboring structures that made radical tumor resection impossible. The gastrectomy was also regarded as "palliative" whenever there was histological demonstration of neoplastic invasion of the surgical border.

This study is based on the detailed analysis of the cases submitted to "curative" resection. Twelve post-operative deaths and 10 cases of severe dysplasia/in situ carcinoma were excluded from the series. Any death occurring within the first month after surgery was considered as "post-operative." Follow-up information was obtained in 227 of the 236 patients (96.1%). Patients were followed until death, loss to follow-up, or end of study (October 1985). Treatment was strictly surgical; no chemotheraphy was used. Operative procedures were recorded as distal, subtotal gastrectomy (n = 176), total gastrectomy (n = 47), and proximal, subtotal gastrectomy (n = 13).

Sex and age of patients were always recorded. The mean age of patients was 55.1 ± 11.7 (mean $\pm$ SD) with a range from 22 to 79 years. The mean age of women (52.2 ± 14.2 years) was significantly lower than that of men (56.3 ± 10.5 years).

The macroscopical appearance of the tumors was classified according to the surgical and pathological descriptions as polypoid and/or fungating (n = 17), ulcerating (n = 62), ulcero-fungating (n = 64), ulcero-infiltrative (n = 54) and infiltrative (n = 26). In 13 cases there was not enough information about the shape of the tumors.

Tumor site was recorded as follows: antrum, including the pyloric region (n = 146), body (n = 50), fundus (n = 23) and cardia (n = 12). Four cases occurred in previously operated stomachs. In one case the bulk of tumor could not be located precisely. Size of the tumors as measured in the surgical specimens was classified in "less than 3 cm" (n = 30), "from 3 to 6 cm" (n = 65) and "6 cm or larger than 6 cm" (n = 96). There was no information on size in 45 cases.

The original descriptions and the microscopic slides from all cases were reviewed for staging purposes. The extent of penetration of gastric wall was evaluated according to the criteria of the A.J.C.[1] Ten cases were classified as T1m (mucosa), 18 as T1sm (submucosa), 84 as T2 (muscularis propria), 94 as T3 (serosa), and 30 as T4a (direct extension of immediately adjacent tissues). An attempt to subdivide T3 tumors according to the extent of penetration of the outer layer of the gastric wall ("invasion of the subserosa," "suspected invasion of the serosa", and "invasion of the serosa") as defined by the WHO International Reference Center[50] was abandoned due to its lack of reproducibility. Cases classified as T4b were excluded from the present series since they were considered as having been submitted to "palliative" resection.

The extent of lymph node involvement was evaluated according to the criteria of the A.J.C.[1] The N0 group was further divided according to the absence or presence of definite signs of lymphatic permeation within the primary tumor (N0 and N01p, respectively), and the N1 group was subdivided in N1(1) (only one lymph node with metastasis) and N1(>1) (two or more than two lymph nodes with metastases). After these criteria, 66 cases were classified as N0, 22 as N01p, 30 as N1(1), 54 as N!(>1), and 54 cases as N2. In 10 cases, lymph node involvement could not be evaluated at all (NX). Cases with metastases to distant, intraabdominal lymph nodes—so-called N3 group—were not included in the present series, since they were regarded as having been submitted to "palliative" resection.

No attempt was made to evaluate the "breach of the capsule of metastatic nodes," which was only found in highly advanced cases (N2-3).

The presence of blood vessel invasion was scrutinized in 206 cases by an experienced histopathologist not aware of the staging and follow-up data. Sections from all these cases were stained with orcein for elastic fibers. A case was regarded as positive for venous invasion (n = 76) only if there were unequivocal clusters of neoplastic cells within the lumina of elastic walled vessels. In some cases the presence of an adjacent artery was useful confirmatory evidence.

Sections stained with hematoxylin-eosin, PAS, and Alcian-blue at pH 2.5 were used for the histological classification of the tumors according to the criteria advanced by Laurén[54] Oota and Sobin (WHO booklet)[55] and Ming.[37]

One hundred and thirty eight carcinomas were classified as intestinal, 59 as diffuse, and 39 as unclassified according to Laurén.[54] In 10 cases there coexisted intestinal and diffuse patterns; in 9 of these cases the intestinal pattern was found on the surface and the diffuse pattern in the deeper portion of the tumors, whereas in the remaining case, both patterns were found "side by side." For statistical purposes these cases were included in the group of diffuse carcinomas.

According to the WHO classification,[55] 88 cases were labeled as well/moderately differentiated (tubular and/or papillary) adenocarcinomas, 64 as poorly differentiated carcinomas, 12 as mucinous carcinomas, and 72 as signet ring-cell carcinomas. Whenever there was more than one pattern, tumors were classified according to the less differentiated pattern.

One hundred and twenty seven carcinomas were classified as expanding and 109 as infiltrative according to Ming criteria.[37]

The reproducibility of Laurén and Ming classifications was evaluated through the comparison of the diagnosis made in 1981 and in the present study by the same observers (MMR and MSS) in a consecutive series of 244 gastric carcinomas. The percentage of disagreement was greater with Laurén classification than with Ming's (15.2% and 9.0%, respectively) (Sobrinho-Simões and Ribeiro, unpublished results).

The degree of desmoplastic reaction was subjectively scored as follows: 157 cases were regarded as having absent/minimal desmoplasia and the remaining 79 cases as having moderate/abundant desmoplasia. The lymphoid infiltration of the primary tumors was semiquantitively evaluated as abundant (n = 42), moderate (n = 68), and minimal or absent (n = 126).

The histological pattern of regional lymph nodes was evaluated according to the degree of sinusal histiocytosis (absent/minimal, 72

TABLE 2-1
Factors Evaluated for their Influence on Survival with Cox Model

Factors	Definition
Stage	1 = T1m N0; 2 = T1sm N0
	3 = T2 N0; 4 = T3 N0
	5 = T1-2 NOLp N1(1); 6 = T3 NOLp N1(1)
	7 = T1-3 N1(>1); 8 = T1-3 N2
	9 = T4a N1-2
Venous invasion	1 = absent; 2 = present
Sex	1 = male; 2 = female
Age	1 = < 40 yr; 2 = 40–59 yr; 3 = ≥ 60 yr
Type of resection	1 = distal; 2 = total; 3 = proximal
Site	1 = antrum; 2 = body; 3 = fundus; 4 = cardia
Histology/Laurén	1 = intestinal; 2 = diffuse; 3 = unclassified
Histology/WHO	1 = mucinous; 2 = well/moderately dif.; 3 = poorly dif.; 4 = signet ring cell
Histology/Ming	1 = expanding; 2 = infiltrative
Desmoplasia	1 = abundant/moderate; 2 = minimal/absent
Lymphoid infiltration	1 = abundant/moderate; 2 = minimal/absent
Follicular hyperplasia	1 = abundant/moderate; 2 = minimal/absent
Sinusal histiocytosis	1 = abundant/moderate; 2 = minimal/absent

cases; and moderate/abundant, 129) and to the number of germinal centers. Cases having the cortex of any regional lymph node occupied by numerous germinal centers were classified as "follicular hyperplasia" (n = 120) according to the criteria advanced by Black et al.[4] This group corresponds grossly to the "germinal center predominance" group of Tsakraklides et al,[56] whereas most of the cases with less numerous germinal centers (n = 81) fit in the groups of "lymphocyte predominance" and "unstimulated nodes" of Tsakraklides et al.[56] In 35 cases there was not enough evidence to label the pattern of nodal response.

The initial prognostic screening of the individual factors was performed using both the death rates and the crude survival curves. Death rates were calculated dividing the number of deaths by the total number of patient months of follow-up ($\times 100$). Survival rates were calculated according to Berkson's actuarial method.[57]

The evaluation of the prognostic significance of several factors acting simultaneously was performed using two different methods: comparison of the survival curves of stratified groups and multivariable regression techniques. The Cox proportional hazards model[58] was employed to evaluate the influence on survival of 13 factors (Table 2-1). The MPLR (maximum partial likelihood ratio) method was employed to perform a linear stepwise multivariate regression of the factors, which are significantly or suggestively related to survival. The assumed limit for significance to enter a term was 0.10 and the limit to remove a term 0.15.

A stepwise procedure was also used to evaluate the prognostic significance of each histological classification alone and in combination with the other ones after adjusting survival for stage and venous invasion.

Results were expressed in percentage or in mean ± standard error. Chi-square method after Yates correction and Student's two sided t test were used to perform statistical analysis. Significance tests relating to the hypothesis that a specific regression coefficient was zero were based on the assumption that the regression coefficient divided by its estimated standard error is distributed according to the Student's t distribution.

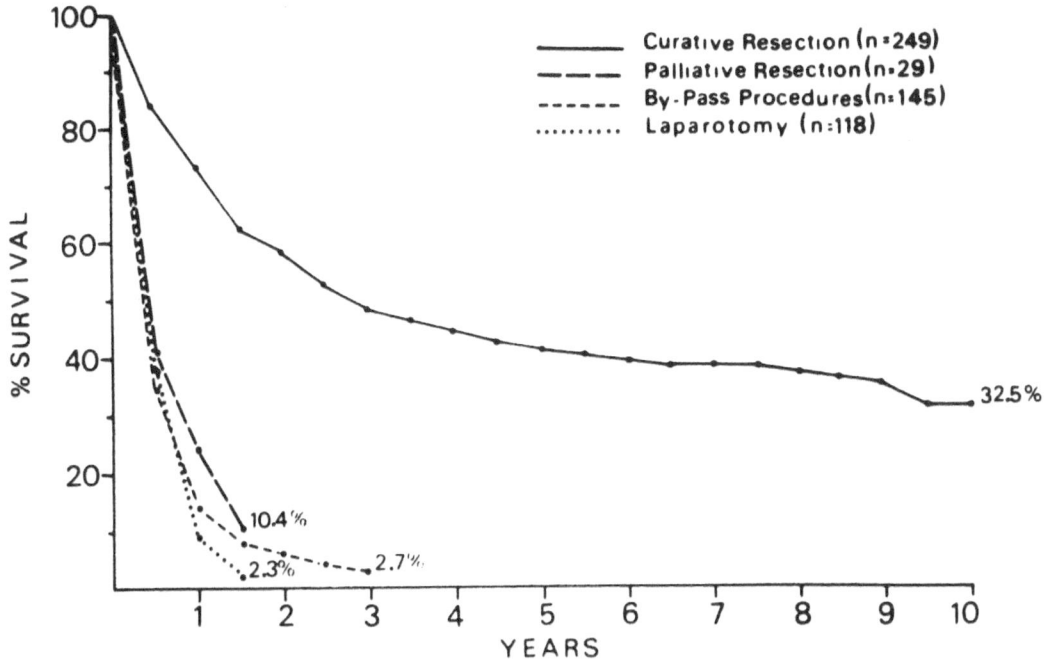

Fig. 2-1. Survival curves of the 541 patients submitted to surgery for gastric carcinoma.

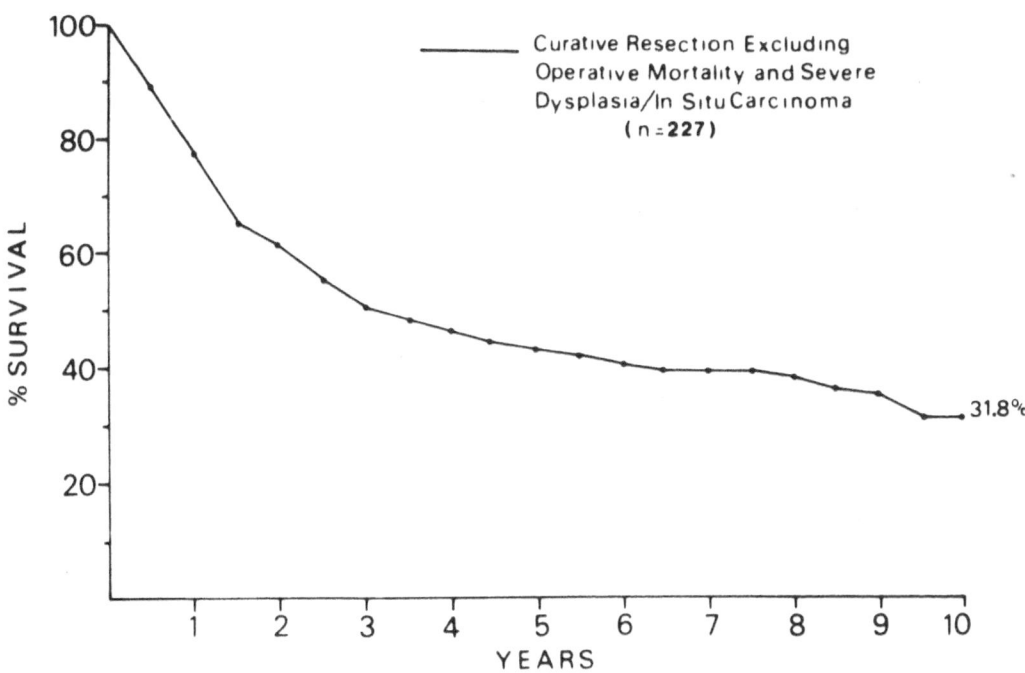

Fig. 2-2. Survival curve of the 227 patients used as basis for the evaluation of the prognostic factors.

TABLE 2-2
Summary of the Results Obtained with the
Multivariate Analysis of Prognostic Factors with
Cox Model

Factors	Regression Coefficient	Coeff/st. error	p value
Stage	0.3647	5.85	p < 0.001
Venous invasion	0.6714	3.18	p < 0.001
Sex	−0.1924	−0.85	NS
Age	0.1431	0.81	NS
Type of resection	−0.1863	−0.55	NS
Site	0.4018	1.97	p < 0.05
Histology/Laurén	0.1930	0.94	NS
Histology/WHO	0.0159	−0.09	NS
Histology/Ming	0.1007	0.32	NS
Desmoplasia	−0.6013	−2.38	p < 0.02
Lymphoid infiltration	−0.0812	0.39	NS
Follicular hyperplasia	0.3807	1.63	p ≃ 0.10
Sinusal histiocytosis	−0.2137	−0.92	NS

TABLE 2-3
Summary of the Results Obtained with the
Stepwise Multivariate Regression of Prognostic
Factors with MPLR Method

Factors	Improvement		
	Log Likelihood	Chi-Square	p Value
0	−472.0		
Stage	−441.8	−60.38	0.001
Venous invasion	−434.8	−14.02	0.001
Desmoplasia	−431.7	−6.24	0.013
Site	−428.5	−6.48	0.011
Follicular hyperplasia	−426.9	−3.14	0.076

RESULTS

As is to be expected, the survival curve of
patients submitted to "curative" resection is
clearly better than those of patients submitted
to other types of surgery (Fig. 2-1). Excluding
post-operative deaths, the 5 and 10-year survival rates of the 227 patients with invasive
carcinomas submitted to curative resection
are 42.3% and 31.8%, respectively (Fig. 2-2).

STAGE AND VENOUS INVASION

The multivariate analysis of prognostic factors shows that stage (extent of neoplastic disease as measured according to the TNM criteria) and venous invasion are, by far, the
most important factors (Tables 2-2 and 2-3).

The prognostic value of both the depth of
tumor invasion (T) and the status of nodal
metastases (N) is shown in Figures 2-3 and 2-
4 and Table 2-4.

The survival experience of patients with
carcinomas lacking nodal metastases and
showing definite signs of lymphatic permeation (NO1p) is much worse than that of patients with NO carcinomas and no signs of
lymphatic permeation (Fig. 2-4) (Table 2-4).
Patients with NO1p carcinomas were, therefore, grouped together with those having me-
tastasized to a single lymph node (N1(1)).
This grouping was used in the evaluation of
the prognostic meaning of the combination of
T and N factors, as well as in the study of the
prognostic value of the other factors (Fig. 2-5)
(Tables 2-1–4).

Most of the patients with carcinomas showing signs of venous invasion have advanced
stages of the neoplastic disease (Table 2-5).
These patients do much worse than those
having similarly advanced carcinomas and
lacking venous invasion (Fig. 2-6) (Table 2-5).
The presence of blood vessel invasion worsens also the survival of patients with less advanced carcinomas, but the difference is, in
these cases, lesser than in the group of advanced carcinomas (Fig. 2-6) (Table 2-5).

SITE, DESMOPLASIA AND PATTERN OF LYMPH NODE RESPONSE

The multivariate analysis shows that site of
tumors and degree of desmoplasia are significantly (p<0.05) correlated with survival (Tables 2-2 and 2-3). The pattern of regional
nodes is also correlated with survival, though

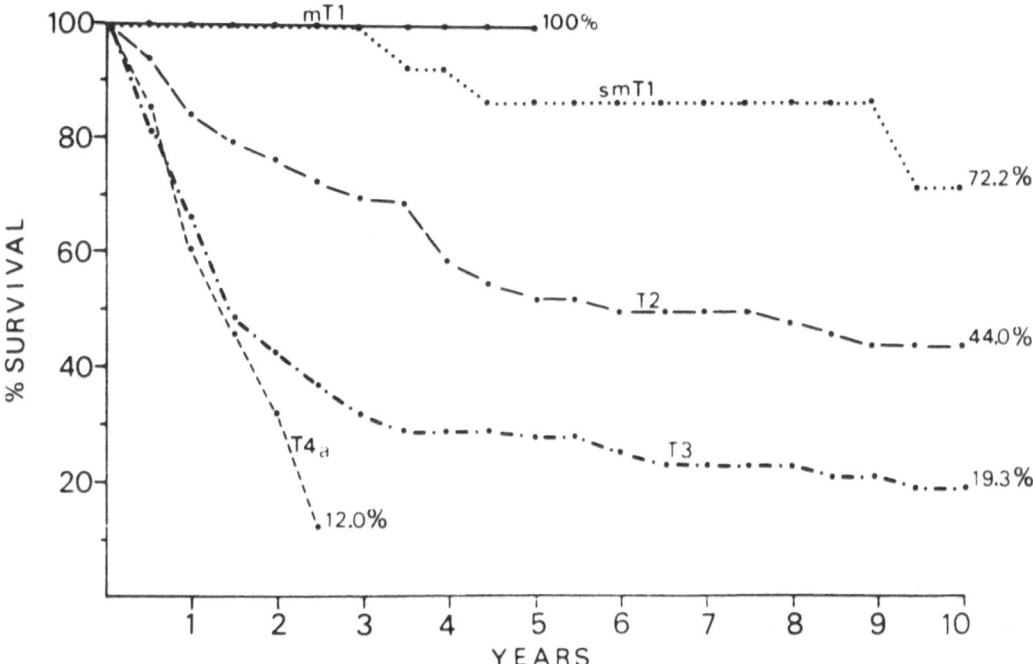

Fig. 2-3. Survival curves of the 227 patients according to the depth of penetration of gastric wall. (Abbrev: m = mucosa, sm = submucosa).

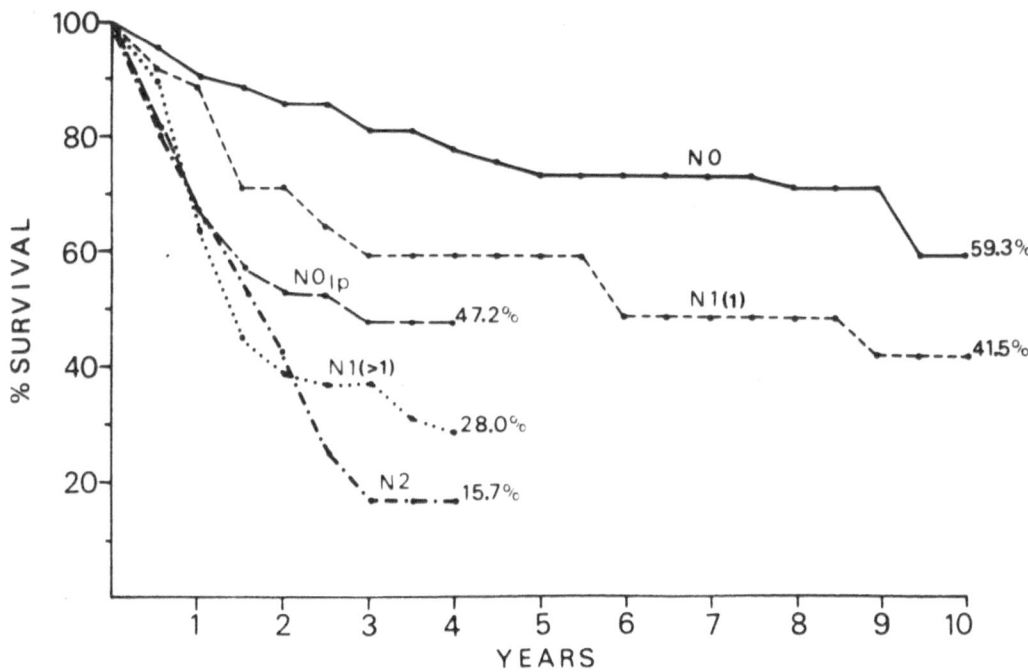

Fig. 2-4. Survival curves of 218 patients according to the status of nodal metastases. (Abbrev: lp = lymphatic permeation). No information was available in 9 patients.

TABLE 2-4
Death Rates According to Depth of Invasion, Nodal Metastases and Stage

Depth of Invasion	Death Rate	Nodal Metastases	Death Rate	Stage	Death Rate
T1m (10)	0.0	NO (64)	0.43	T1m NO (8)	0.0
T1sm (18)	0.33	NOLp (21)	1.59	T1sm NO (7)	0.37
T2 (80)	0.83	N1 (1) (29)	0.86	T2 NO (30)	0.30
T3 (91)	2.02	N1 (>1) (52)	2.48	T3 NO (18)	0.79
T4a (28)	4.13	N2 (52)	3.82	T4a NO (2)	6.45
		Nx (9)	0.69	T1-2 NOLp N1(1) (24)	0.68
				T3 NOLp N1 (1) (18)	1.60
				T1-3 N1 (>1) (44)	2.34
				T1-3 N2 (41)	3.78
				T4a NOLpN1-2 (26)	4.0

The number of patients is recorded in parentheses.

only at a suggestive (p<0.10) level (Tables 2-2 and 2-3).

Site

Patients with tumors located in the antrum have better prognosis (5 and 10-year survival rates of 48.3% and 36.3%, respectively) than those with tumors originating in the body of the stomach (39.2% and 28.2%, respectively). The prognosis worsens clearly when the bulk of the tumor is located in the fundus or in the cardia (2-year survival rates of 36.1% and

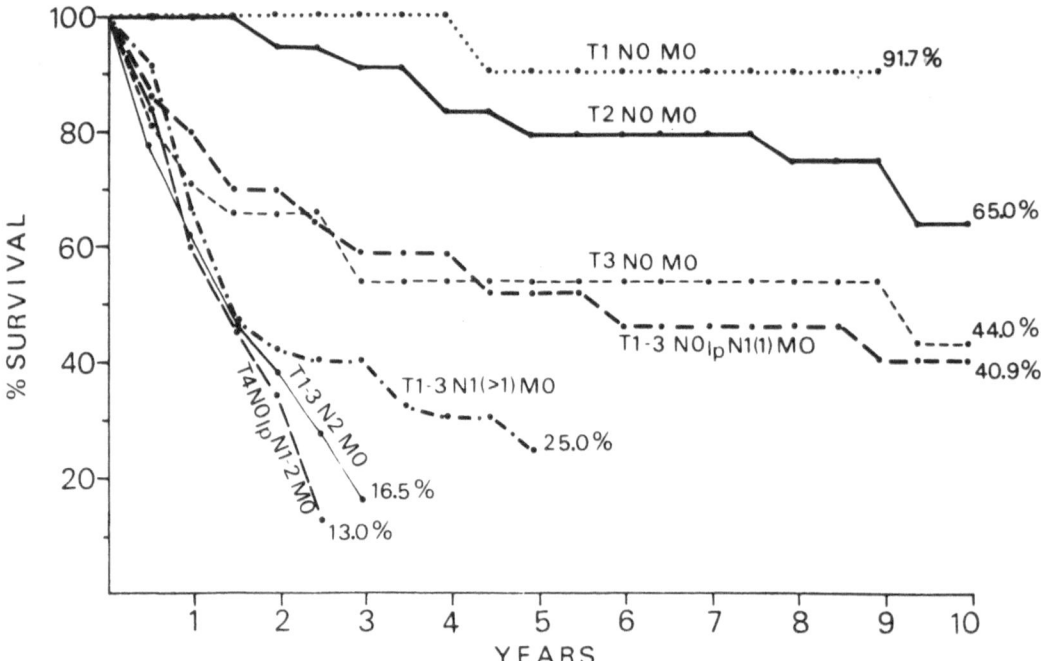

Fig. 2-5. Survival curves of 216 patients according to the TNM stage. (Abbrev: lp = lymphatic permeation). Two T4NOMO cases and 9 NX cases were excluded.

TABLE 2-5
Death Rates According to Stage and Venous Invasion

T1-3 N0		T1-3 N0Lp N1 (1)		T1-4a N1 (> 1)N2	
Venous Invasion	Death Rate	Venous Invasion	Death Rate	Venous Invasion	Death Rate
Absent (46)	0.29	Absent (20)	0.88	Absent (54)	2.33
Present (8)	1.04	Present (13)	1.21	Present (46)	5.40

The number of patients is recorded in parentheses.

45.5%, respectively). This worse prognosis is confirmed by the evaluation of death rate (Table 2-6).

The prognostic significance of the site of tumors depends upon the type of resection. The putative influence of other factors (technical problems related to the operative procedures, topography of the upper part of the abdomen, and "special" routes of lymphatic drainage in the proximal stomach) will be discussed in detail elsewhere (Ribeiro et al in preparation).

Desmoplasia

Patients with carcinomas showing moderate to abundant desmoplastic reaction do worse (5 and 10-year survival rates of 21.7% and 17.4%, respectively) than those with tumors lacking this histologic feature (51.8% and 38.6%, respectively). The analysis of death rate provides similar results (Table 2-6). The presence of moderate to abundant desmoplasia is significantly correlated with the size and shape of tumors, being particularly frequent in large tumors displaying an infiltrative or ulcero-infiltrative macroscopical appearance.

Pattern of Lymph Node Response

The 5 and 10-year survival rates of patients with "follicular hyperplasia" of regional

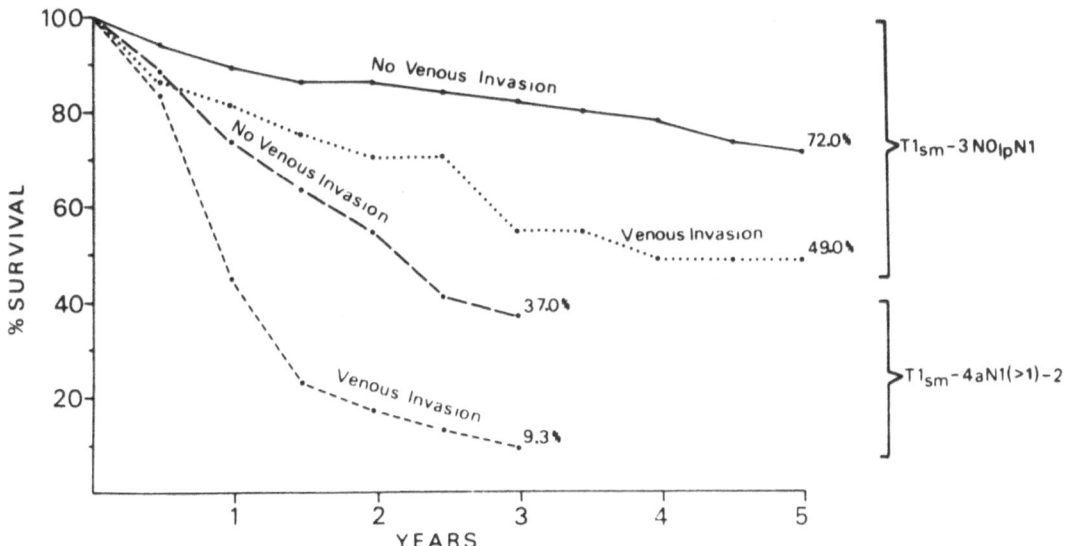

Fig. 2-6. Survival curves of 184 patients according to TNM stage and venous invasion (Abbrev: sm = submucosa, lp = lymphatic permeation). Ten intramucosal (T1m) carcinomas, 2 T4N0M0 carcinomas, 9 NX carcinomas, and 22 cases without information on venous invasion were excluded.

TABLE 2-6

Death Rates According to Site, Desmoplasia and
Pattern of Regional Lymph Nodes (Follicular
Hyperplasia)

	Factors	No of Patients	Death Rate
Site	Antrum	142	1.02
	Body	47	1.36
	Fundus	22	2.66
	Cardia	11	2.80
Follicular Hyperplasia	Abund./Moderate	119	0.97
	Min./Absent	77	1.80

nodes (53.8% and 38.1%, respectively) are
higher than those of patients lacking this feature (25.8% and 21.7%, respectively). These
results were confirmed by death rate analysis
(Table 2-6). Follicular hyperplasia is significantly correlated with the presence of moderate to abundant sinusal histiocytosis and independent from the degree of lymphoid

infiltration of the tumors and extent of neoplastic disease.

Histology

The multivariate analysis reveals that none
of the histological classifications is significantly correlated with survival (Tables 2-2
and 2-3). This lack of prognostic significance
does not depend upon the presence of desmoplasia as a covariate, since similar results
were obtained when desmoplasia was removed from the regression equation.

The evaluation of the prognostic value of
each histological classification shows that, *per
se*, Ming[37] classification appears to be the
most discriminating (Figs. 2-7–2-9) (Table 2-
7). The combined use of WHO[55] and Ming
classifications reveal that patients with poorly
differentiated carcinomas of expanding pattern do better than those with well/moder-
ately differentiated carcinomas of infiltrative
pattern (Fig. 2-10).

Ming classification also provides better
prognostic information than Laurén[54] and

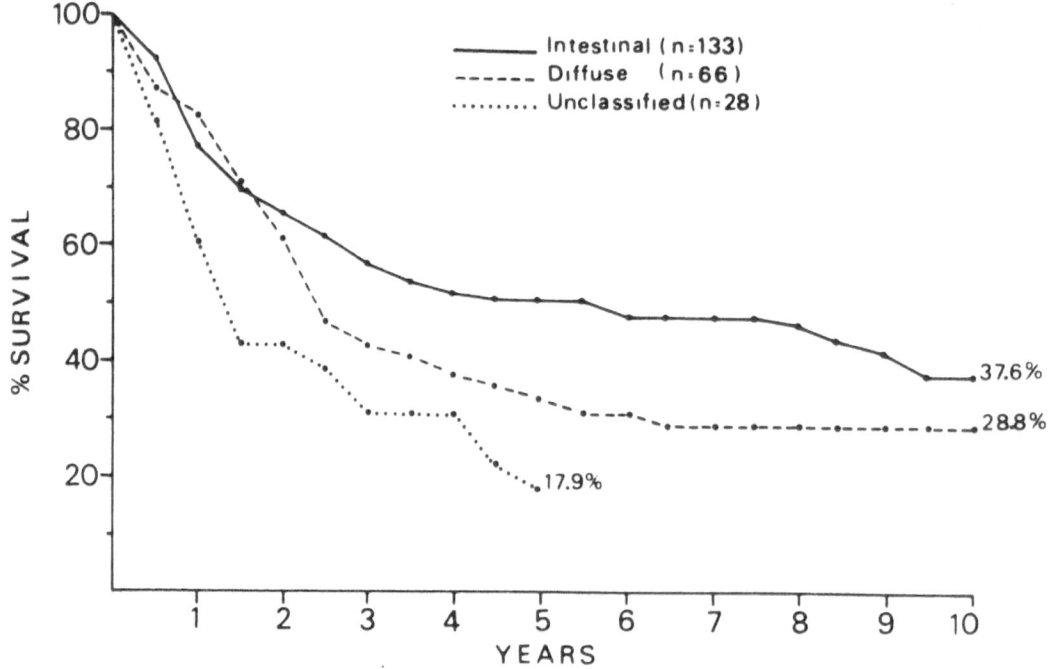

Fig. 2-7. Survival curves of the 227 patients according to Laurén classification.

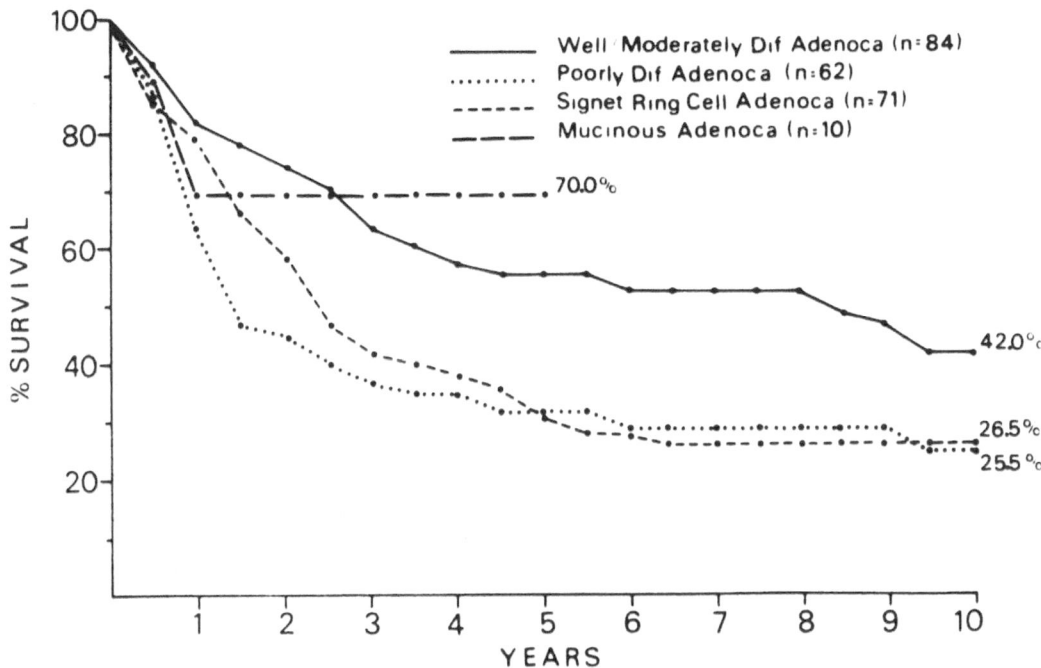

Fig. 2-8. Survival curves of the 227 patients according to WHO classification.

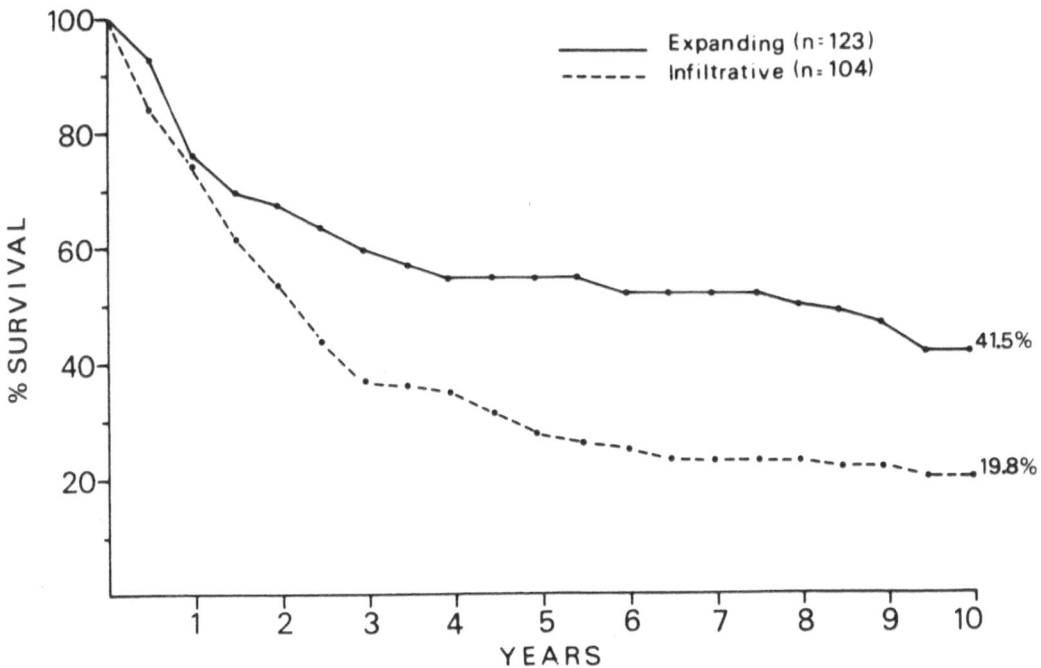

Fig. 2-9. Survival curves of the 227 patients according to Ming classification.

TABLE 2-7

Death Rates According to Histological
Classification

	Factors	No of Patients	Death Rate
Laurén	Intestinal	133	0.97
	Diffuse	66	1.53
	Unclassified	28	2.74
WHO	Mucinous	10	1.07
	Well/Moderately dif.	84	0.79
	Signet ring cell	70	1.66
	Poorly dif.	63	1.77
Ming	Expanding	122	0.87
	Infiltrative	105	1.88

WHO classifications when stage and venous invasion are kept as the sole covariates of the regression equation (Table 2-8). Using this model, no further improvement is obtained when two classifications are used instead of one (Table 2-8).

Other Factors

Sex and Age of Patients

The 5 and 10-year survival rates of women (44.9% and 34.9%) are slightly better than those of men (40.0% and 29.7%, respectively). Death rate is also slightly lower in women than in men (Table 2-9).

The 5-year survival rate of patients less than 40 years (38.2%) is slightly lower than those of patients from 40 to 60 years (42.3%) and older than 60 years (43.4%). The analysis of death rate shows the worse prognosis of the youngest patients (Table 2-9). The multivariate analysis demonstrates that neither sex nor age are significantly correlated with survival (Tables 2-2 and 2-3).

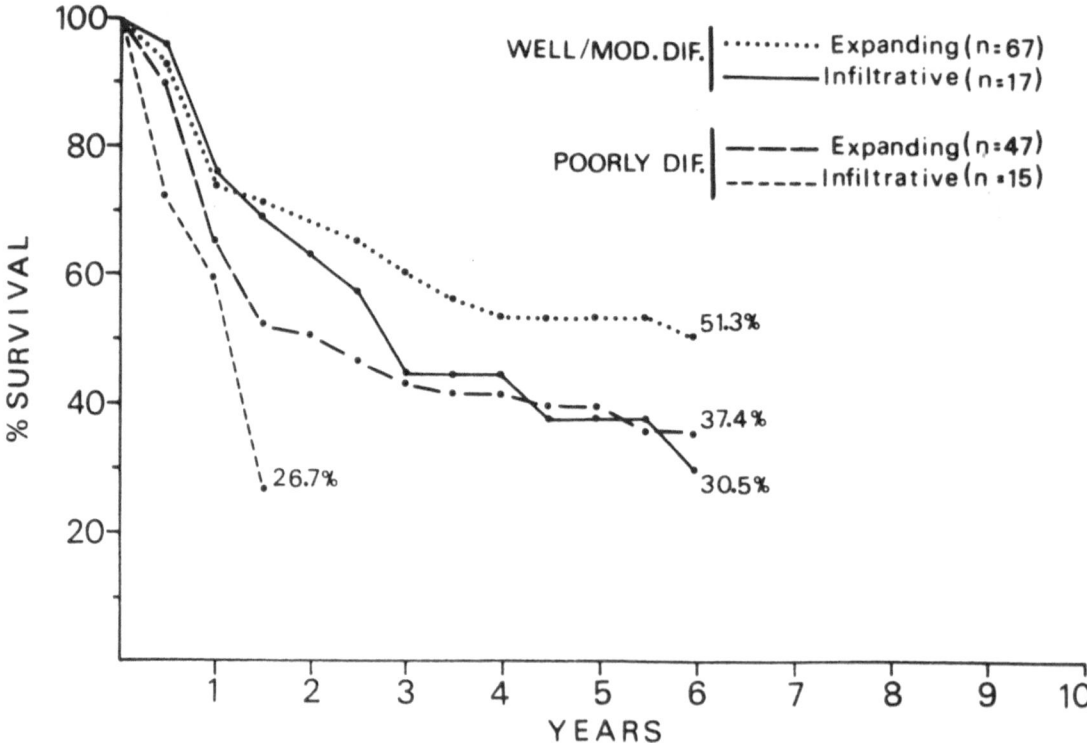

Fig. 2-10. Survival curves of 146 patients according to Ming and WHO classifications. Ten mucinous carcinomas and 71 signet ring cell carcinomas were excluded.

TABLE 2-8
Summary of the Results Obtained with the Multivariate Analysis of
the Prognostic Significance of Histological Classifications

Factors	Improvement Log Likelihood	p Value
Stage + Ven. Inv.	−515.8	
Stage + Ven. Inv. + Laurén	−515.3	NS
+ WHO	−515.6	NS
+ Ming	−514.2	p < 0.10
Stage + Ven. Inv. + Laurén + WHO	−515.3	NS
+ Laurén + Ming	−514.1	NS
+ WHO + Ming	−514.1	NS

TABLE 2-9
Death Rates According to Sex, Age, Type of
Resection, Shape, Size, Lymphoid Infiltration,
and Sinusal Histiocytosis

Factors		No of Patients	Death Rate
Sex	Women	85	1.18
	Men	142	1.28
Age	< 30	7	2.10
	30–39	16	1.13
	40–49	42	0.96
	50–59	68	1.29
	60–69	71	1.42
	70–79	23	1.19
Type of Resection	Distal	170	1.10
	Total	45	1.70
	Proximal	12	3.66
Shape	Polyp./Fungating	17	0.82
	Ulcerative	57	0.86
	Ulc./Fungating	61	0.91
	Ulc./Infiltrative	53	2.19
	Infiltrative	26	2.76
Size	< 3 cm	29	0.70
	≥ 3 < 6 cm	64	0.94
	≥ 6 cm	92	1.74
Lymphoid Infiltration	Abundant	40	0.97
	Moderate	67	1.22
	Min./Absent	120	1.36
Sinusal Histiocytosis	Abundant/Moderate	125	0.87
	Min./Absent	70	1.51

Type of Resection

Patients submitted to distal gastrectomy do better (5-year survival of 46.0%) than those submitted to total gastrectomy (5-year survival of 32.8%) and proximal gastrectomy (2-year survival of 41.7%). The 10-year survival rate of patients submitted to distal gastrectomy (33.0%) is, however, similar to that of patients submitted to total gastrectomy (32.8%). The analysis of death rate also demonstrates the worse prognosis of patients submitted to proximal gastrectomy (Table 2-9). The prognostic value of this factor is closely related to that of "tumor site" as mentioned previously and does not stand when the multivariate analysis is performed (Tables 2-2 and 2-3).

Shape and Size of Tumors

The 5 and 10-year survival rates of patients with polypoid/fungating tumors (59.3% and 48.5%, respectively) are similar to those of patients with ulcerating (68.5% and 52.4%) and ulcero-fungating tumors (63.6% and 48.9%). The prognosis is clearly worse in patients with ulcero-infiltrative tumors (5 and 10-year survival rates of 23.4% and 14.9%, respectively) and even much worse in those bearing infiltrative carcinomas (3-year survival rate of 27.0%). These results are confirmed by death rate analysis (Table 2-9).

Patients with tumors 6 cm, or larger than 6 cm, do worse (5 and 10-year survival rates of 35.0% and 21.9%, respectively) than those with smaller tumors (3 to 6 cm, 49.0% and 38.4%; less than 3 cm, 58.6% and 51.7%, respectively). Death rate analysis provides similar results (Table 2-9).

The prognostic value of both the macroscopical appearance and the size of tumors almost disappears when the influence of stage, venous invasion, and desmoplasia is controlled.

Lymphoid Infiltration of the Tumors and Histiocytosis of Regional Nodes

The 5 and 10-year survival rates of patients with carcinomas showing abundant lymphoid infiltration (55.6% and 38.9%, respectively) do better than those with carcinomas displaying moderate (44.2% and 33.9%, respectively) and minimal/absent lymphoid infiltration (38.6% and 29.9%, respectively). These results are confirmed by death rate analysis (Table 2-9). Lymphoid infiltration is independent of the stage of tumors and correlates negatively with mucin producing carcinomas (so-called mucinous and signet ring cell carcinomas).

Patients with abundant/moderate nodal histiocytosis do better (5 and 10-year survival rates of 46.5% and 32.7%, respectively) than those with minimal/absent histiocytosis (34.0% and 27.0%, respectively). Death rate analysis provides similar results (Table 2-9).

The multivariate analysis demonstrates that neither lymphoid infiltration nor nodal histiocytosis are significantly correlated with survival (Tables 2-2 and 2-3).

DISCUSSION

As it usually happens with papers dealing with statistical analysis of interrelated clinicopathological variables, our study offers a number of conclusions that will be tentatively discussed in a stepwise fashion.

The first of such conclusions concerns the major prognostic significance of the evaluation of the extent of neoplastic disease as measured according to the TNM criteria defined by the American Joint Committee.[1] This finding might be anticipated from most of the results obtained elsewhere[1,9,12,16,17,20,22,26,28,29,38,40,41,45,51] and does not justify, therefore, any special comment.

Our second conclusion regards the advantage of adding the evaluation of lymphatic permeation and status of nodal metastases to the traditional TNM criteria. In fact, the survival experience of patients with "N0 carcinomas plus lymphatic permeation" is sufficiently bad to advise the inclusion of these cases, for staging purposes, in the group of N1 carcinomas. The subdivision of N1 carcinomas according to the number of positive nodes was also found to provide additional and valuable prognostic information.

These results reinforce the concept of neoplastic development, which forms the rational basis for the TNM method and demonstrate that the predictive value of this method can still be improved. It is likely that further improvement would have been achieved if more detailed information on the number and localization of metastatic lymph nodes had been available. However, the possibility of testing this hypothesis, which has already been confirmed in several other models (e.g., breast carcinoma), rests beyond the limits of a retrospective study like this.

The exceedingly important prognostic role played in our series by the presence of unequivocal signs of venous invasion within the primary tumors also deserves a special mention. The search for venous invasion is easily performed in slides stained with orcein and does not require the study of extramural veins unlike what happens in colorectal carcinoma.[59] It seems, therefore, quite surprising that most authors apparently ignore the study of this factor.

The major predictive value of venous invasion had been previously reported.[18,32,38,44] Kodama et al[27] obtained similar results in a study of early gastric carcinoma, thus supporting our assumption that venous invasion worsens the outcome of patients regardless of the extent of neoplastic disease. The negative findings of Bedikian et al[3] may reflect different criteria in judging blood vessel invasion which, in our experience, should only be affirmed if clusters of neoplastic cells are seen within the lumina (often distending the walls) of elastic walled vessels.

Desmoplasia was the third most important prognostic factor disclosed in our series. This finding is in keeping with the dreadful prognosis that is generally linked to the well-known "linitis plastica" and to its histological counterpart, the so-called scirrhous carcinoma.[4,8,11,18,21,30,36,44] The predictive value of the desmoplastic reaction goes far beyond those of signet ring cell carcinomas and diffuse carcinomas. Desmoplasia correlates with size and macroscopical appearance of tumors. One can therefore assume that the predictive value of the presence of desmoplastic reaction may be due, partly at least, to the large size and the infiltrative (or ulcero-infiltrative) growth of the tumors displaying such reaction.

The site of carcinomas was also found to carry significant prognostic information. This is particularly obvious in what concerns the poor outcome of patients with high-seated tumors and has been repeatedly reported in the literature.[7,10,12,13,17,23,31,33] This worse prognosis cannot be merely ascribed to a more advanced extent of the neoplastic disease. It expresses probably the concurrence of several "negative" factors related to the anatomy and topography of the cardioeosophageal junction and to some specific problems of the surgical approach to such tumors (Ribeiro et al, in preparation).

The pattern of regional lymph nodes as measured through the evaluation of the degree of follicular hyperplasia was the last factor carrying some prognostic value, though at a suggestive level only. Our findings support therefore those of Black et al[4] who claim the superiority of follicular hyperplasia over nodal histiocytosis for prognostic purposes. They clearly contradict, on the other hand, those authors that stress the prognostic significance of nodal histiocytosis.[3]

The absence of any predictive value of the lymphoid infiltration of the tumors also contradicts many previous reports.[4,15,17,30,35,49] This does not mean, however, that we question the existence of a special type of tumor successively coined as "blue cell carcinoma," "medullary carcinoma with lymphoid infiltration," and "gastric carcinoma with lymphoid stroma" (for a thorough review see Watanabe et al[49]). This type of carcinoma, which is slightly more prevalent in our series (5.4%) than in Watanabe et al[49] series (4%), indeed carries an excellent prognosis.[15,35,49]

Such benign behavior should not be ascribed in our opinion to the abundance of lymphoid infiltrate, since our cases, like those of Watanabe et al,[49] have such limited extent of the neoplastic disease that this fact might, per se, explain their good prognosis (as it does in similarly well circumscribed carcinomas lacking moderate to abundant lymphoid infiltration). Most of these carcinomas are well circumscribed tumors with pushing margins that do not infiltrate deeply the gastric wall and do not have nodal metastases. It is of course impossible to decide whether or not the lymphoid infiltration plays any decisive role in the limitation of the neoplastic extension in these tumors.

It is also difficult to draw any definite conclusions from the contradictory prognostic results obtained in the study of the factors admittedly linked to the so called host-immunologic "response" that suggest positive findings with follicular hyperplasia and negative findings with nodal histiocytosis and lymphoid infiltration. The study of this "response" with other methods did not provide conclusive results either,[5] and the problem rests, therefore, unsolved, namely in what concerns advanced carcinomas.[5] Our attitude in this area remains pragmatic: the use of follicular hyperplasia as a prognostic factor is justified by its suggestive influence on the outcome of the patients without necessarily implying any specific relationship with the host-immunologic response.

Our last conclusions will concentrate on the most impressive negative finding of the study—the lack of prognostic significance of any of the most well-known histological classifications. In fact, our results demonstrate that none of them provides valuable prognostic information. They demonstrate also that no additional information is obtained when two histological classifications are used in combination. This lack of predictive value cannot be ascribed to the presence of desmoplasia as a covariable, since the results were almost the same when desmoplasia was removed from the regression equation. Our results confirm, therefore, those[8,31] who stressed the lack of prognostic significance of histology when the influence of staging was controlled. They contradict, on the other hand, most of the papers published so far on the subject in which the prognostic value of histology in general, or of some histological types of carcinoma in particular (e.g. signet ring cell carcinoma), is stressed.[3,8,12,15,19,41,42,46]

We feel somewhat embarrassed with these results since one of the main goals of the study was actually to decide the best classification for prognostic purposes. This lack of prognostic significance does not mean, however, that histological classifications of gastric carcinoma are useless and should be abandoned. Several reasons support this opinion. First, the three classifications provide valuable information for the study of the neoplastic transformation of gastric epithelium. In this field Laurén classification appears to be, in spite of its relatively low reproducibility,[37,60] Sobrinho-Simões and Ribeiro, (unpublished results), the most rewarding as it has been repeatedly proven in epidemiological studies.[41,54] Second, all of them provide the indispensable morphologic basis for further histochemical and immunocytochemical characterization of gastric carcinoma cells. Finally, and this is probably the most interesting conclusion of our study within this area, all of them are closely related with the extent of neoplastic disease. That is the reason why they lose their prognostic significance when survival is adjusted for stage and venous invasion.

The existence of a significant correlation between histology and extent of disease means that these classifications do indeed "measure" some biological properties of the neoplastic cells. In our hands, as well as in others, Ming classification was found to be, per se, the most discriminating. It is also noteworthy that the combination of Ming and WHO classifications were found the best "pair" under these circumstances (read: no adjustment for stage and venous invasion). One might anticipate this result from the fact that Ming and WHO "measure" two quite different morphological variables (pattern of growth and differentiation, respectively), whereas both of them more or less overlap Laurén classification.[15,37,55,41]

CONCLUSIONS

Staging together with the assessment of lymphatic permeation and venous invasion is, by far, the most valuable prognostic factor in gastric carcinoma. The evaluation of the tumoral desmoplasia and pattern of regional lymph node response also provides significant prognostic information.

None of the available histological classifications seems to add any meaningful information regarding prognosis.

High seated tumors carry a worse prognosis, whereas the remaining factors (age and sex of patients, type of resection, tumor shape, tumors size and lymphoid infiltration of the tumors, and histiocytosis of the regional nodes) do not influence significantly the outcome of the patients.

ACKNOWLEDGMENT

This work was supported by Instituto Nacional de Investigacão Científica (Centro MbP3). The authors thank Dr. Carlos Menezes for his help in the statistical analysis of the results, and Mrs. Olga Ferreira, Miss Fatima Magalhães and Mrs. Odete Ferreira da Costa for technical assistance.

REFERENCES

1. American Joint Committee for Cancer Staging and End-Results Reporting, In: Manual for Staging of Cancer, Chicago, American Joint Committee, 1978, pp 71–76
2. Barber Jr K.W., Gage R.P., Priestley J.T.: Significance of duration of symptoms and size of lesion in the prognosis of gastric carcinoma. Surg Gynecol Obstet 113:673–676, 1961
3. Bedikian A.Y., Chen T.T., Khankhanian N., Heilbrun L.K., McBride C.M., McMurtrey M.J., Bodey G.P.: The natural history of gastric cancer and prognostic factors influencing survival. J Clin Oncol 2:305–310, 1984
4. Black M.M., Freeman C., Mork T., Harvei S., Cutler S.: Prognostic significance of microscopic structure of gastric carcinomas and their regional lymph nodes. Cancer 27:703–711, 1971
5. Blanca I., Grases P.J., Matos M.V., Contreras C.E., Ochoa M., Wright H., Bianco N.C.: Immunology of human gastric cancer: a preliminary report. Cancer 49:1810–1816, 1982
6. Bloss R.S., Miller T.A., Copeland III EM: Carcinoma of the stomach in the young adult. Surg Gynecol Obstet 150:883–886, 1980
7. Brookes V.S., Waterhouse J.A.H., Powell D.J.: Carcinoma of the stomach: a 10-year survey of results and of factors affecting prognosis. Br Med J 1:1577–1583, 1965
8. Curtis R.E., Kennedy B.J., Myers M.H., Hankey B.F.: Evaluation of AJC stomach cancer staging using the Seer Population. Semin Oncol 12:21–31, 1985
9. Douglass H.O., Nava H.R.: Gastric adenocarcinoma: management of primary disease. Semin Oncol 12:32–45, 1985
10. Dupont J.B., Lee J.R., Burton G.R., Cohn I.: Adenocarcinoma of the stomach: review of 1,497 cases. Cancer 41:941–947, 1978
11. Eker R., Efskind J.: The pathology and prognosis of gastric carcinoma. Acta Chir Scand, suppl 264, 1960
12. Gennari L., Bonfanti G., Salvadori B.: Prognostic factors in gastric cancer. In: International Congress on Diagnosis and Treatment of Upper Gastrointestinal Tumors, International Congress Series 542, Mainz, Excerpta Medica, 1980, pp 173–184
13. Goldenberg I.S., Cohen J.M., Skinner D.G.: A study of survival patterns in patients with gastric carcinoma. Surg Gynecol Obstet 124:241–250,, 1967
14. Grabiec J., Owen D.A.: Carcinoma of the stomach in young persons. Cancer 56:388–396, 1985
15. Hoat J., Degels M.A.: Cancer gastrique. Classification anatomopathologique des tumeurs épithéliales malignes de l'estomac. Acta Gastro-Enterol Belg 42:433–449, 1979.
16. Hautefeuille P., Valleur P., Castaing D., Piel J.-L., Gérum A., Houdart R., Villet R., Galian A.: Influence de l'extension ganglionnaire sur la survie après resection de cancers gastriques infiltrants. Gastroenterol Clin Biol 6:849–856, 1982
17. Hawley P.R., Westerholm P., Morson B.C.: Pathology and prognosis of carcinoma of the stomach. Br J Surg 57:877–883, 1970
18 Higgins Jr G.A., Serlin O., Amadeo J.H., McElhinney J., Keehn J: Gastric cancer: factors in survival. Chir Gastroenterol 10:393–398, 1976
19. Hillon P., Faivre J., Milan C., Justrabo E., Piard F., Michiels R., Klepping C.: Traitement et pronostic des carcinomes gastriques. Étude de la population du département de la Côte-d'Or. Gastroenterol Clin Biol 7:585–590, 1983
20. Hoerr S.O.: Prognosis for carcinoma of the stomach. Surg Gynecol Obstet 137:205–209, 1973
21. Hoerr S.O., Hazard J.B., Bailey D.: Prognosis in carcinoma of the stomach in relation to the microscopic type. Surg Gynecol Obstet 122:485–494, 1966
22. Huguier M., Lacaine F.: Cancer de l'estomac. Facteurs de survie. La Nouv Presse Méd 9:231–234, 1980
23. Inberg M., Laurén P., Viikari S.J.: Factors influencing survival after radical operation for gastric carcinoma. Acta Chir Scand 132:195–199, 1966
24. Inberg M.V., Vuori J., Viikari S.J.: Carcinoma of the stomach. A follow-up study of 1963 patients. Acta Chir Scand 138:195–201, 1972
25. Inlow R.P., Dockerty M.B., Priestley J.T.: Large gastric cancers. Surg Gynecol Obstet 120:725–730, 1965
26. Kennedy B.J.: TNM classification for stomach cancer. Cancer 26:971–983, 1970
27. Kodama Y., Inokuchi K., Soejima K., Matsusaka T., Okamura T.: Growth patterns and prognosis in early gastric carcinoma. Superficially spreading and penetrating growth types. Cancer 51:320–326, 1983
28. Kodama Y., Sugimachi K., Soejima K., Matsusaka T., Inokuchi K.: Evaluation of extensive lymph node dissection for carcinoma of the stomach. World J Surg 5:241–248, 1981
29. Lambert R.: Les bases rationnelles du pronostic du cancer gastrique opéré. Arch Fr Mal App Dig 64:679–696, 1975
30. Larmi T.K.I., Saxén L.: "Host Reactions" in gastric cancer. A preliminary study of 119 cases of gastrectomy. Acta Chir Scand 125:144–146, 1963
31. Lawrence W.T., Lawrence Jr W.: Gastric cancer: The surgeon's viewpoint. Semin Oncol 7:400–414, 1980
32. Lewin E.: Gastric cancer. Acta Clin Scand Suppl 262, 1960
33. Lumpkin W.M., Crow R.L., Hernandez C.M., Cohn I.: Carcinoma of the stomach: Review of 1,035 cases. Ann Surg 159:919–932, 1964
34. MacDonald W.C.: Clinical and pathologic features of adenocarcinoma of the gastric cardia. Cancer 29:724–732, 1972
35. Martin C., Kay S.: The prognosis of gastric carcinoma as related to its morphologic characteristics. Surg Gynecol Obstet 119:319–322, 1964
36. Mehrotra M.L., Gupta I.M., Khanna S., Vaidya M.P.: Host response and tumor biological behaviour in the two histological types of gastric carcinoma. Histopathology 2:373–382, 1978
37. Ming S.-C.: Gastric carcinoma: a pathobiological classification. Cancer 39:2475–2485, 1977
38. Öhman U., Wetterfors J., Moberg A.: Primary gastric cancer and its prognosis. Acta Chir Scand 138:378–383, 1972
39. Papachristou D.N., Agnanti N., D'Agostino H., Fortner J.G.: Histologically positive esophageal margin in the surgical treatment of gastric cancer. Amer J Surg 139:711–713, 1980
40. Remine W.H., Gomes M.M.R., Dockerty M.B.: Long-term survival (10 to 56 years) after surgery for carcinoma of the stomach. Amer J Surg 117:177–184, 1969
41. Ribeiro M.N., Sarmento J.A., Sobrinho-Simões M.A.,

Bastos J.: Prognostic significance of Laurén and Ming classifications and other pathologic parameters in gastric carcinoma. Cancer 47:780–784, 1981

42. Ribeiro M.M., Sobrinho-Simões M.A., Bastos J.: Analysis of 242 cases of gastric carcinoma. World J Surg 5:97–102, 1981

43. Roux M., Vayrè P., Lassau J.-P., Chevallard A.: Une série de 100 cancers de l'estomac opérés avec un recul de 5 ans. Commentaires et réflexions. J Chir (Paris) 101:377–388, 1971

44. Serlin O., Keehn R.J., Higgins G.A. Jr, Harrower H.W., Mendeloff G.L.: Factors related to survival following resection for gastric carcinoma: analysis of 903 cases. Cancer 40:1318–1329, 1977

45. Soga J., Kobayashi K., Saito J., Fujimaki M., Muto T.: The role of lymphadenectomy in curative surgery for gastric cancer. World J Surg 3:701–708, 1979

46. Stemmermann G.N., Brown C.: A survival study of intestinal and diffuse types of gastric carcinoma. Cancer 33:1190–1195, 1974

47. Teglbjaerg P.S., Vetner M.: Gastric carcinoma: an analysis of morphological and prognostic parameters correlated to the classification proposed by Masson, Rember & Mulligan. Acta Path Microbiol Scand (A) 85:528–534, 1977

48. Wanke M., Schwan H.: Pathology of gastric cancer. World J Surg 3:675–684, 1979

49. Watanabe H., Enjoji M., Imai T.: Gastric carcinoma with lymphoid stroma. Its morphologic characteristics and prognostic correlations. Cancer 38:232–243, 1976

50 WHO International Reference Center to evaluate methods of diagnosis and treatment of stomach cancer. Report of the Meeting National Cancer Center Publ., Tokyo, 1972

51. Yamada E., Miyaishi S., Nakazato H., Kato K., Kito T., Takagi H., Yasue M., Kato T., Morimoto T., Yamauchi M.: The surgical treatment of cancer of the stomach. Internat Surg 65:387–399, 1980

52. Zacho A., Cederovist C., Fishermann K.: Surgical treatment of gastric malignancies: a twenty-year series comprising mainly far advanced and high-seated tumors. Ann Surg 1:94:101, 1974

53. Zacho A., Fischermann K., Sorensen B.L.: Prognostic role of breach of lymph node capsule in nodal metastases from gastric carcinoma. Acta Chir Scand 125:365–369, 1963

54. Laurén P.: The two histological main types of gastric carcinoma: diffuse and so-called intestinal-type carcinoma. An attempt at a histo-clinical classification. Acta Path Microbiol Scand 64:31–49, 1965

55. Oota K., Sobin L.H.: Histological Typing of Gastric and Oesophageal Tumours. International Histological Classification of Tumours no 18, World Health Organization, Geneva, 1977

56. Tsakraklides V., Anastassiados O.T., Kersey J.H.: Prognostic significance of regional lymph nodes histology in uterine cervical cancer. Cancer 31:860–868, 1973

57. Berkson J., Gage R.P.: Calculation of survival rates for cancer. Mayo Clin Proc 25:270, 1950

58. Cox D.R.: Regression models and life tables. J Roy Soc Stat, Series B, 34:187–220, 1972

59. Talbot I.C., Ritchie S., Leighton M., Hughes A.O., Bussey H.J.R., Morson B.C.: Invasion of veins by carcinoma of rectum: method of detection, histological features and significance. Histopathology 5:141–163, 1981

60. Pagnini C.A., Rugge M.: Gastric cancer: problems in histological diagnosis. Histopathology 6:391–398, 1982

3

Varioliform Gastritis Revisited

J.P. van Spreeuwel M.D., Ph.D.
C.J.L.M. Meijer M.D., Ph.D.
J. Lindeman M.D., Ph.D.

Gastritis is very commonly encountered in both asymptomatic individuals and in patients with upper abdominal discomfort; its frequency increases with age. It is the result of various endogenous and exogenous and often poorly defined noxes to the gastric mucosa. It represents a diagnostic and therapeutic problem for the clinician, since correlation between symptoms and histologically proven gastritis is poor, correlation between endoscopic and histological findings is poor, and there is no effective therapy.

Several classifications of gastritis have been proposed and attempts have been made to discriminate certain more or less specific forms of gastritis. One of these is the so called varioliform gastritis, alternatively known as chronic erosive gastritis, dellen gastritis, superficial hypertrophic gastritis, aphthous ulcers, or complete erosions, which has been claimed to be an entity characterized by an increased number of IgE containing cells in the gastric mucosa and requiring specific treatment.[1] Varioliform gastritis, especially whether or not it represents a specific entity, will be the subject of this paper.

CLINICAL FEATURES

Varioliform gastritis is characterized by usually multiple, round, or oval lesions of the gastric mucosa, 5–10 mm in diameter, consisting of a central erosion surrounded by an elevated border (Fig. 3-1). Varioliform or chronic erosions as opposed to acute erosions have elevated margins and are predominantly located in the gastric antrum along the greater curvature.[2,3] They may, on the other hand, occur diffusely throughout the stomach and be accompanied by congested swollen rugae. The name gastritis has been argued because the surrounding gastric mucosa may be entirely normal. Although they have already been described in autopsy studies in the 18th century,[4] the first demonstration by gastroscopy and radiology dates back to 1933.[5]

The diagnosis varioliform gastritis has become relatively common since the 70s when endoscopy became widely available in the workup of patients with upper abdominal complaints. The prevalence in patients subjected for some reason to diagnostic gastroduodenoscopy varies from 0.3 to 12.7% with an average of 3%.[3,6–13] It is three-fold more common in males than in females, and its frequency reaches a maximum in the 5th and 6th decades, thereby resembling very much the age profile of gastric and duodenal ulcer disease.[14] Although varioliform gastritis has been diagnosed in asymptomatic persons during cancer screening procedures the majority of patients reported have periodic symptoms reminiscent of peptic ulcer disease such as epigastric pain, pyrosis, nausea, and food intolerance often of many years standing. Atypical complaints and considerable weight loss

Fig. 3-1. Endoscopic view of a varioliform erosion.

have also been reported especially in patients with the diffuse type.

In a considerable number, 30–40% of the patients, peptic ulceration of the duodenum or the stomach is diagnosed simultaneously[3] or during follow-up.[3,6,15] Gastrointestinal

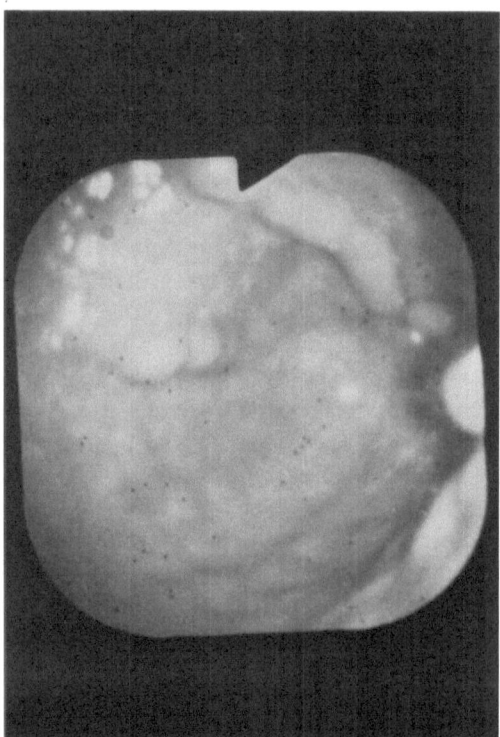

Fig. 3-2. Endoscopic view of the gastric antrum showing a swollen mucosal fold as a result of fusion of varioliform erosions.

bleeding, common in acute erosions, is rare. Occasionally, varioliform gastritis is complicated by protein losing enteropathy.[9,12,17] Association with recurrent oral aphthous ulcers has been described.[19] Long-term observations in 64 patients with varioliform gastritis[3] showed that the condition remained stable in 26, deteriorated in 12, improved in 13; whereas in 13 other patients the lesions healed completely. In 16 patients a gastric or duodenal ulcer developed during follow-up but this was not shown to arise from a varioliform erosion. In some patients erosions fuse together to form hypertrophic folds in the gastric antrum (Fig. 3-2). Evolution to gastric polyps has been suggested, but this was not confirmed.[3] Although varioliform erosions have been shown to heal in several days, most authors have confirmed the persistent or recurrent nature of the lesions.[1,12,16,20]

HISTOPATHOLOGICAL FEATURES

Histologically varioliform gastritis is characterized by a central epithelial defect not penetrating the muscularis mucosae (Fig. 3-3). The lamina propria is infiltrated by mononuclear cells: plasma cells, lymphocytes, macrophages, and eosinophilic and neutrophilic granulocytes. The latter often infiltrate both surface and glandular epithelium. Marked foveolar hyperplasia and sometimes cystic dilatation of glands in the margins of the lesion explain the macroscopical appearance. Metaplasia of the intestinal type may be found, as well as atrophy of the glandular layer of the epithelium. Specific histological features such as a marked preponderance of eosinophils or granulomas are absent. The surrounding gastric epithelium, may likewise show features of chronic nonspecific gastritis (Fig. 3-4) or be completely normal.

Immunohistochemically Rösh and colleagues[21] found a decrease of IgM and an increase of IgG containing cells, whereas André and colleagues demonstrated a marked increase of IgE containing cells (Fig. 3-5), both plasma cells and activated mast cells, in gastric biopsies of patients with varioliform gastritis.[22] Other studies, however, failed to confirm this.[23-25] Ultrastructural examination failed to reveal specific abnormalities, especially no virus particles could be detected.[14,26] Sometimes microorganisms can be observed in the mucus overlying the gastric mucosa. Recently the presence of campylobacter-like microorganisms in upper gastrointestinal biopsies from patients with gastritis and peptic ulcer disease was given much attention in the literature. These organisms could also be found in 4 of 10 patients with varioliform gastritis.[25] In one histological study of chronic gastric erosions, completely removed by diathermy, a greatly thickened muscularis mucosae, dissociated by fibrous bundles, was observed as well as thickening of vessel walls in the submucosa and occasional cystic gastric glands penetrating the submucosa.[15]

ination, the latter probably being more sensitive.[16,25] Varioliform erosions can be differentiated from acute erosions by their elevated margins. Otherwise they differ from true ulcers, since they do not penetrate the muscularis mucosae and, therefore, do not interfere with the peristalsis of the gastric wall.

Crohn's disease may produce varioliform or aphthous erosions in the stomach as well.[29] Differentiation relies both on the demonstration of granulomas in the gastric mucosa, which can be found in two-thirds of patients, as well as the demonstration of Crohn's disease elsewhere in the gastrointestinal tract, as this is invariably present. This, however, applies only to those patients in whom on clinical grounds more extensive disease of the intestine is suspected, and in our experience this is a rare occasion.

Varioliform erosions sometimes fuse to form enlarged folds of the gastric mucosa, and in such cases multiple forceps biopsies should be obtained to exclude other disorders such as infiltrating gastric carcinoma or lymphoma. Other hypertrophic gastropathies such as Menetrier's disease or the Zollinger-Ellison syndrome present with more diffuse abnormalities, but they can be confused with diffuse varioliform gastritis. Large sized biopsies, as well as serum gastrin determination (normal levels are found in varioliform gastritis)[1] should allow differentiation from the Zollinger-Ellison syndrome. A differentiation from Menetrier's disease that relies on histological examination showing hyperplasia of the foveolar layer of the gastric mucosa in the presence of inflammation may be more difficult.

DIFFERENTIAL DIAGNOSIS

The differential diagnosis of varioliform gastritis should not pose too big a problem. It can reliably be diagnosed by radiological examination,[26,28] preferably by the double contrast method, and by endoscopical exam-

IS VARIOLIFORM GASTRITIS A SPECIFIC ENTITY?

Arguments to consider varioliform gastritis as a specific entity have been put forward by André and coworkers.[22] They found increased

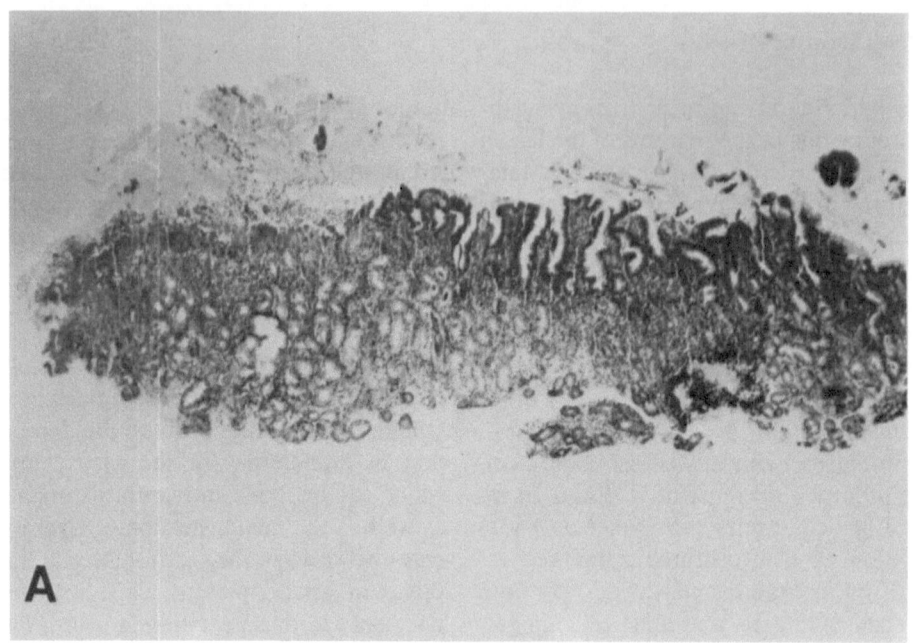

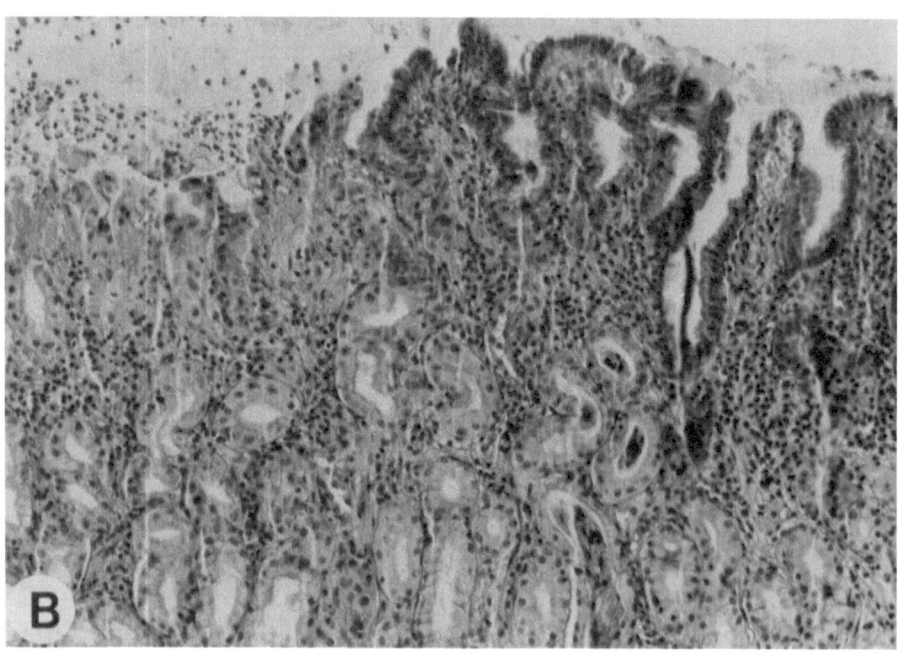

Fig. 3-3. Biopsy of a varioliform erosive lesion of the antrum. (a) Low power view. (×10)
Note the fibrinoid necrosis of the surface epithelium on the left part of this biopsy. (b) Detail
of the transitional area of the erosion (left) and the inflamed adjacent foveolar layer. (×100)
(c) Detail of the fibrinoid necrosis of the surface epithelium. (×250)

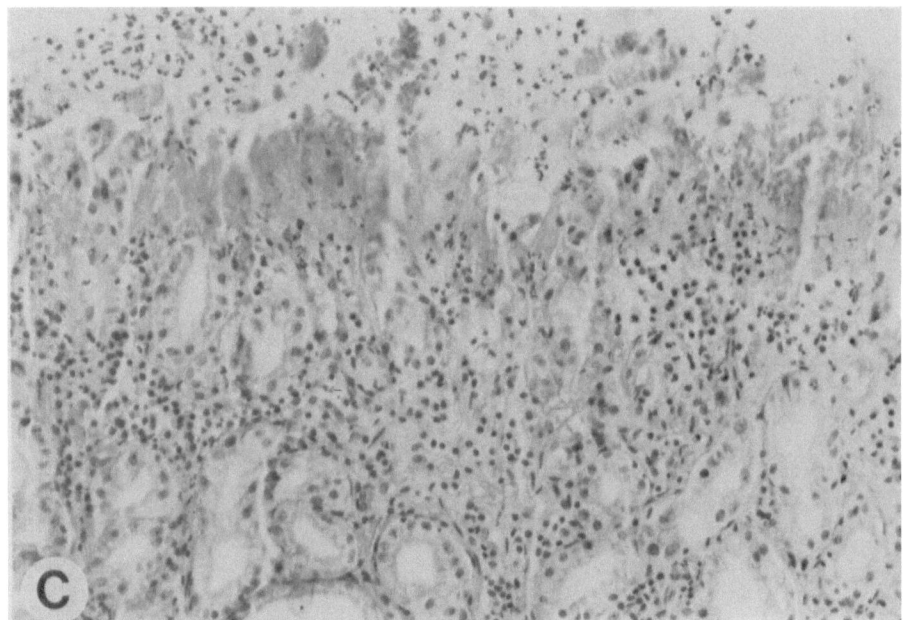

Fig. 3-3. *(continued)*

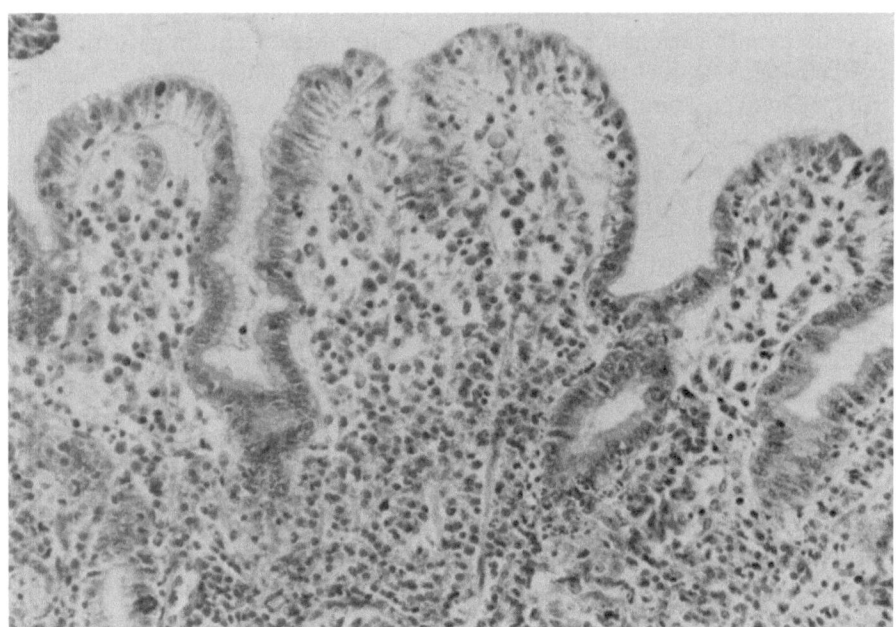

Fig. 3-4. Biopsy from the margin of a varioliform erosion of the antrum. (×250) Note the hyperplastic foveolar layer and several interepithelial lymphocytes in the surface epithelium. Locally the neck region is invaded by a neutrophilic infiltrate.

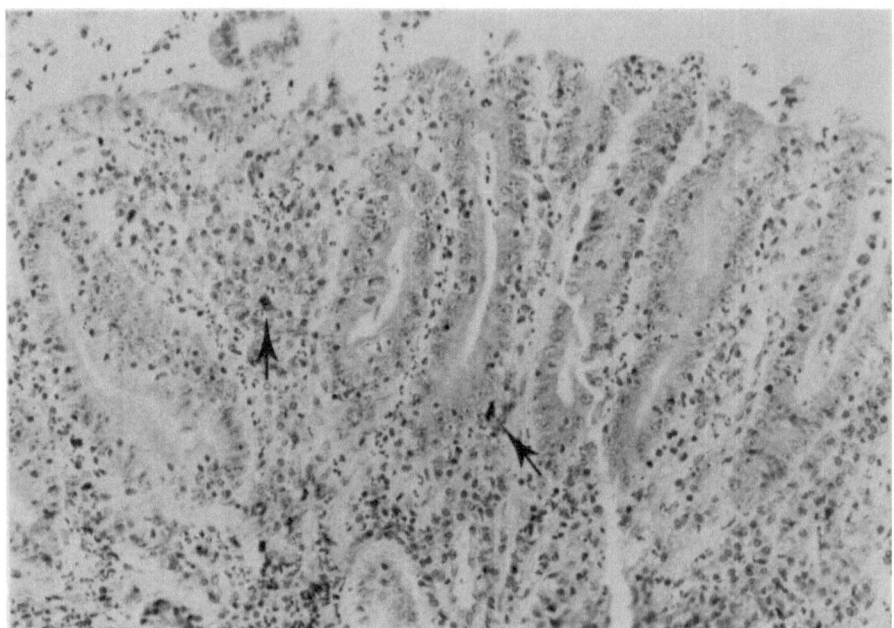

Fig. 3-5. Biopsy from a varioliform erosion of the antrum. Note two IgE-containing plasma cells (arrows). (×250)

numbers of IgE-containing cells in gastric biopsies of patients with varioliform gastritis, as compared to patients with chronic nonspecific gastritis. Moreover, some patients had raised serum IgE levels and those who were treated with disodium cromoglycate showed a favorable response.[1,22] Therefore, they proposed an allergic (type I, IgE-mediated hypersensitivity) immune reaction as the pathophysiological mechanism. This hypothesis was further substantiated by the demonstration of anaphylaxis producing gastric ulceration,[30,31] and the successful treatment of varioliform gastritis with disodium cromoglycate[1] and prednisolone.[32]

Increased numbers of IgE-containing cells have been shown in the jejunal mucosa of patients with food allergy[33,34] and in the tonsils of patients with atopy[36] and are, therefore, associated with type I IgE-mediated hypersensitivity. As far as the stomach is concerned, however, an increased number of IgE-containing cells in the mucosal biopsies specimens has, besides in varioliform gastritis, also

been demonstrated at the base of gastric and duodenal ulcers[37] and in gastritis[38] especially gastritis due to biliary reflux.[39]

Moreover, in a survey of gastric biopsies of 2543 patients IgE-containing cells were increased in 2.6% of the patients who suffered from a variety of chronic inflammatory disorders of the stomach of various etiology.[24] This finding was fairly reproducible in time within the same patient. Since an increase of IgE-containing cells in mucosal biopsies was observed in various disorders it was considered unlikely that type I IgE-mediated hypersensitivity played a primary role and suggested that it could be an epiphenomenon, reflecting allergy probably towards food constituents, secondary to chronic non-specific inflammation as a result of increased antigen exposure to the intestinal mucosa. Therefore, increased numbers of IgE containing cells in mucosal biopsies cannot be considered to be definite proof of an allergic type I IgE-mediated immune reaction as the primary mechanism. Moreover, an increase of IgE-containing cells in gastric biopsies of patients with varioliform gastritis has not been confirmed in other studies.[23,24]

It should be stated, however, that André et al[22] initially made their observations in patients with diffuse varioliform gastritis. In the other studies the type of varioliform gastritis was not further specified in one[23] and concerned antral varioliform gastritis in the other.[24] Therefore, varioliform gastritis of the diffuse type may be different from antral varioliform gastritis.

André and coworkers, however, have subsequently extended their observation of an increase of IgE-containing cells to antral varioliform gastritis. Uncontrolled therapeutic trials with either disodium cromoglycate or prednisolone[22,32] that showed a favorable response of the gastritis have their obvious drawbacks in a disorder, which may have spontaneous remissions. The one placebo-controlled trial in varioliform gastritis, however, exploring the effect of disodium cromoglycate and cimetidine, showed a favorable response to disodium cromoglycate.[1] Again it concerned patients with diffuse varioliform gastritis. Studies of gastric acid production failed to show a distinct pattern.[6,7,9,26] Gastric acid production ranged from hyper- to normo-acidity, whereas in one study even some patients with anacidity were described. The age distribution of patients with varioliform gastritis is very similar to that of patients with peptic ulcer disease.[3,14] Moreover, benign gastric and duodenal ulcers are frequently associated with varioliform erosions, suggesting that the two disorders are related. Therapy with cimetidine, ranitidine, or pirenzipine, however, has been shown to produce healing of the peptic ulcers, whereas the co-existing varioliform erosions persisted.[15] Furthermore, it has never been documented that peptic ulcers arose from varioliform erosions and indeed both lesions have a different topographical distribution in the stomach.

Other associated and possibly etiological factors observed in varioliform gastritis are the use of coffee and tea, smoking as well as corticosteroids.[14] The same author failed to show an association with acetylsalicylic acid that by interfering with local prostaglandin synthesis may damage the mucosal barrier.

Finally, based upon histological similarities with solitary rectal ulcers and colitis cystica profunda an ischemic origin of varioliform erosions has been suggested.[15]

Summarizing the available data on varioliform gastritis, it appears the clinical and histological features are nonspecific, whereas various etiological mechanisms have been incriminated. Therefore, since evidence is lacking to support the statement that varioliform gastritis is a specific entity, varioliform gastritis should be considered as a heterogeneous disorder. Probably it merely represents a morphological variant of chronic nonspecific gastritis.

SUMMARY

Varioliform gastritis has been claimed to represent a specific entity, characterized by an increased number of IgE-containing cells in the gastric mucosa, which requires specific therapy. The clinical and histological features of varioliform gastritis are reviewed and considered nonspecific. It is argued that the increase of IgE-containing cells in mucosal biopsies cannot be considered as definite proof for a type I IgE-mediated immune mechanism and may represent an epiphenomenon. Moreover, other etiological factors have been incriminated. It is, therefore, concluded that varioliform gastritis is a heterogeneous disorder that probably merely represents a morphological variant of chronic nonspecific gastritis.

ACKNOWLEDGMENT

The authors express their gratitude to Mrs. W. van Golde who prepared the manuscript.

REFERENCES

1. André G., Gillon J., Moulinier B., Martin A., Fargier M.C.: Randomised placebo-controlled doubleblind trial of two dosages of sodium cromoglycate in the treatment of varioliform gastritis: comparison with cimetidine. Gut 23:348–352, 1982
2. Roesch W.: Erosions of the upper gastrointestinal tract. Clinics in Gastroenterology Vol 7, nr. 3:623–634, 1978
3. Freise J., Hofmann R., Gebel H., Huchzermeyer M.: Follow-up study of chronic gastric erosions. Endoscopy 1:13–17, 1979
4. Morgagni G.B.: De sedibus et causis morborum per anatomem indagatis. Tomus II. Vet EP Anat Med 30:20, 1756
5. Henning N., Schatzki R.: Gastrophotographisched und roentgenologisches Bild der Gastritis erosiva. Fortschr Roentgenstrahle 48:177–182, 1933
6. Kawai K., Shimamoto K., Misaki F., Hurakami K., Masuda M.: Erosions of gastric mucosa: Pathogenesis, incidence and classification of the erosive gastritis. Endoscopy 3:168–174, 1970
7. Roesch W., Ottenjahn R.: Gastric erosions. Endoscopy 2:93–98, 1970
8. Seifert E., Paul F., Schmidt W.C.: Akute und chronischen Magenerosionen. Med Klin 3:83–87, 1971
9. Filippini L., Isliker K. Gastritis varioliformis mit Proteinverlust. Dtsch Med Wrschr 98:1892–1894, 1973
10. Bosseckert H., Koppe P., Heid R. Die endoskopische Diagnostik von Magenerosionen und ihre klinische Bedeutung. Z inn Med 29:888–891, 1974
11. Hauzeur F., Arendt R., Leithauser W.: Die kompletten Magenerosionen—ein relativ haufiger gastroskopischer Befund. Z inn Med 30:353–355, 1975
12. Krentz K., Gohrband G. Klinik und Verlauf gastraler Erosionen. Med Klin 71:156–162, 1976
13. Green P.H.R., Feure D.I., Barrett P.J., Hunt J.H., Gillespie P.E., Nagy G.S.. Chronic erosive (verrucous) gastritis. A study of 108 patients. Endoscopy 9:74–78, 1977
14. Walinga H. Varioliforme erosies. Thesis, Amsterdam, 1985
15. Franzin G., Manfrini C., Musola R., Rodella S., Fratton A. Chronic erosions of the stomach. A clinical, endoscopic and histological evaluation. Endoscopy 16:1–5, 1984
16. Roesch W. Erosions of the upper gastrointestinal tract. Clinics in Gastroenterology 7:623–634, 1978
17. Clarke A.C., Lee S.P., Nicholson G.I. Gastritis varioliformis. Chronic erosive gastritis with protein-losing gastropathy Am J Gastroenterol 68:599–602, 1977
18. Walk L. Polyps caused by gastric erosions. Radiologe 15:354–355, 1975
19. O'Brian T.K., Saunders D.R., Templeton F.E. Chronic gastric erosions and oral aphthae. Am J Dig Dis 17:447–454, 1972
20. Walk L. Long-term prognosis of idiopathic gastric erosions. Radiologe 15:356–359, 1975
21. Rösch W., Warnatz H. Immunofluorescenzmikroskopische Untersuchungen bei Magenerosionen, in: Lindener H. Fortschritte in der gastroenterologische

Endoskopie, 1974 Baden-Baden, Witztrock, 194–251.
22. André C., Moulinier B., Lambert R., Bugnon B.: Gastritis varioliformis, allergy and disodium cromoglycate. Lancet I:964–965, 1976
23. Dekker W., Walinga H., Balk T., Tytgat G.N.J.: Chronische varioliforme laesies van de maag: een onderzoek naar de aethiologie, Ned Tijdschr v Geneeskd 127:240–244, 1983
24. Spreeuwel van J.P., Lindeman J., Maanen van J., Meijer C.J.L.M.: Increased numbers of IgE containing cells in gastric and duodenal biopsies, 1984 J Clin Pathol 37:601–606.
25. Price A.B., Levi J., Dolby J.N., Dunscombe P.L., Smith A., Clark J., Stephenson M.J.: Campylobacter pyloridis in peptic ulcer disease: Microbiology, pathology and scanning electron microscopy. Gut 26:1183–1188, 1985
26. Morgan A.G., Mc Adam W.A.F., Pypah R.D., Tinsley E.G.F.: Multiple recurring gastric erosions (aphthous ulcers). Gut 17:633–637, 1976
27. Laufer I., Hamilton J., Mullens J.E.: Demonstration of superficial gastric erosions by double contrast radiography. Gastroenterology 68:387–391, 1975.
28. Op den Orth J.O., Dekker W.: Gastric erosions: radiological and endoscopical aspects. Radiol Clin 45:88–99, 1976
29. Rutgeerts P., Ponette E., Vantrappen G., Geboes K., Broeckaert L., Taleven L.: Crohn's disease of the stomach and duodenum: a clinical study with emphasis on the value of endoscopy and endoscopic biopsies. Endoscopy 12:288–294, 1980
30. André F., André C.: Gastric ulcer induced by mucosal anaphylaxis in ovalbumin-sensitized Proamys (Mastomys) natalensis. Am J Pathol 102:133–135, 1981
31. André F., André C., Vialard J.L.: Role of homocytotrophic antibodies in the pathogenesis of gastric ulcer. Digestion 19:175–179, 1979
32. Farthing M.J.G., Fairclough P.D., Hegarthy J.E., Swarbrick E.T., Dawson A.M.: Treatment of chronic erosive gastritis with prednisolone. Gut 22:759–762, 1981
33. Shiner M., Ballard, J., Smith M.E.: The small intestinal mucosa in cows with intolerance. Lancet I; 136–140, 1975
34. Rosekrans P.C.M., Meijer C.J.L.M., Cornelisse C.J., Wal van der A.M., Lindeman J.: Use of morphometry and immunohistochemistry of small intestinal biopsy specimens in the diagnosis of food allergy. J Clin Pathol 33:155–130, 1980
35. Spreeuwel van J.P., Meijer C.J.L.M., Rosekrans P.C.M., Lindeman J.: Immunoglobulin containing cells in gastrointestinal pathology. Diagnostic applications. Pathol Ann 1986, 21:(Part 2)295–310, 1985
36. Feltkamp Vroom T.M., Stallman P.J., Aalbers R.C., Reerink Brongers E.E.: Immunofluorescence studies on renal tissue, tonsils, adenoids, nasal polyps and skin of atopic and non-atopic patients with special reference to IgE. Clin Immunol Immunopathol 4:392–404, 1975
37. Brown W.R., Borthistle V.K., Chen S.T.: Immunoglobulin E (IgE) and IgE-containing cells in human gastrointestinal fluids and tissues Clin Exp Immunol 20:227–237, 1975.
38. Niedobitek F., Volkheimer G., Dumke K., Schlecht

Martine: Zur Haufigkeit and Verteilung IgE-haltiger Zellen in der Magenschleimhaut. Pathologe 5:212–215, 1984

39. André C., Vilart J.L., Fargier M.C.: IgE mediated reactions in inflammation of the stomach, in: Pepys J., Edward A.M., The Mast Cell, its Role in Health and Disease. Kent, Pitman Medical Publishing Comp Ltd 642–646, 1980

40. André C., Moulinier B., André F., Daniere S.: Evidence for anaphylactic reactions in peptic ulcer and varioliform gastritis. Ann Allergy 51:325–328, 1983

4

Aminergic and Peptidergic Innervation of the Gastric Mucosa—Its Possible Relevance to Ulcerogenesis

Masaya Oda M.D.
Masahiko Nakamura M.D.
Kotaro Kaneko M.D.
Masaharu Tsuchiya M.D.

A number of studies on the relationship between autonomic nervous abnormalities and gastric ulcer formation were performed since the pioneering reports of Cushing[1] and Bergamann.[2] However, further investigation of this pathognomonic relationship from a different angle or using a newly developed technique is still warranted in order to clarify the mechanism of gastric ulceration.

Recently, a balance theory was proposed,[3] whereby peptic ulcer formation is dependent upon an equilibrium between aggressive and defensive factors. The former comprise acid and pepsin, the latter mucus, HCO_3^- and the gastric mucosal microcirculatory system.[4]

It is proposed that ulcer formation occurs mainly due to the hypersecretion of gastric acid as an aggressive factor, possibly triggered by stress-induced overactivity of the sympathetic and/or parasympathetic (vagal) nerves.[5] On the other hand, disruption of the gastric mucosal barrier,[6] which is caused or aggravated by disturbances of the mucosal microcirculation[4,7] and H^+ back-diffusion[8] are considered to be crucial in gastric ulcerogenesis.

It is established that the mucosal microcirculation supporting the defensive mechanism of the stomach is regulated by sympathetic and parasympathetic nerves.[9,10] Thus both aggressive and defensive factors in the stomach are directly or indirectly influenced by the functional state of the autonomic nerves.

The gastrointestinal tract is richly innervated by the enteric or peptidergic nervous system,[11,12,13] which is partly independent of the central autonomic nervous system and is supposed to act as "gut brain." These enteric autonomic nerves possess a variety of neurotransmitters. It is well known that the classical neurotransmitters, acetylcholine[14] and noradrenaline,[15] are widely distributed in the nervous system throughout the gastrointestinal wall. However, since a pioneering immunohistochemical study demonstrating the existence of substance P in the intramural plexuses in mammalian intestine,[16] a variety of the gastrointestinal peptides such as vasoactive intestinal polypeptide (VIP)[17,18] and gastrin releasing peptide (GRP)[19,27a] are also found to exist in the enteric nervous system, and they are considered to play an important

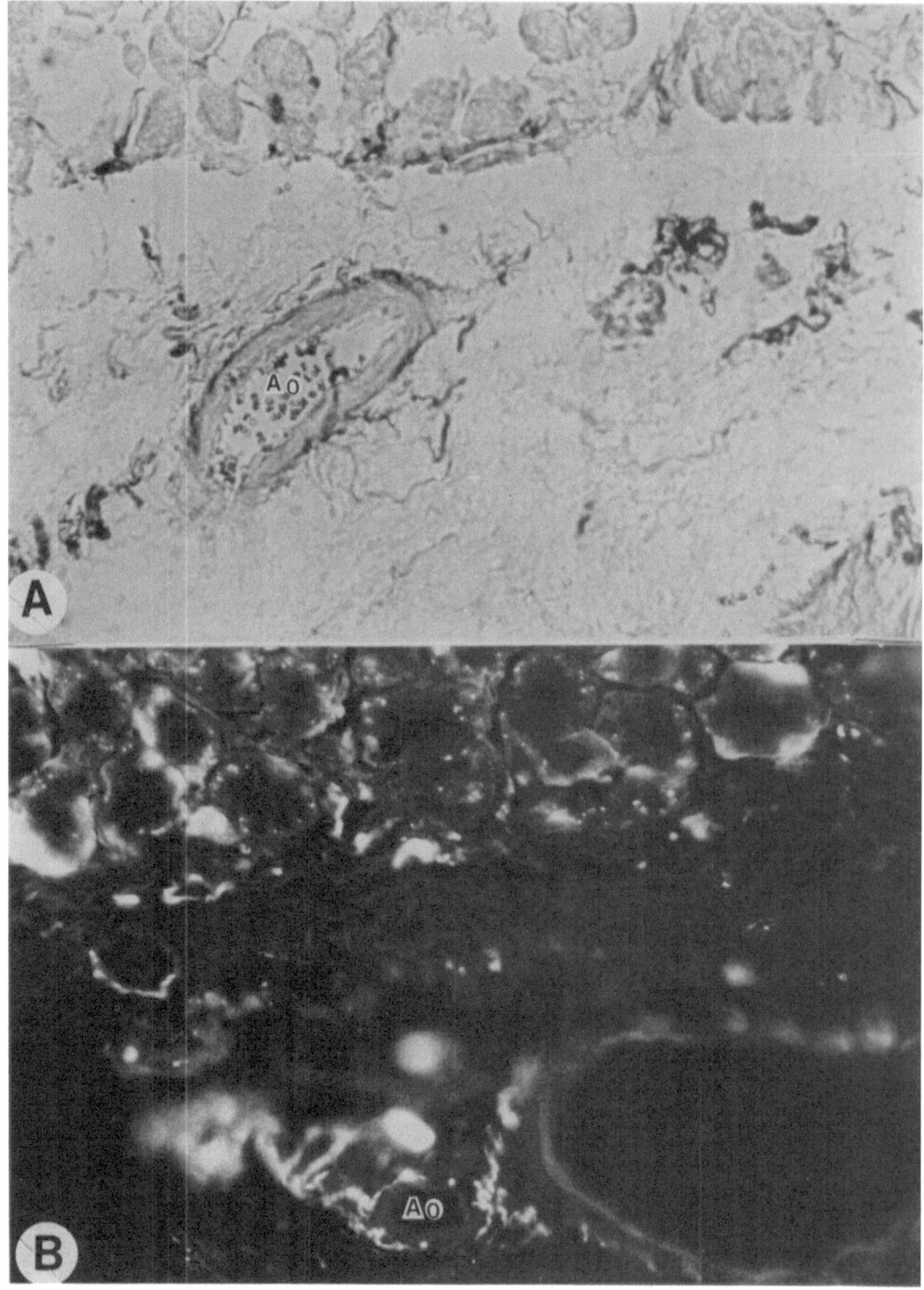

Fig. 4-1. The autonomic nerve plexuses in the submucosal layer of the rat fundic mucosa. (a) Karnovsky-Roots stain. The AChE-positive nerve fibers are noted in the submucous plexuses near the arterioles (Ao). ×800. (b) A modification of Falck-Hillarp method. The noradrenaline-specific fluorescence is seen in the perivascular plexuses of the arterioles (Ao). ×800.

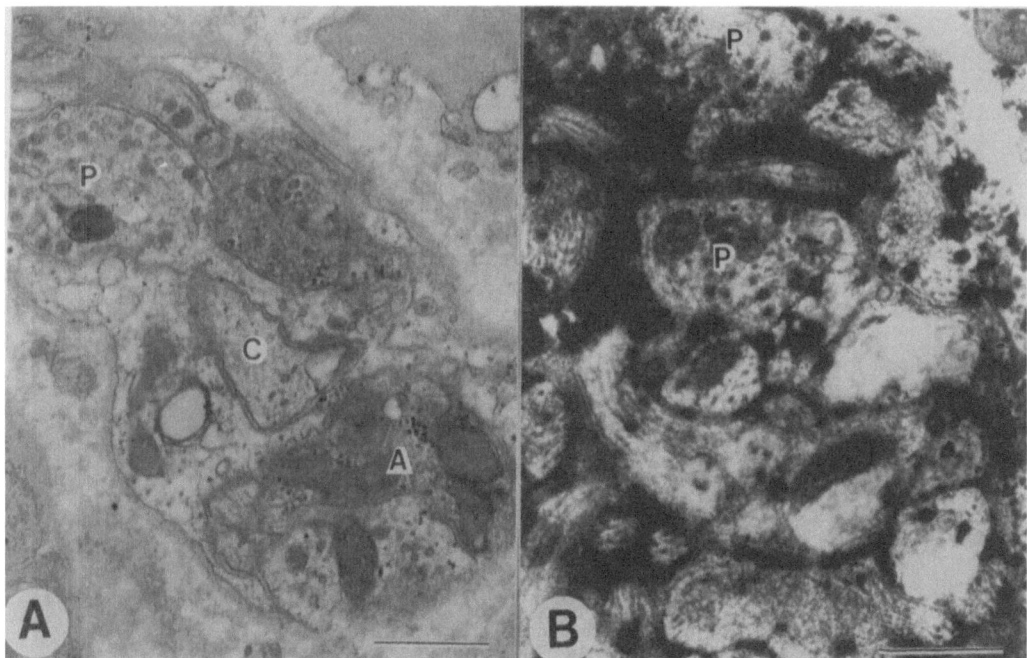

Fig. 4-2. Electron micrographs of the unmyelinated nerve endings in the submucosal layer of the rat stomach. (a) A typical plexus composed of adrenergic (A), cholinergic (C) and peptidergic (P) nerve endings. Routine fixation. Most of the nerve fibers in these plexuses include agranular small synaptic vesicles, corresponding to the cholinergic nerves. Some of these nerves contain small granular vesicles characteristic to adrenergic nerves and large granular vesicles probably corresponding to peptidergic nerves. ×18,000. (b) On the axonal membranes of the peptidergic nerve endings (P), AChE reaction products are also recognized. × 20,000.

role in the regulation of gastrointestinal functions.[20] The existence of histaminergic,[21] serotonergic,[22] dopaminergic[23] and purinergic nerves[24] are also postulated. There is little known about the detailed innervation of epithelial cells and microvessels in the mucosal layer of the stomach. It is essential for better understanding of pathophysiology of the stomach, particularly ulcerogenesis, to clarify the morphological and functional properties of these aminergic and peptidergic nerves in the stomach.

In this chapter, the distribution of cholinergic, adrenergic, VIP-ergic and histaminergic nerves, and the localization of their receptors in the gastric mucosa in the rat are described according to our recent studies. Functions of these nerves are also discussed.

DISTRIBUTION OF THE CHOLINERGIC NERVES AND THEIR RECEPTORS

The parasympathetic nerve supply to the stomach is via the vagal nerves. The histochemical localization of the cholinergic nerves was identified by acetylcholinesterase (AChE) activity[25,26] and choline acetyltransferase (ChA) immunoreactivity.[27]

In the submucosal layer, the AChE-positive nerves are recognized in the submucous plexuses (Meissner plexuses) near the arterioles (Fig. 4-1A). Most of the nerve fibers in these plexuses include agranular small synaptic vesicles specific for cholinergic nerves. Some of these nerves also contain small granular vesicles characteristic of adrenergic nerves and

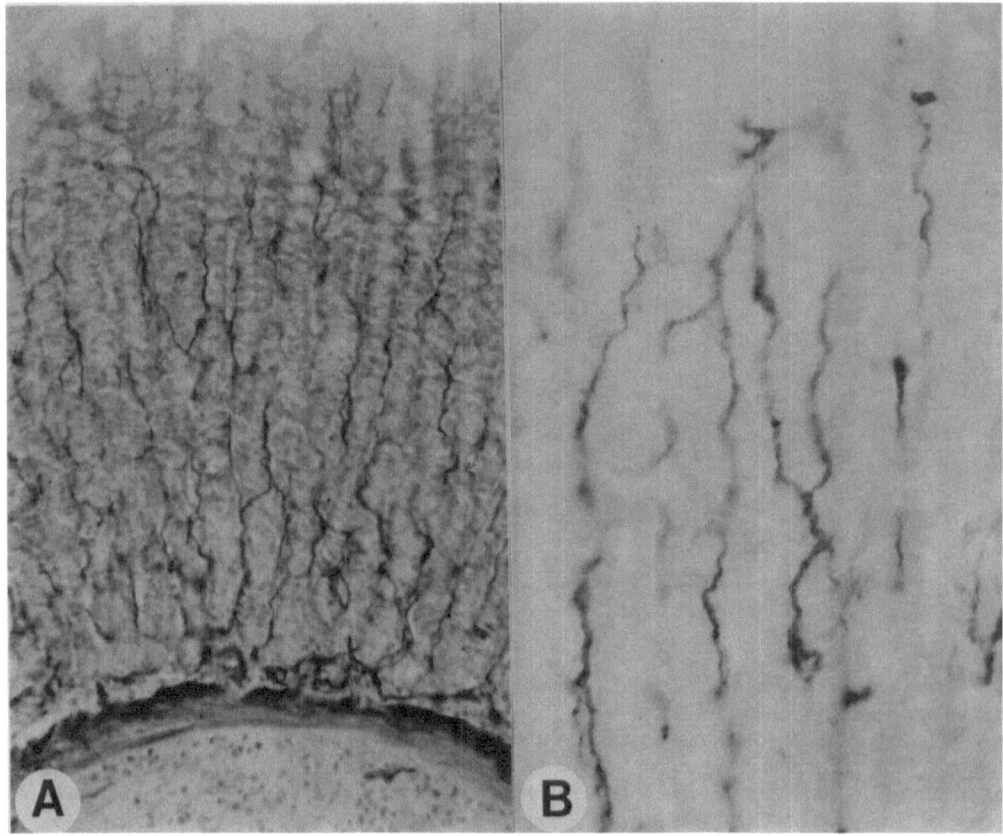

Fig. 4-3.. Histochemical distributions of the AChE-positive nerve fibers in the rat fundic mucosa. (a) In the vertical section of the gastric mucosa, cholinergic nerves are noted in the lamina propria mucosae between the gastric epithelial cells. ×400. (b) At high magnification, the AChE-positive nerve fibers are observed up to the top por-tion of the gastric mucosa. ×800. (c) In the cross section, cholinergic nerves are noted in dot form between the epithelial cell columns. ×400. (d) Fluorescence micrographs obtained by the indirect immunofluorescence antibody method using the anti-ChA serum. ChA-positive nerve fibers and cell bodies are seen between the gastric epithelial cells. ×400.

large granular vesicles probably corresponding to peptidergic nerves (Fig. 4-2A&B).

The nerve fibers arising from the submucosa extend to the basal part of the gastric mucosa and then form plexuses near the terminal arterioles. They are noted in linear form in the longitudinal section (Fig. 4-3A&B) and some in dot form in the cross-sections (Fig. 4-3C) between the gastric epithelial cell columns.[28] According to the AChE histochemical findings, only linear nerve fibers are recognized in the adult rat stomach. By the histofluorescence study using anti-ChA antiserum, however, these cholinergic nerves are found

to consist of the nerve cell body and nerve fibers (Fig. 4-3D).

Recent embryological studies using isolated cultured cells show that autonomic nerve cells and their effectors affect each others' differentiation.[29] In an attempt to clarify a relationship between the activity of autonomic nerves and the differentiation of parietal cells, histochemical studies were performed in the rat in the embryonic and postnatal periods.

The AChE-positive nerve cells appeared in the rat glandular stomach by the 14th day of the embryonic period (Fig. 4-4A), and ganglia formed on the 18th to 20th day. The ganglia,

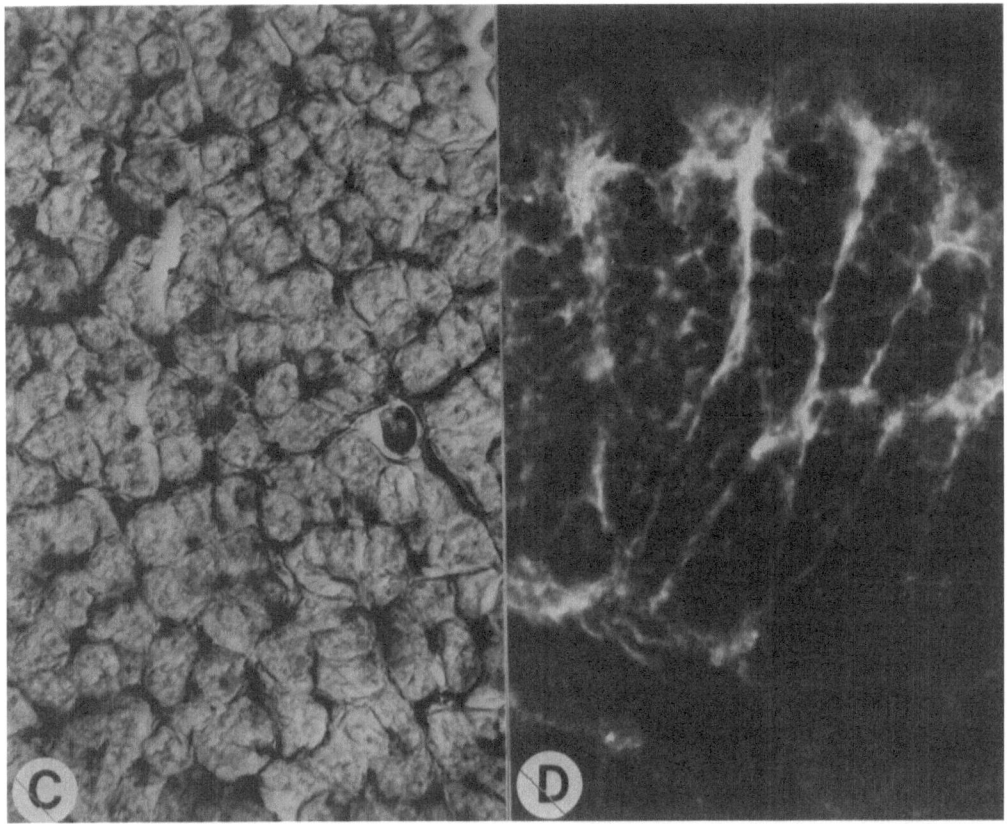

which were very large on the fourth day after birth, became reduced in size during the third postnatal week, largely corresponding to those found in adult rat stomach. AChE-positive nerve cells and their neural processes are clearly demonstrated between the gastric epithelial cells (Fig. 4-4B), and electron microscopically, the huge AChE-positive nerves are seen just under the epithelial cells (Fig. 4-4C&D).[30]

Regarding the regulation of differentiation of effectors by peripheral nerves, there is a report that differentiation of striated muscle cells is enhanced by noradrenaline released from adrenergic nerves, while it is suppressed by acetylcholine from cholinergic nerves.[31] Hence the chronological observations described above suggest that differentiation of parietal cells may be induced by cholinergic nervous activity. Further studies on neural degeneration or using appropriate inhibitors are needed to establish this possibility.

These observations suggest that cholinergic nerves may induce both the proliferation of the epithelial cells such as parietal and chief cells and the development of microcirculatory system comprising arterioles, true capillaries and collecting venules, leading to the hypothesis of dual action of cholinergic nerves in the gastric mucosa, (i.e., direct regulation of gastric mucosal microcirculation as well as acid and pepsinogen secretion).[32,33] By histochemical studies, the distribution pattern of the autonomic nerves is found to be largely similar to that in human stomach and in rat stomach.[32,34]

In an attempt to determine the effectors of the cholinergic nerves morphologically in the stomach wall, it is useful to clarify the localization of the AChE reaction products, since AChE is released from the nerve terminals to the effector cell plasma membrane. It is also essential for the determination of the cholinergic effector cells to identify the localization

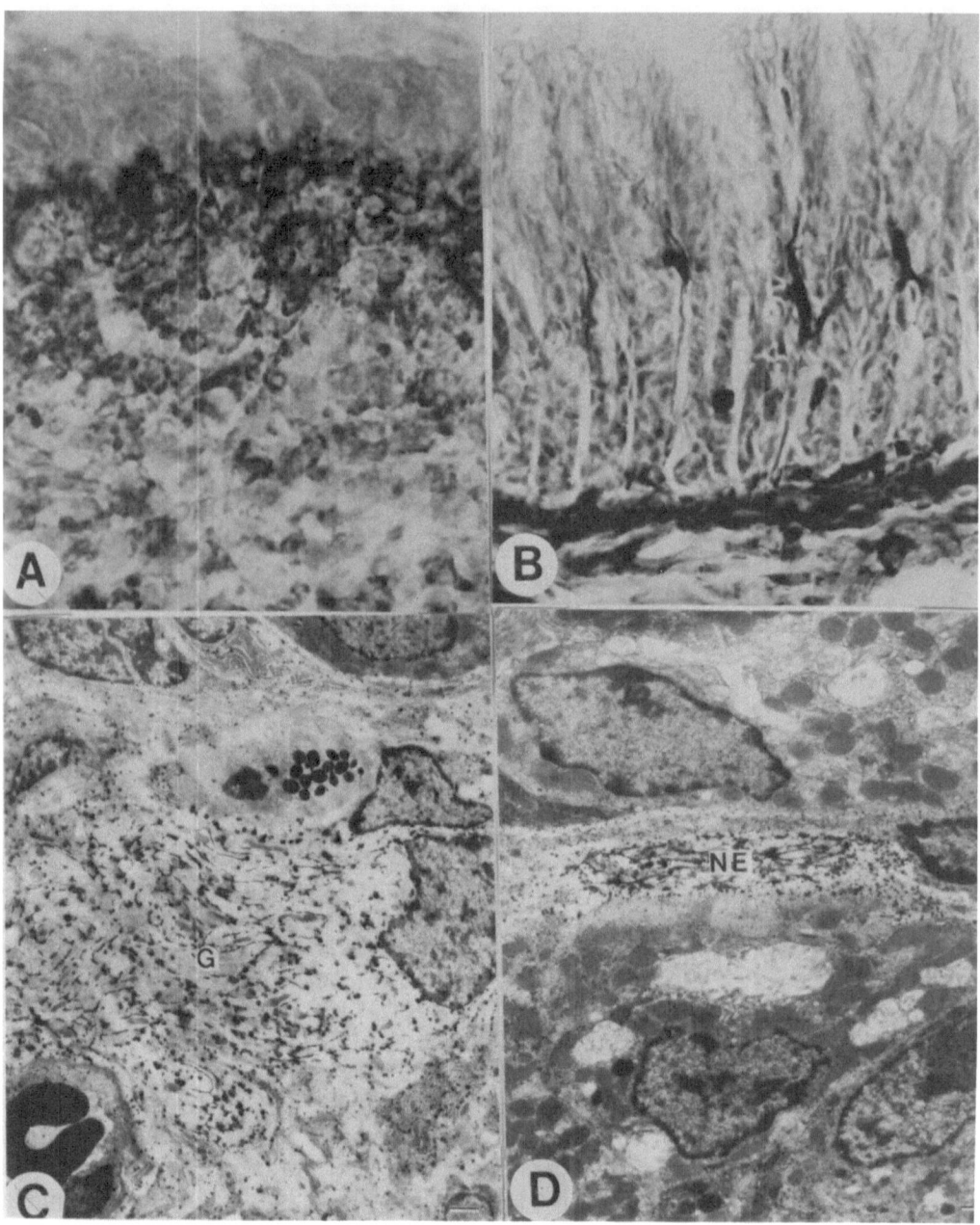

Fig. 4-4. Embryological observations of the AChE-positive nerves in the rat fundic mucosa. (a) In the 14-day-old rat embryo, the AChE-positive cells are clustered under the epithelial cells. ×160. (b) In the 4-day-old rat, the AChE-positive nerve cells and their neural processes are clearly observed between the gastric epithelial cells. ×400. (c) Elec-

tron microscopically, the huge AChE-positive ganglion (G) is seen just under the epithelial cells in the 4-day-old rat. ×5,000. (d) Unmyelinated nerve endings between the parietal cells in the 18-day-old rat. AChE reaction products are located on the axonal membrane of the unmyelinated nerve endings (NE). ×5,000.

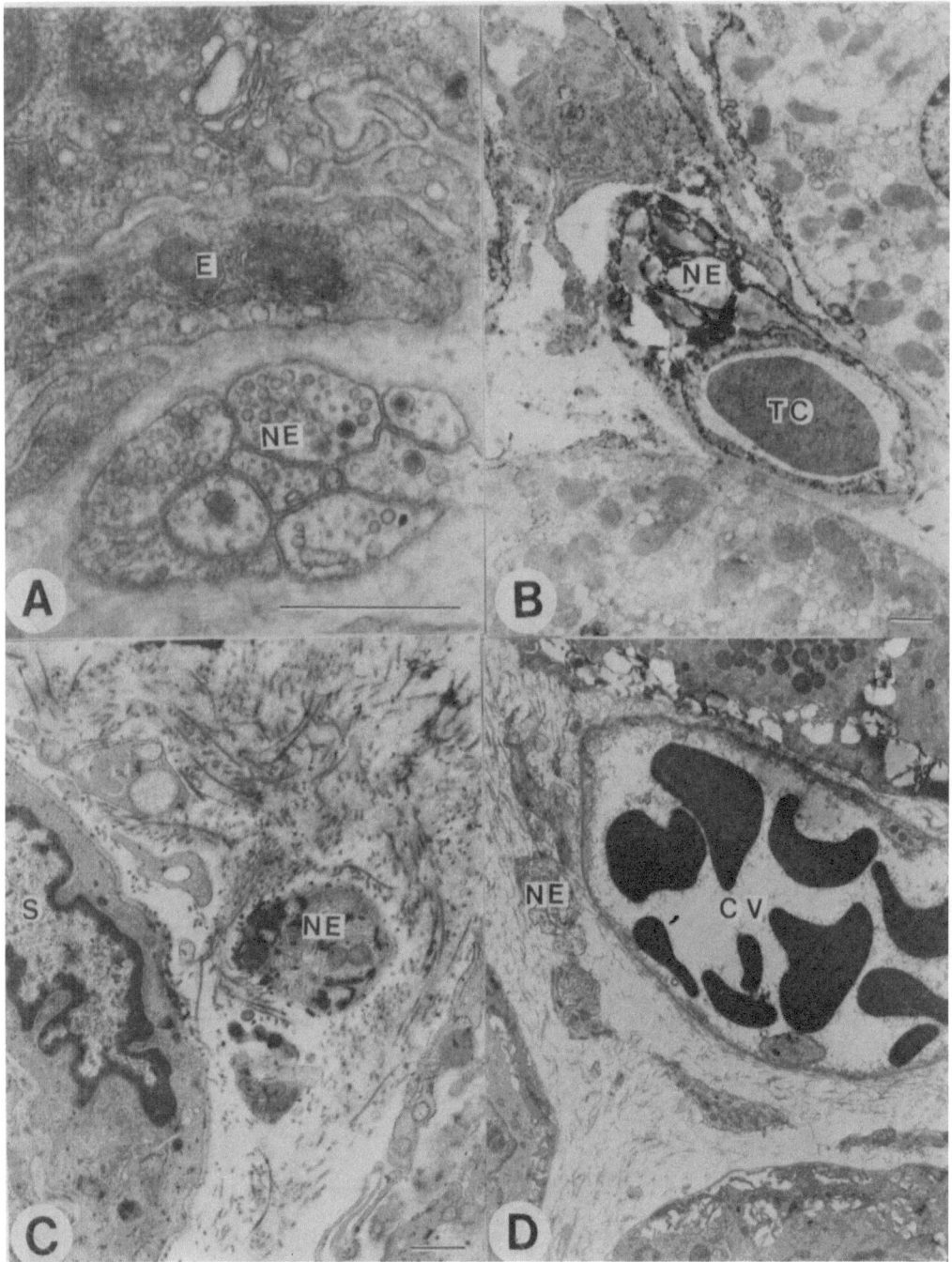

Fig. 4-5. Electron micrographs of the unmyelinated nerve endings near the microvessels. (a) Unmyelinated nerve endings (NE) near the true capillary endothelium (E). Synaptic vesicles in this nerve are small agranular, corresponding to the cholinergic nerves. ×30,000. (b) AChE reaction products are seen on the axonal membranes of the unmyelinated nerve endings (NE) as well as on the abluminal surface of the endothelial plasma membrane. TC: true capillary ×8,000. (c) Unmyelinated nerve endings (NE) near the smooth muscle cell (S) of the arteriole. The AChE reaction products are present on the smooth muscle cell. × 10,000. (d) Unmyelinated nerve endings near the collecting venule (CV). ×7,000.

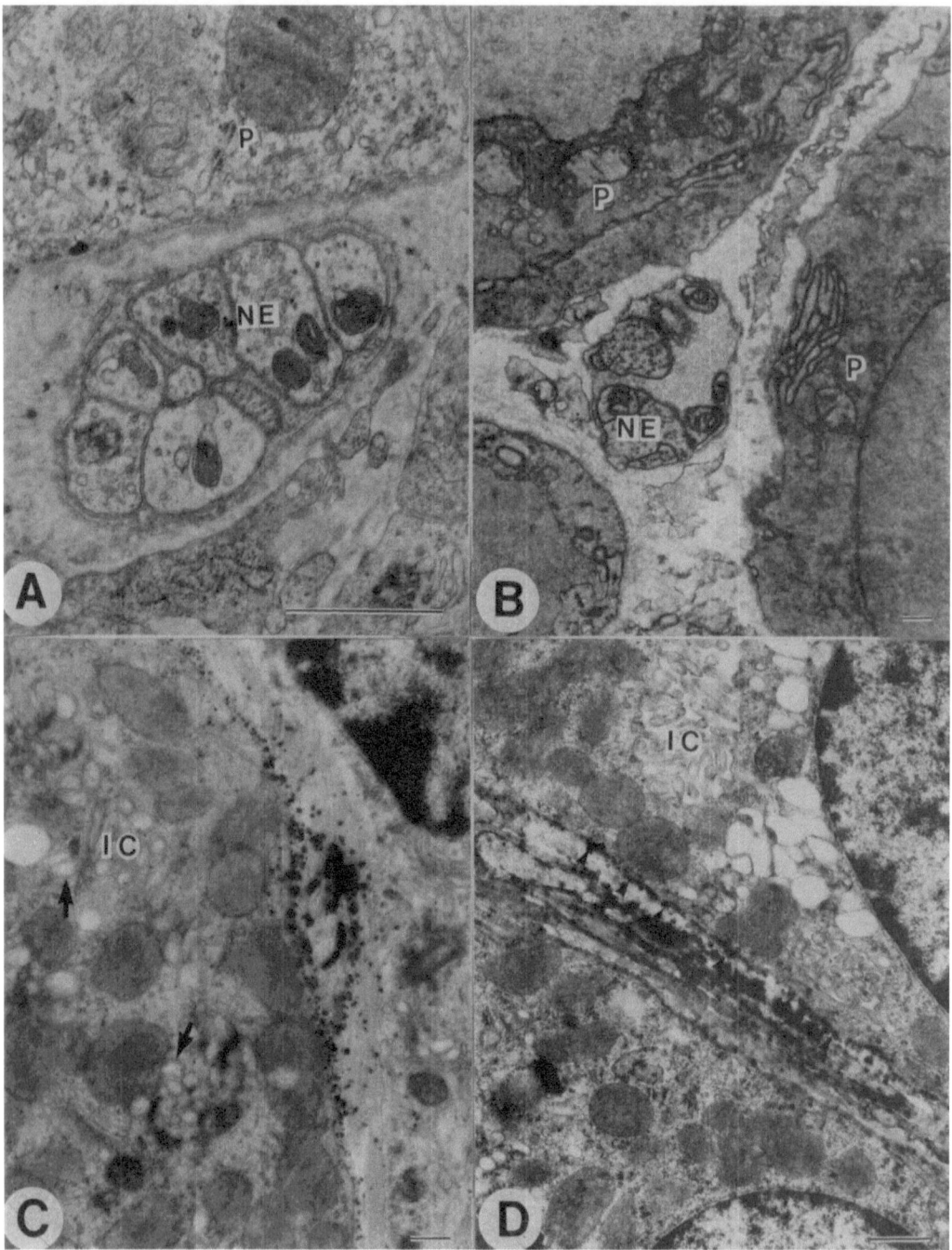

Fig. 4-6. Electron micrographs of the nerve endings near the parietal cells. (a) Unmyelinated nerve endings (NE) near the parietal cell (P). Routine fixation. ×26,000. (b) The synaptic vesicles of these nerve endings are agranular, corresponding to the cholinergic nerves. KMnO₄ fixation. ×5,000. (c) The AChE reaction products surrounding the nerve endings are decreased by truncal vagotomy. The tubulovesicles are clearly increased (arrows). IC: intracellular canaliculi. ×7,000. (d) In the control, the AChE reaction products are normally present on the axonal membrane of unmyelinated nerve endings. IC:intracellular canaliculi. ×7,000.

of muscarinic acetylcholine receptors (m-AChRs) on the cell plasma membrane in the close vicinity of the nerve terminals.

The AChE reaction products are demonstrated both on the axonal membranes of the unmyelinated nerve endings containing small agranular synaptic vesicles and on the plasma membrane of the true capillary endotherium (Fig. 4-5A–D). Also the AChE reaction products are noted on the basal plasma membrane of the parietal cell and on the smooth muscle cell plasma membrane (Fig. 4-6A–D). These distributions of the AChE reaction products suggest the direct cholinergic innervation of the mucosal capillaries, parietal cells, and arterioles.

The radioautographic study using the tritium-labelled muscarinic antagonist, ^{3}H-quinuclidinyl benzilate (QNB), and ^{3}H-pirenzepine (PZ) is very useful for proving the localization of m-AChRs in the gastric mucosa.[37] Under light anesthesia with intraperitoneal injection of sodium pentobarbital, aqueous solutions of ^{3}H-QNB were infused for 30 min through an aortic catheter by an infusion pump at a constant rate, followed by an infusion of saline to wash out the unbound ligand. Immediately after the infusion, the small tissue blocks of the stomach were quickly frozen in isopentane cooled with liquid nitrogen, and were freeze-dried at $-50°C$ and evacuated at 9×10^{-3} Torr. The freeze-dried tissue blocks were then exposed to osmium vapor, followed by infiltration of Epon in a dripping unit. Thereafter, the tissue blocks were embedded in Epon.

Semithin or ultrathin sections were cut with LKB ultramicrotome using ethylene glycol instead of water.[35] The emulsion film (Sakura NR-H2 or M2) was then applied to the glass plates or meshes on which sections were mounted. They were exposed in a refrigerator in the dark for 4 to 8 weeks. After development, they were examined with light or electron microscopy. As shown in Figs. 4-7 and 4-8, the silver grains indicating the ^{3}H-QNB-binding sites (i.e., the localization of m-AChRs) are mainly located in the basal two-thirds of the gastric mucosa, coinciding with the localization of the cholinergic nerves in the gastric mucosa. Electron microscopically the silver grains indicating the presence of m-AChRs are recognized on the parietal cells as well as on the endothelial cell plasma membranes of the true capillaries.[36] (Figs. 4-9A-C, 4-10A-C). The cellular ulstrastructures in these radiographs are not well maintained, since the radioautographic method for soluble compounds[35] applied in this study avoids fixation to prevent the migration of radiolabelled receptor antagonists defining the receptor sites. These silver grains were significantly increased in number after truncal vagotomy, while they were diminished by atropine pretreatment, supporting the specificity of these radioautographic reactions. Moreover, these grains were not noticed in the rat stomach infused with unlabelled QNB. The localization of the silver grains is therefore thought to be specific for the m-AchRs. The radioautography using ^{3}H-PZ reveals that the localization sites of a high dose of ^{3}H-PZ showing the distribution of m-AchRs are almost the same as those of ^{3}H-QNB (Fig. 4-11A-C).[37]

GASTRIC MUCOSAL MICROCIRCULATION AND CHOLINERGIC CONTROL

In vivo microscopy revealed the hemodynamics in the microvasculature of the gastric mucosal surface in the control rat.[34,38] Blood is seen flowing rapidly and uniformly in the anastomosing capillary network surrounding the gastric pits, and ultimately draining into the collecting venules, forming a functional unit in the mucosal microvasculature. In the rat restrained by the plaster bandage method,[34] the blood flow is not uniform in the mucosal capillaries, and a variety of vasomotor disturbances such as sludge, regurgitation, and stasis are observed concomitant with hemorrhagic changes, particularly in the area surrounding the hemorrhagic erosive lesions induced by the restraint stress.[33,34,39]

In an experimental model of stress ulcer induced by restraint using a plaster bandage,[34]

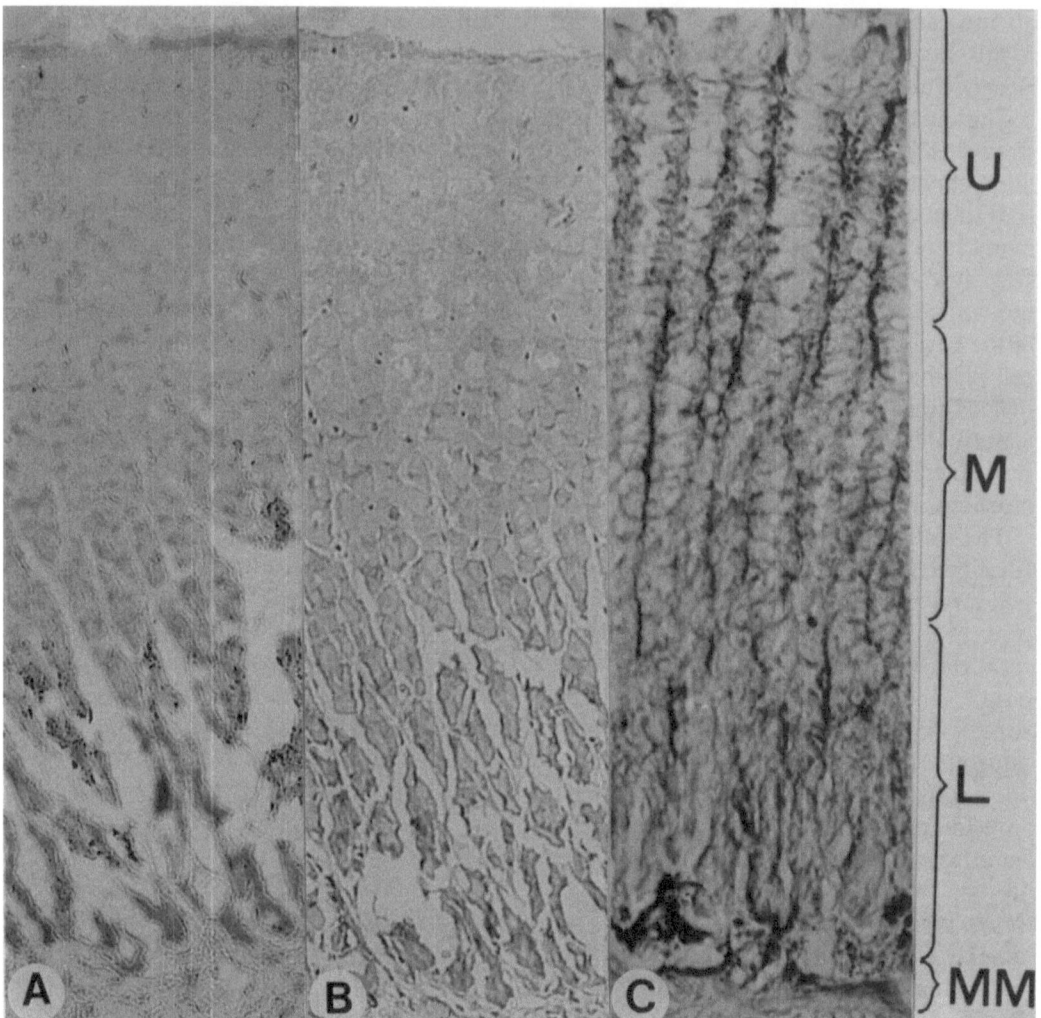

Fig. 4-7. Light microscopic radioautographs of the ³H-QNB-binding sites in the fundic mucosa. The silver grains are mainly found in the basal two-thirds of the gastric mucosa. U: upper, M: middle, L: lower gastric mucosa; MM: muscularis mucosae. (a) control group. ×400. (b) In the atropine-treated group, few grains are seen compared with control group. ×400. (c) AChE stain. ×400.

hemorrhagic erosions were formed in the glandular stomach of the rat eight hours after starting the restraint. The AChE reaction products were increased, both on the axonal membranes of the unmyelinated nerve endings and on the basal site of the plasma membrane of the parietal cell, implying an enhanced transmission of ACh from the former to the latter via m-AChRs demonstrated on the parietal cell plasma membrane under restraint stress.[36] On the other hand, the nora-drenaline fluorescence, indicating sympathetic nervous activity, was decreased in the mucosal layer.[34] The dye-4% pontamine sky blue, or horseradish peroxidase (HRP), administered via an aortic catheter, had permeated remarkably from the collecting venules and capillaries in the mucosal layer, particularly around the hemorrhagic erosions where AChE activity was greatly activated. Electron microscopic observation revealed a widening of the gaps between the capillary en-

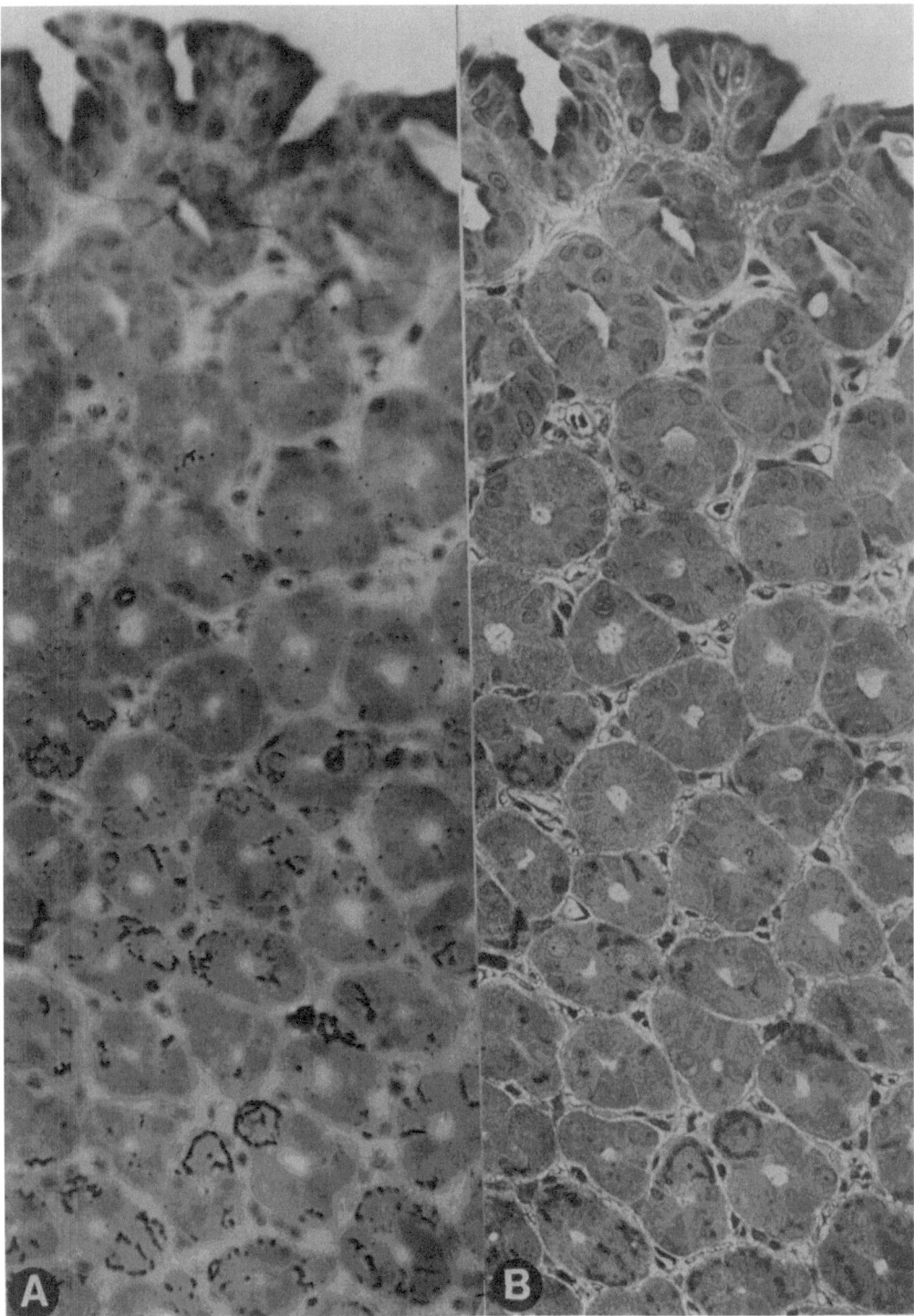

Fig. 4-8. Light microscopic radioautograph of the ^{3}H-PZ-binding sites in the fundic mucosa. The silver grains are mainly seen on the parietal cells. (a) focused on the grain. ×800. (b) focused on the underlying tissue. ×800.

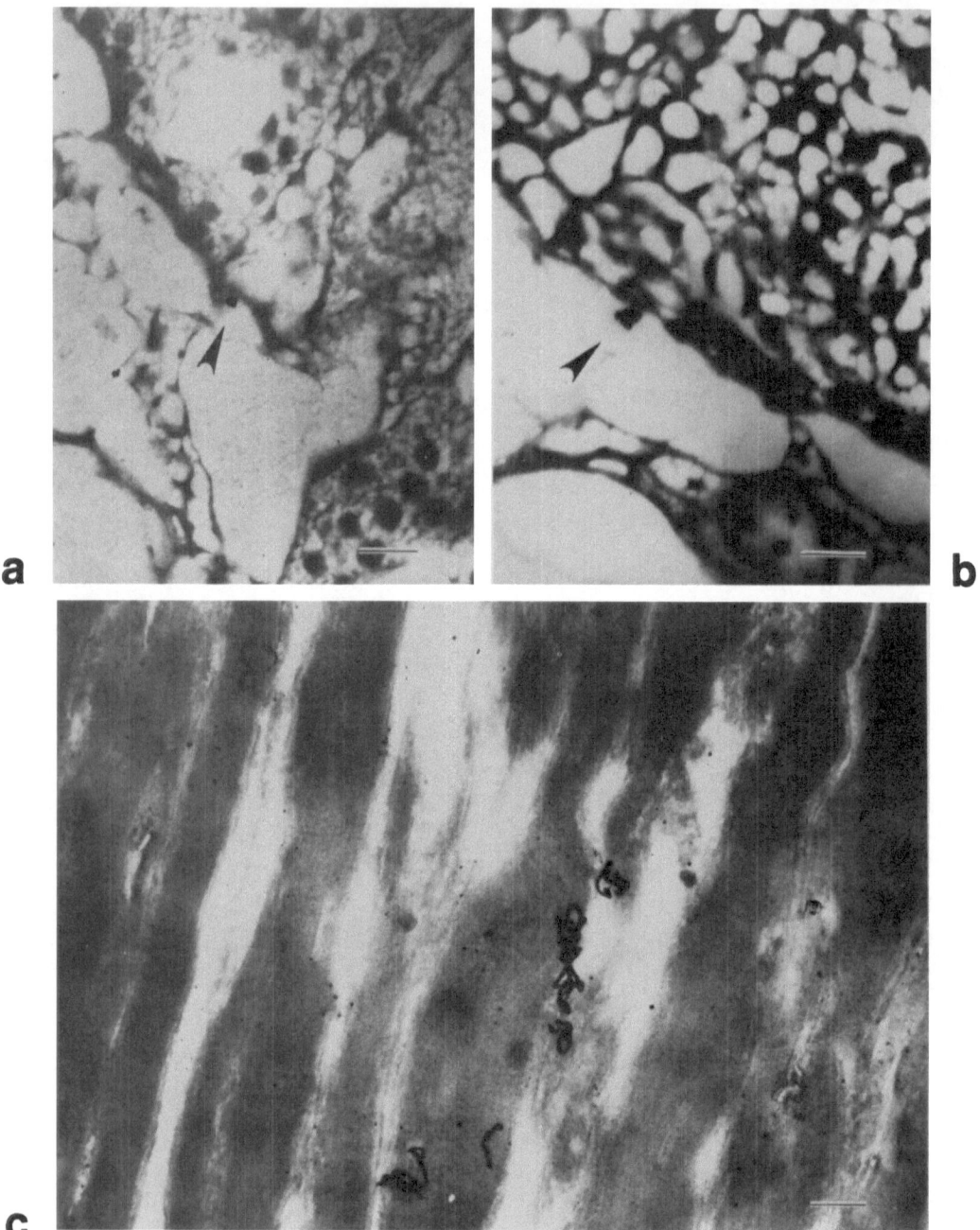

Fig 4-9. Electron microscopic radioautographs of the 3H-QNB-binding sites (a), (b). The grains (arrowheads) are found near the plasma membrane of the parietal cells. ×8,000. (c) In the smooth muscle layer, 3H-QNB is found to bind to the smooth muscle cells. The cellular ultrastructure in these radioautographs are not maintained well since the radiographic method for soluble compounds avoids fixation for preventing migration of radiolabelled receptor antagonists. ×8,000

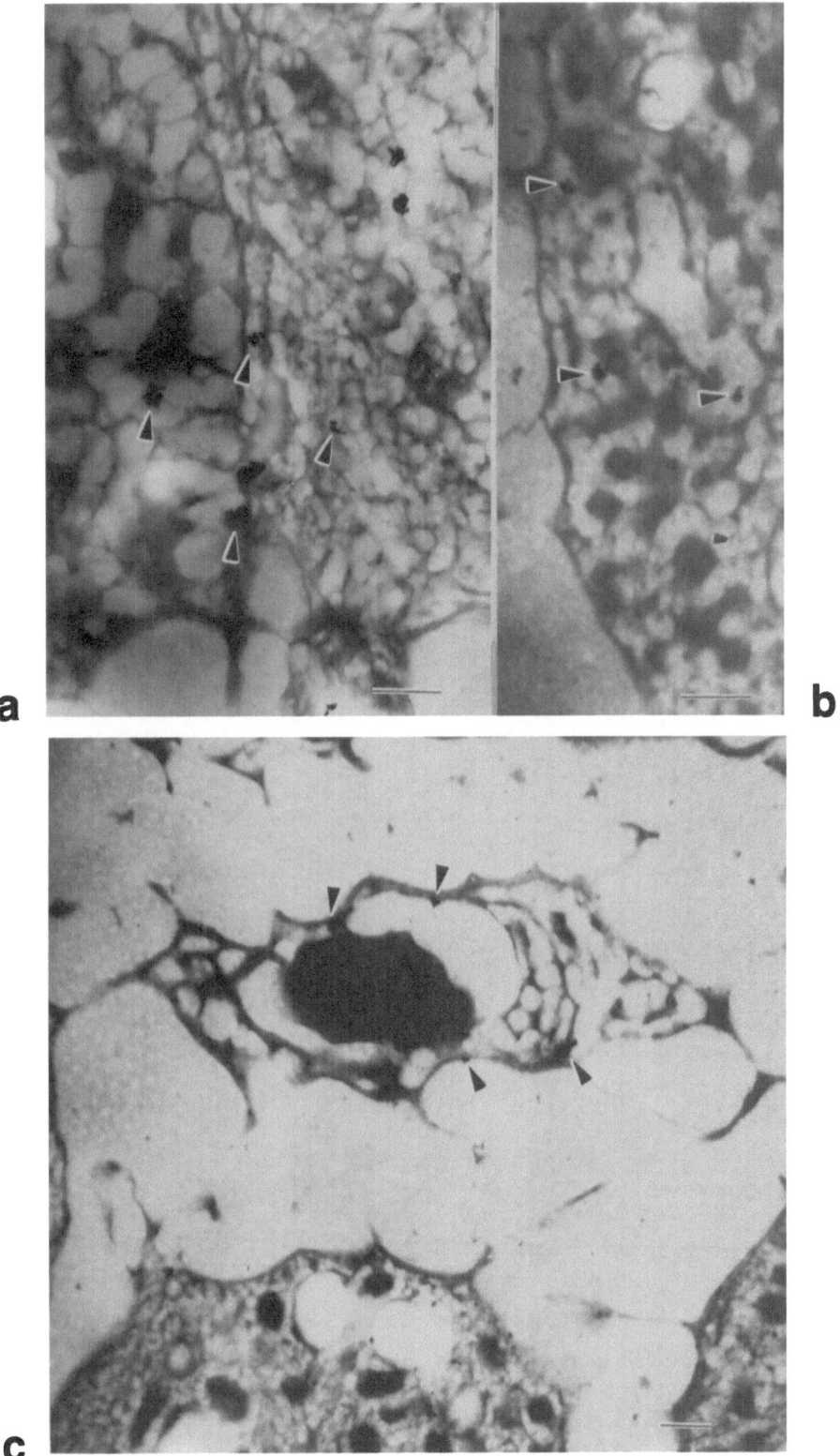

Fig 4-10. Electron microscopic radiographs of the 3H-QNB binding sites of the vagotomized rat. (a)(b). The silver grains on the parietal cells are re- markably increased. ×10,000 (c) The grains are seen in large numbers on the true capillary endo- thelium. ×8,000

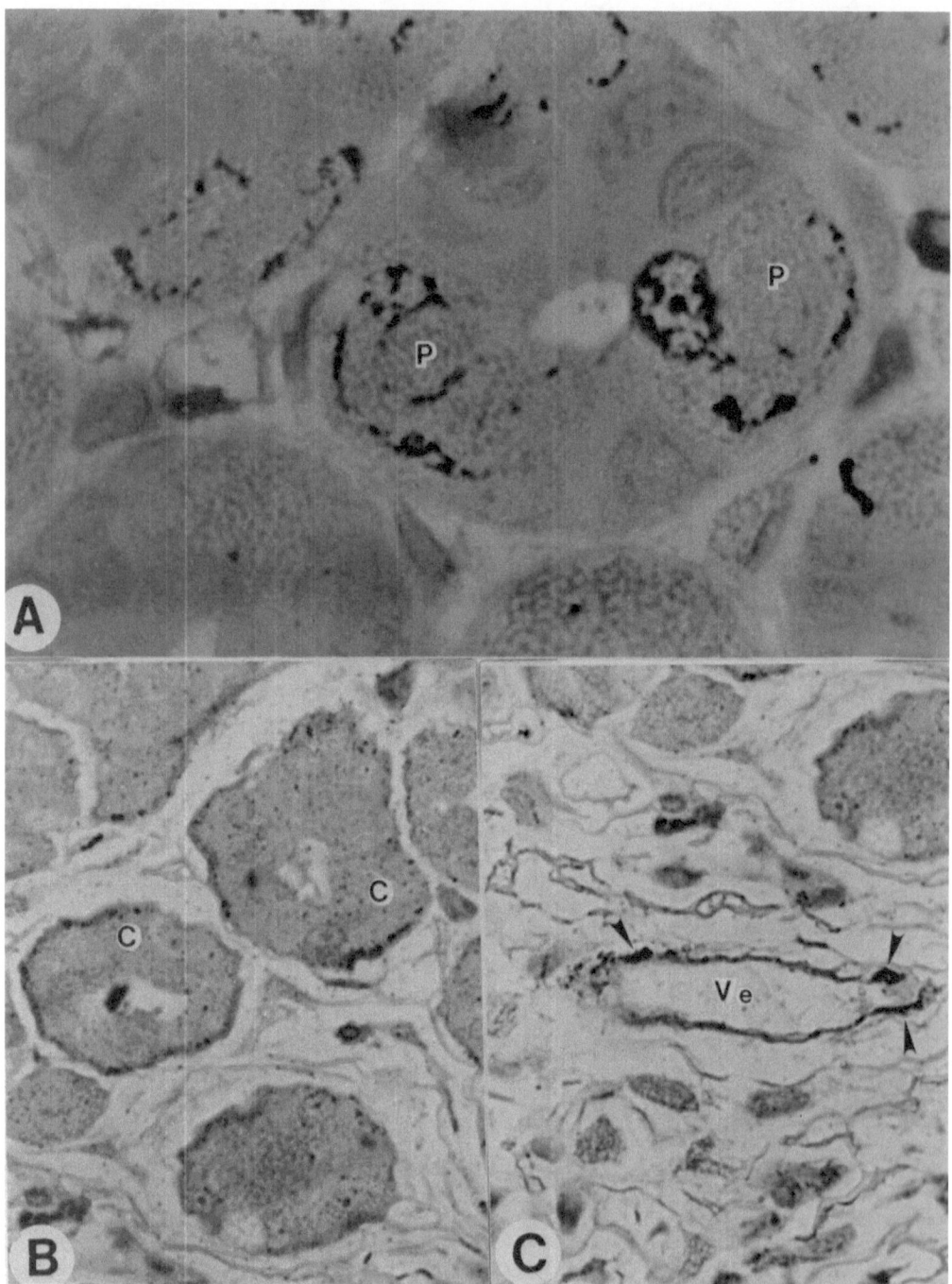

Fig. 4-11. Light microscopic radioautographs of the ³H-PZ binding sites in the gastric mucosa. (a) In the middle portion of the gastric mucosa, a large number of silver grains showing the ³H-PZ binding sites are deposited on the parietal cells (P). ×800. (b) In the lower portion of the gastric mucosa, the grains are seen on the chief cells (C). ×400. (c) The ³H-PZ-binding sites are found on the endothelium of the venules (Ve) and the arterioles. ×400.

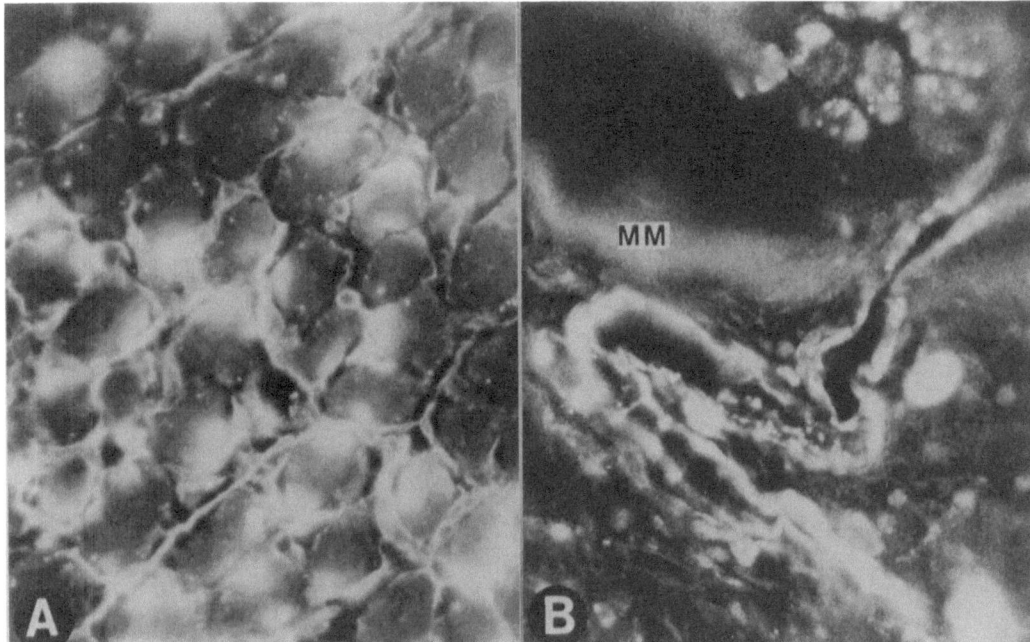

Fig. 4-12. Fluorescent micrographs of noradrenaline by the Falck-Hillarp methods. (a) In the mucosal layer, specific fluorescence of noradrenaline, corresponding to the adrenergic nerve fibers, is seen between the epithelial cells. ×400. (b) In the submucosal layer, the arterioles are found to be constricted in the muscularis mucosae (MM). ×400.

dothelial cells, possibly due to contraction of the endothelia and/or enhancement of vesicular and vacuolar transport across the capillary endothelium, leading to an increased permeability of the capillary vessels, concomitant with a variety of vasomotor disturbances in the gastric mucosal microcirculation.[33]

In biopsy specimens of the human gastric mucosa obtained from a patient with gastric ulcer, AChE activity is progressively increased the nearer it is to the hemorrhagic erosions. Using electron microscopy, the increased AChE reaction products are found both on the unmyelinated nerve endings and on the capillary endothelium or on the parietal cell plasma membrane.[33]

According to these studies, it is tentatively speculated that an excessive transmission of ACh to the capillary endothelium would directly cause an increased permeability of the mucosal capillaries around collecting venules, comcomitant with a variety of vasomotor dis-

turbances in the capillary blood flow, leading to ischemic lesions in the gastric mucosa. There is an intimate relation between the autonomic nerve endings and the capillaries in the human gastric mucosa, suggesting that the pathogenesis of acute gastric ulcers (acute gastric hemorrhagic lesions) in humans could be explained, at least in part, by a mechanism similar to that of stress-induced experimental ulcer formation.

DISTRIBUTION OF THE ADRENERGIC NERVES AND THEIR ACTION ON THE MICROCIRCULATORY SYSTEM

The sympathetic nerve supply to the rat stomach is derived from spinal nerves and terminates in the celiac ganglia. From these ganglia, the postganglionic adrenergic fibers reach the stomach as discrete nerves, as

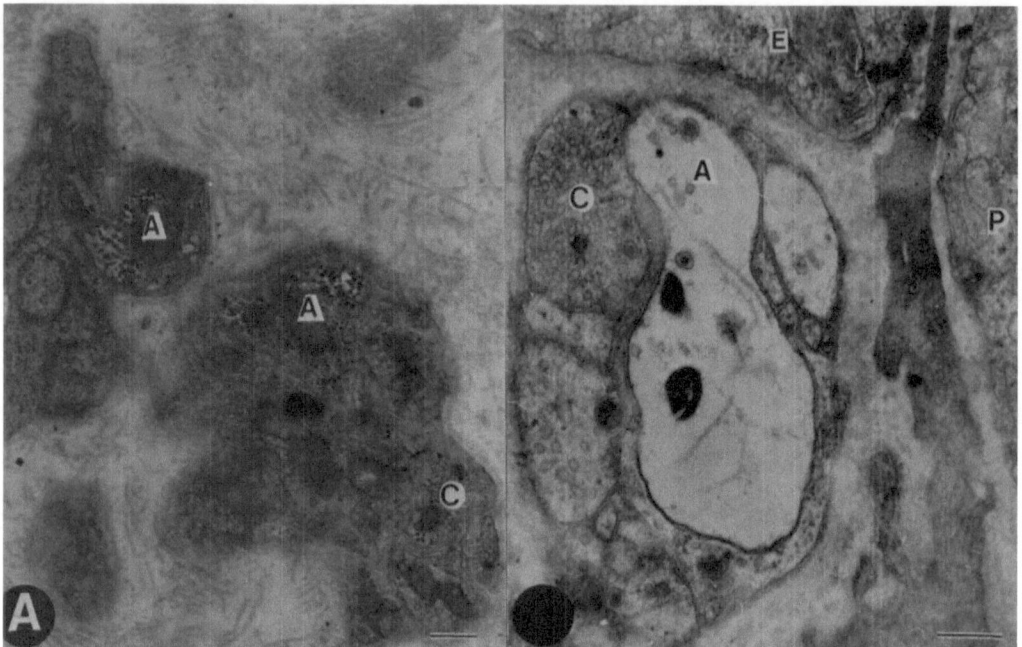

Fig. 4-13. Electron micrographs of the adrenergic nerve endings (A) in the mucosa. (a) The granular small synaptic vesicles, specific for noradrenaline, are clearly seen. Chromaffin fixation. ×7,000. (b) Transmission electron micrograph demonstrating the coexistence of the sympathetic and parasym-pathetic nerve endings in the fundic mucosal layer of rat stomach. The sympathetic nerve endings (A) are selectively degenerated by α-hydroxydopamine administration, while parasympathetic nerve endings (C) remain unaltered. P: parietal cell E: true capillary endothelium. ×7,000.

nerves closely associated with vagal nerves or as nerves accompanying the arterial vessels.

Using a fluorescent histochemical method,[40,41] the nerve endings showing the specific noradrenaline fluorescence are located mainly in the perivascular plexuses of the arterioles and some in the myenteric and submucous plexuses of the nerve fibers in the basal portion of the gastric mucosa (Figs. 4-1B, 4-12A&B).[10,42] Electron microscopically, the nerve fibers possessing small electron-dense synaptic vesicles clearly demonstrated in the chromaffin-fixed preparations, probably corresponding to the adrenergic fibers, are found mainly along the terminal arterioles in the basal part of the mucosa as well as along the arterioles in the submucosa (Fig. 4-13A&B), while those in the superficial part of the mucosa are almost devoid of the adrenergic fluorescence.

From the evolutional point of view, a large number of intramural adrenergic neurons are present in the gut of amphibians and reptiles, but few in mammals.[43] In the gut of mammals, peptidergic nerves are thought to act as a counterpart. Therefore, the adrenergic nerves would not be involved in the contraction of the nonvascular smooth muscle layer, but rather in the regulation of the mesenteric blood flow.

The significance of the peripheral dopaminergic nerve has been re-evaluated by a study using anti-dopamine β-hydroxylase antibody.[23] There are some studies suggesting that most of the adrenergic nerves may belong to the dopaminergic fibers.

To clarify the functional significance of the adrenergic innervation, the effects of noradrenaline, isoproterenol and dopamine on the gastric mucosal microcirculatory system were examined by the infusion of horseradish peroxidase (HRP: Sigma type II) as a marker[44] for microvascular permeability. By the infusion of α-agonist noradrenaline, the arterioles in the basal portion of the gastric mucosa are constricted and the permeability of the capil-

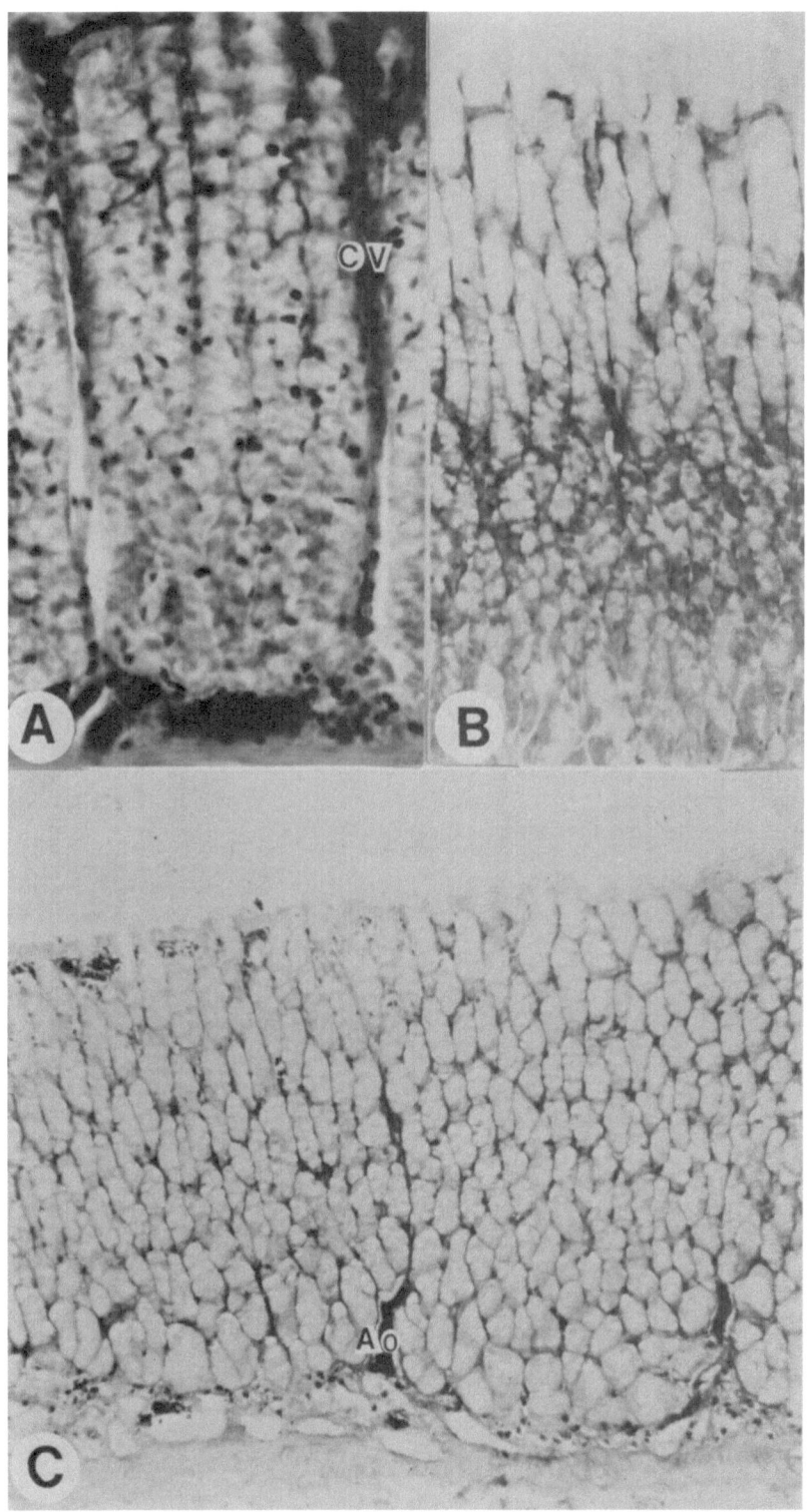

Fig. 4-14. The microcirculatory alterations induced by various adrenergic agents. (a) Control group. The upper half of the capillary network and the collecting venules (CV) are seen. ×400. (b) The capillary permeability is clearly increased by noradrenaline infusion. ×400. (c) The arterioles (Ao) in basal portion become enlarged after isoproterenol infusion. ×300.

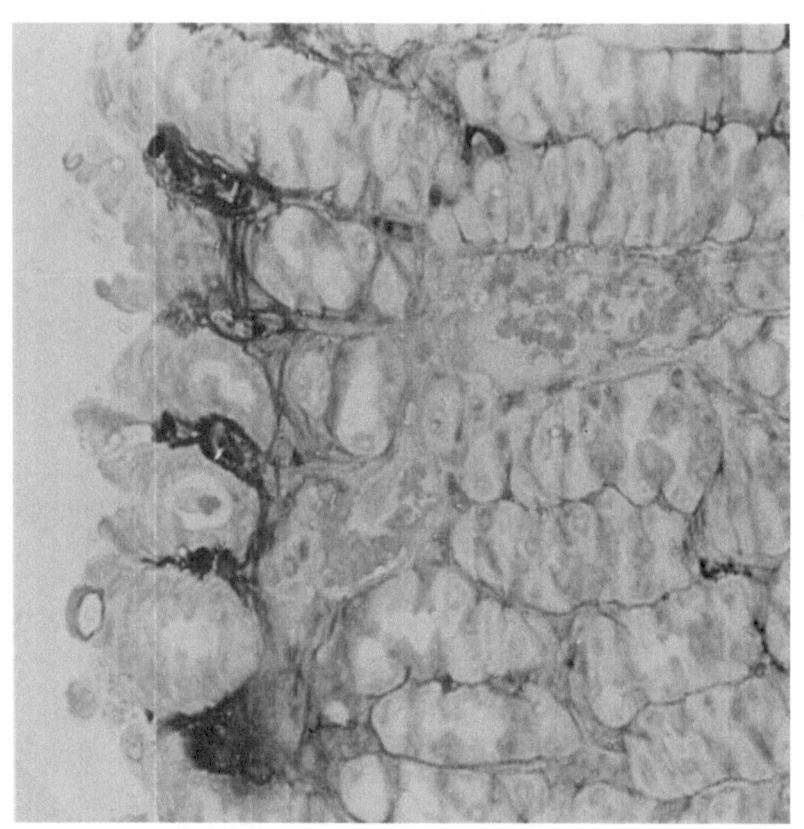

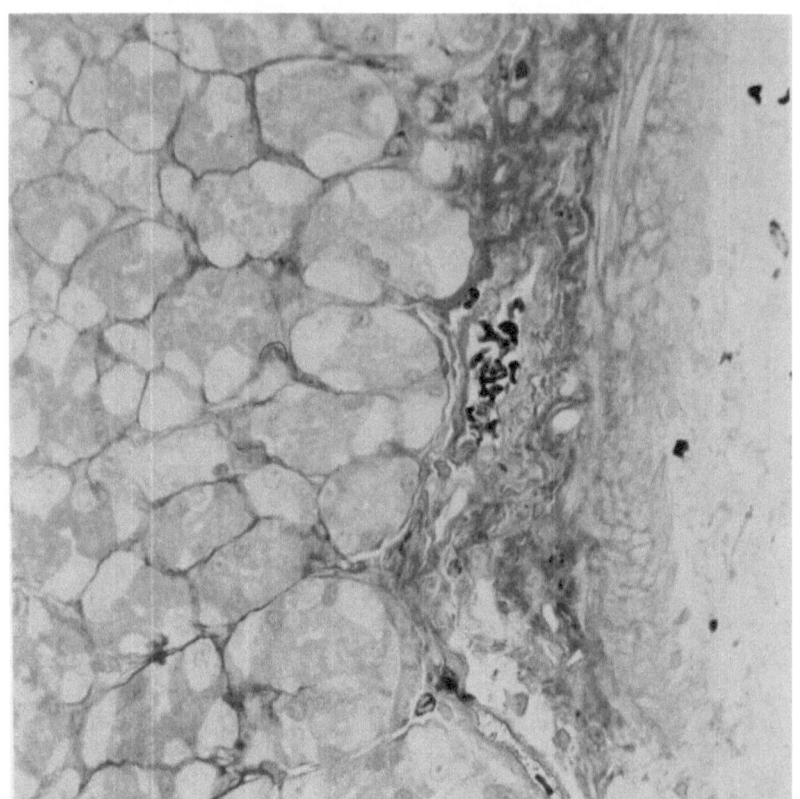

Fig. 4-15. Microcirculatory alterations induced by L-dopa administration. The HRP reaction is exclusively found in arterioles and venules (a) ×300 (b) ×1,200.

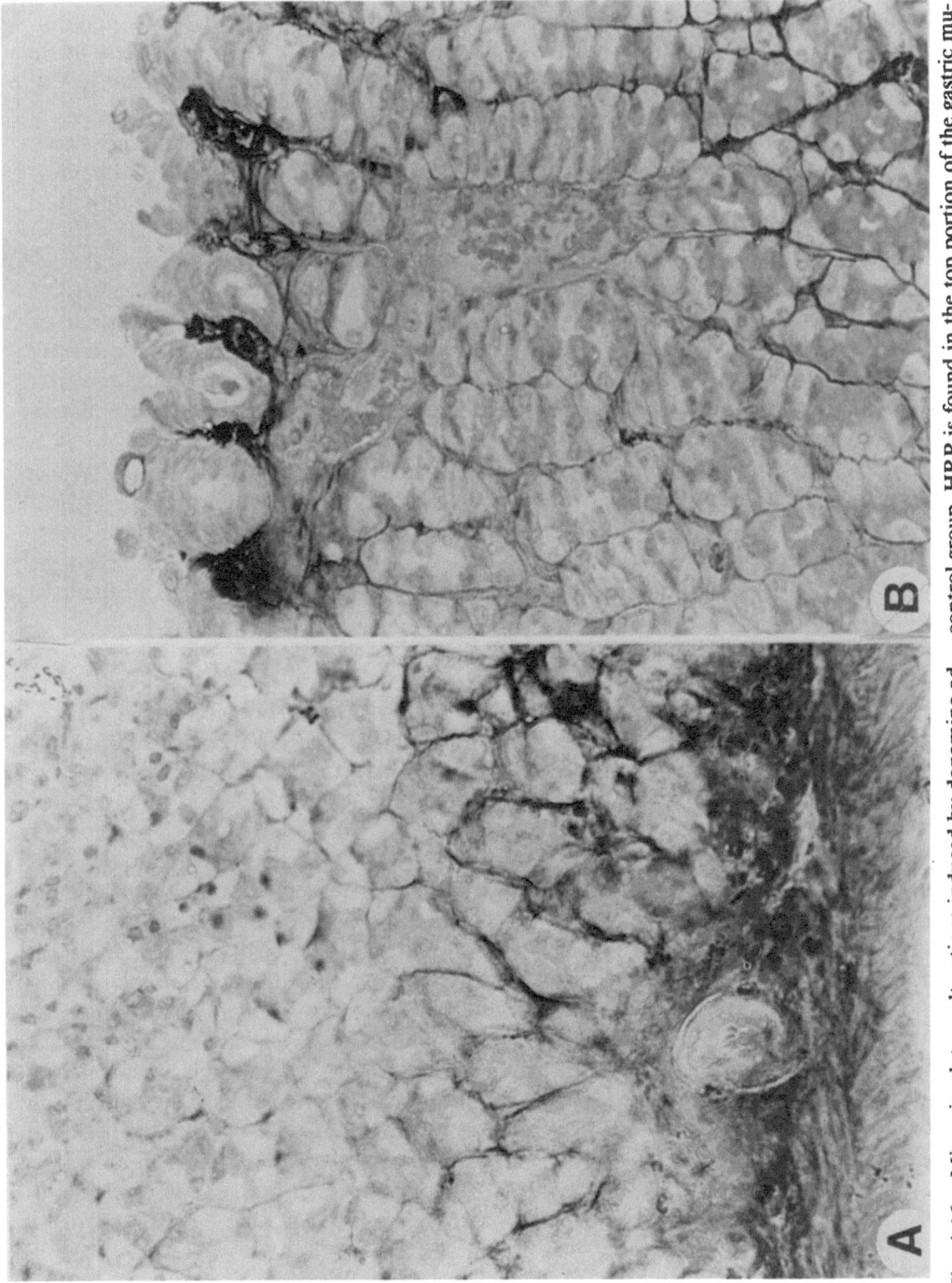

Fig. 4-16. Microcirculatory alterations induced by dopamine administration. (a) HRP is present only in the basal portion of the gastric mucosa after dopamine administration. ×1200. (b) In the control group, HRP is found in the top portion of the gastric mucosa. ×1,200.

laries in the middle portion of the gastric mucosa is found to be markedly increased (Fig. 4-14A&B). By the infusion of β-agonist isoproterenol, small arterioles located just above the muscularis mucosae, possibly corresponding to the terminal arterioles or metarterioles, are dilated compared with those in the control group (Fig. 4-14C). By the infusion of L-dopa or dopamine, the upper half of the gastric mucosa becomes ischemic, resembling the mucosal alterations observed in the process of the plaster bandage restraint-induced ulcer formation (Figs. 4-15A&B, 4-16A&B).[34] These observations suggest that dopamine may open the arteriovenous (A-V) anastomoses, causing mucosal ischemia. This would be supported by the report that dopaminergic nerve fibers may regulate the opening of A-V shunts in the dog paw pad.[45]

There is, however, a dispute as to whether A-V anastomosis is present in the gastric microcirculatory system in the rat stomach. It has been postulated that opening the submucosal A-V anastomoses is a important factor for gastric microcirculatory disturbances in stress-induced ulcerogenesis.[46,47] On the contrary, in vivo fluorescence microscopy revealed no A-V anastomosis in normal and sympathetic nerve-stimulated rat stomach,[48,49] implying that A-V shunts play no significant role in the mucosal blood flow responses to sympathetic nerve stimulation. In the restrained rats, the intensity of the specific fluorescence for adrenergic nerves is decreased in the mucosal layer, indicating that cholinergic nerves are excessively overstimulated in the gastric mucosa in the process of restraint-induced ulcerogenesis as described above.[34]

DISTRIBUTION OF VIP-ERGIC NERVE FIBERS AND THE LOCALIZATION OF VIP RECEPTORS

The VIP-immunoreactivity-positive nerve fibers (i.e., VIP-ergic nerve fibers) show a distribution almost like that of the cholinergic nerve fibers in the gastric mucosa. Electron

microscopically, the large cored vesicle-containing nerves are thought to be peptidergic in nature (Fig. 4-17A&B).[17] Some of these nerve fibers are shown to be immunoreactive to VIP in the rat stomach.

The localization of VIP-binding sites in the gastric mucosa was observed by radioautography for soluble compounds, as described above, using ^{125}I-VIP as a ligand.

The receptors of VIP are found on the parietal cells in the gastric mucosa (Fig. 4-18A). Some VIP receptors are also visualized on the endothelia of the arterioles (Fig. 4-18B), suggesting that VIP may have some direct effects on the mucosal microcirculatory system.

There is a possibility that some of VIP-positive nerve fibers extending to the inferior mesenteric ganglia may correspond to sensory fibers.[50] Some of the nerves like VIP-ergic nerves may act as afferent fibers in the local reflex circuit.

HISTAMINE-CONTAINING CELLS, HISTAMINERGIC NERVES AND THE LOCALIZATION OF HISTAMINE H_1 AND H_2 RECEPTORS

There is increasing evidence that histamine functions as a neurotransmitter in the central and peripheral nervous system.[21,51] In recent years, it was revealed that histamine-containing nerves are located mainly in the ganglia in the submucosal layer, not in the mucosal layer of the gastrointestinal tract.[21] Histamine-containing nerve fibers are present in the external muscle layer. In the mucosal layer of the rodent stomach, histamine is synthesized and stored in mast cells and enterochromaffin-like cells, but not in the nerve fibers.[21]

It is generally accepted that histamine H_1 receptors[52] located on smooth muscles and blood vessels are involved in the regulation of blood flow, while histamine H_2 receptors[53] specifically located on parietal cells are involved in the regulation of acid secretion.

In the stomach histamine is considered not

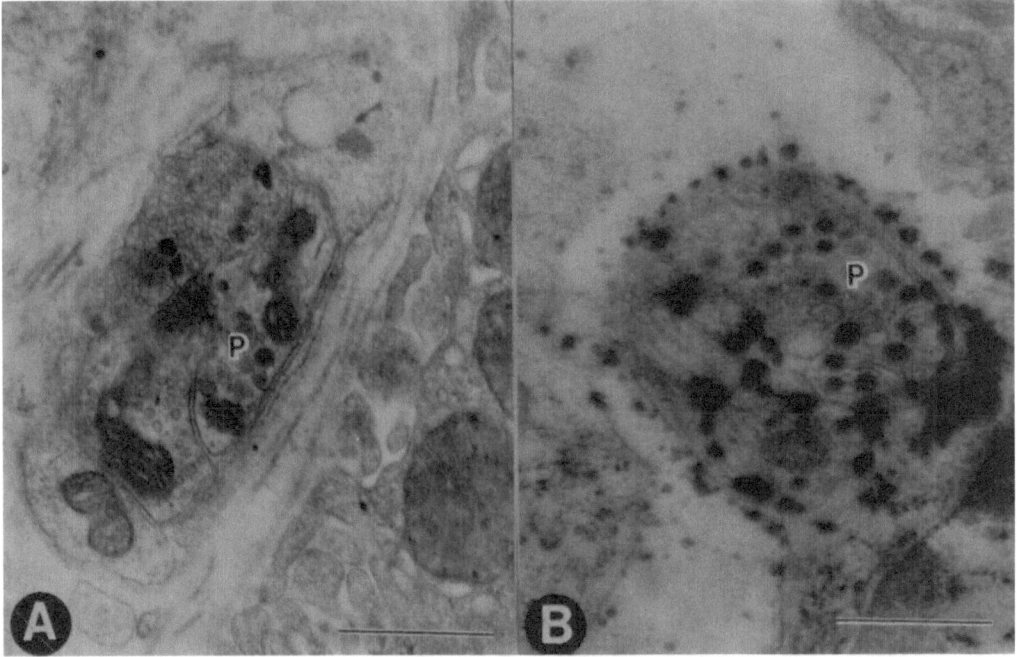

Fig. 4-17. Electron micrographs of the nerve endings composed of peptidergic (P) and cholinergic (C) nerve endings. (a) Some nerve fibers contain large granular vesicles probably corresponding to peptidergic nerves. ×25,000. (b) In the AChE staining, few reaction products are found on the axonal membranes of the peptidergic nerve endings. ×25,000

only to induce acid secretion from the parietal cells through H_2 receptors,[54] but also to dilate the submucosal arterioles through H_1 and H_2 receptors.[55]

H_1 receptor antagonist, diphenhydramine, decreases the gastric mucosal blood flow enhanced by the specific receptor agonist, 2-methylhistamine, while it hardly increases acid secretion, suggesting that H_1 receptors may play a possible physiological role in the control of the mucosal blood flow, regardless of acid secretion.[53] Histamine receptor antagonists suppress an increase in the gastric mucosal blood flow induced by H_2 receptor agonist but also inhibit acid secretion.[56] Therefore it still remains equivocal whether H_2 receptors directly regulate the mucosal blood flow, or indirectly affect the blood flow via acid secretory responses.[53]

The localization of both types of histamine receptors in the gastric mucosa was clarified by radioautography using the tritium-labelled histamine H_1 antagonist, ^3H-pyrilamine and H_2 antagonist, ^3H-cimetidine, as described above.[57] H_1 receptors are distributed mainly on the endothelial cells of the collecting venules, and H_2 receptors are chiefly present both on the parietal cells and on the collecting venules (Fig. 4-19A–C).

The presence of both H_1 and H_2 receptors on the collecting venules and their capillaries implies that direct interaction of both receptors may regulate the gastric mucosal microcirculation.[57] In particular, H_2 receptors located on the collecting venules and capillaries would be involved in the regulation of vascular permeability in the mucosal microcirculatory system. This is supported by evidence that H_2 receptors may regulate capillary permeability, whereas H_1 receptors may control arteriolar dilatation.[58] Increased microvascular permeability induced by histamine in the gastric mucosa is one of the factors causing a variety of vasomotor disturbances in the mucosal microcirculatory system, leading to the impairment of mucosal defensive mechanisms. Histamine is released from mast cells and enterochromaffin-like

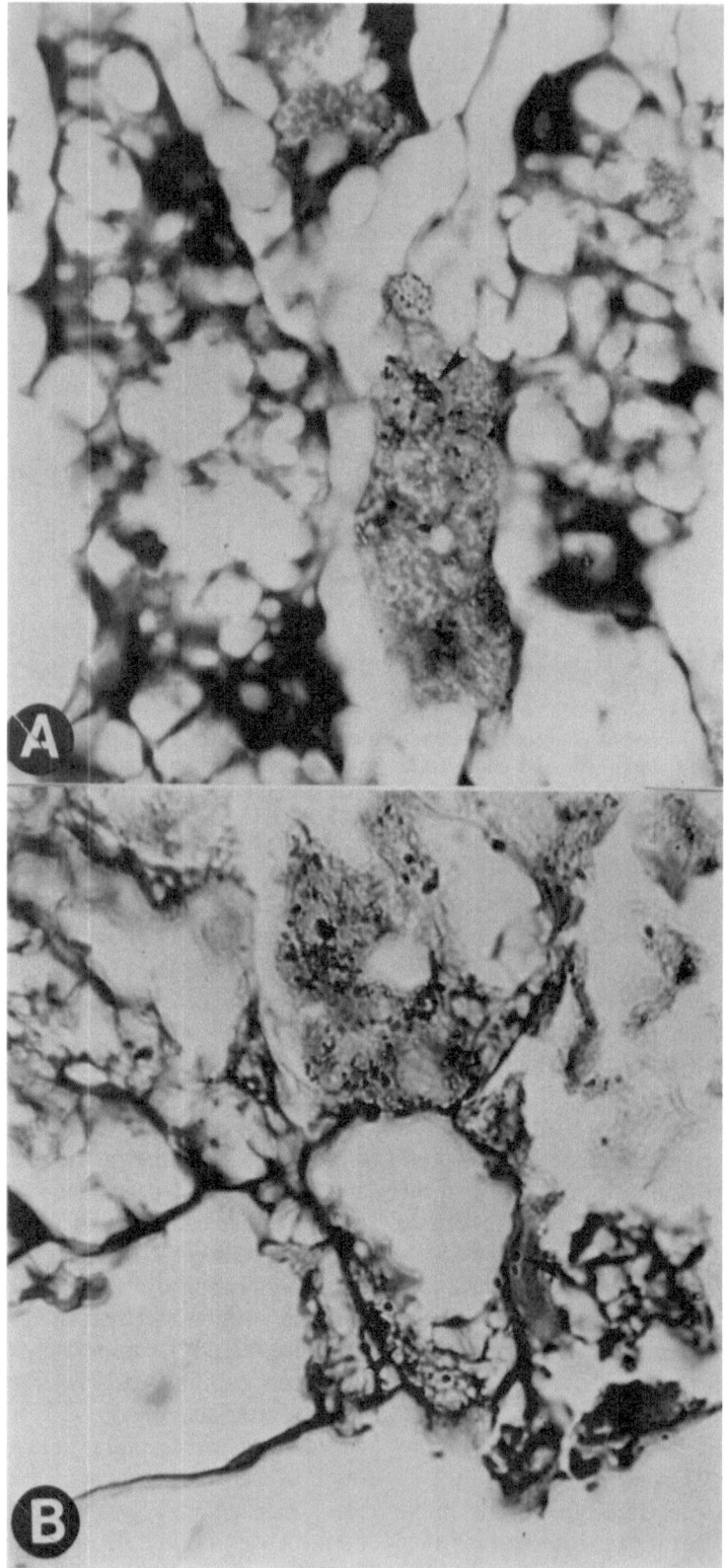

Fig. 4-18. Light microscopic radioautographs of the ^{125}I-VIP binding sites in the gastric mucosa. (a) In the middle portion of the gastric mucosa, the grains are mainly found on the parietal cells (arrowhead). $\times 2,000$. (b) In the basal portion of the gastric mucosa the grains are found on the smooth muscle cells of the arterioles (arrowheads). $\times 200$.

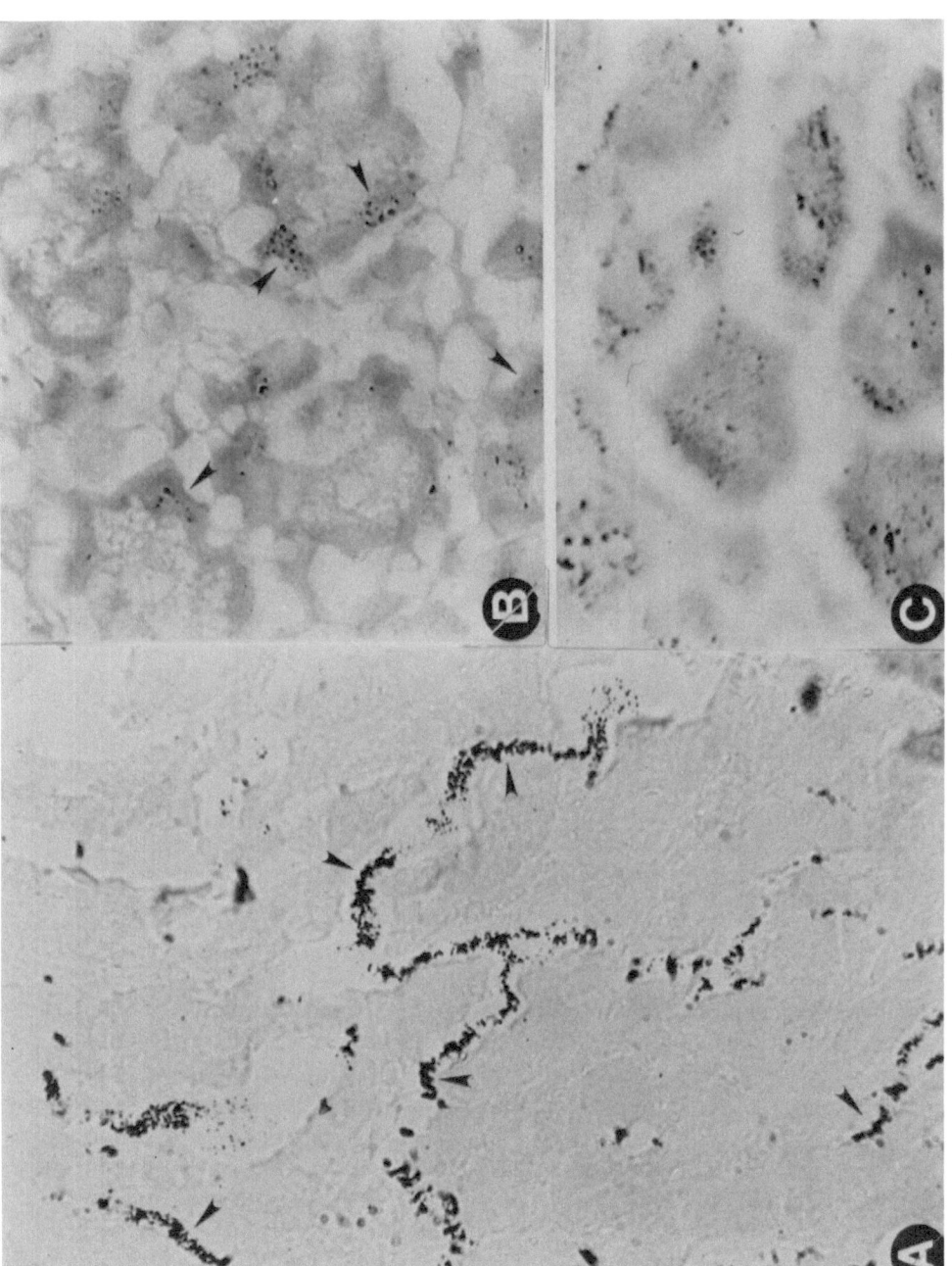

Fig. 4-19. Light microscopic radioautographs showing the H_1 and H_2 receptor antagonists in the gastric mucosa. (a) The H_1 receptor antagonist, ^{3}H-pyrilamine, is binding to the endothelial cells of the true capillaries and the collecting venules (arrowheads). ×2,000. (b) The H_2 receptor antagonist, ^{3}H-cimetidine, is binding to the parietal cells in the middle portion of the gastric mucosa (arrowheads). ×2,000. (c) ^{3}H-cimetidine is also binding to the endothelial cells of the collecting venule and true capillaries. ×2,000.

DISTRIBUTION OF AUTONOMIC NERVES AND THEIR RECEPTORS

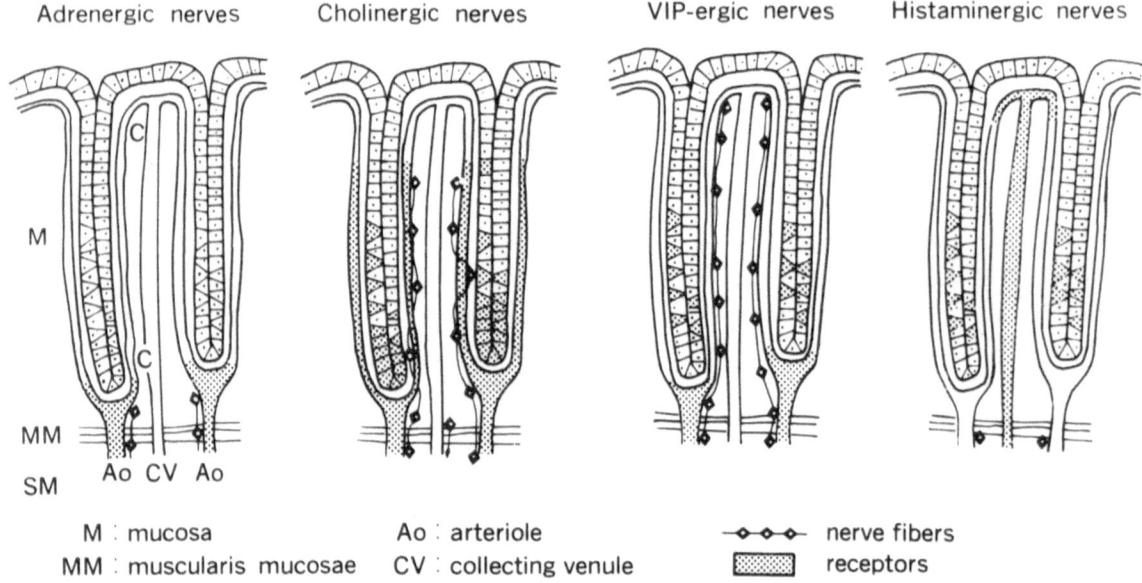

Adrenergic nerves   Cholinergic nerves   VIP-ergic nerves   Histaminergic nerves

M : mucosa   Ao : arteriole   ⬦–⬦–⬦ nerve fibers
MM : muscularis mucosae   CV : collecting venule   ▦▦▦   receptors
SM : submucosa   C : capillary

Fig. 4-20. Schematic illustration of adrenergic, cholinergic, VIP-ergic and histaminergic innervation of the gastric mucosa in the rat. The dotted area denotes the localization of adrenaline α-receptors, muscarinic acetylcholine receptors, VIP receptors or histamine receptors on the effector cells and shows the areas innervated by each type of aminergic nerve fibers.

cells, and possibly from histamine-containing nerves in the gastric wall. Histamine release from mast cells is partly enhanced by cholinergic stimulation.

SUMMARY

Adrenergic, cholinergic, VIP-ergic, and histaminergic innervation of the gastric mucosa in the rat is schematically illustrated in Fig. 4-20. Adrenergic α-receptors, muscarinic acetylcholine receptors and VIP receptors are present on the mucosal effector cells in close vicinity of the autonomic peripheral nerves containing respectively each neurotransmitter noradrenaline, acetylcholine, and VIP. The distribution of cholinergic nerve fibers is similar to that of VIP-ergic nerve fibers, extending up to the upper portion of the mucosa and innervating the mucosal microvessels and epithelial cells such as parietal cells. Cholinergic and VIP-ergic innervation is predominant throughout the mucosa. The adrenergic nerve fibers extend to the basal portion of the mucosa partly in coexistence with cholinergic nerve fibers, also innervating the mucosal microvessels and possibly the epithelial cells. Dopamine would contribute to the opening of arteriovenous anastomoses, just above the muscularis mucosae. Histamine H_2 receptors are located mainly in the upper and middle portions of the gastric mucosa, while histaminergic nerve fibers are localized in the submucosa, suggesting that histaminergic fibers may not be directly involved in the regulation of a variety of gastric mucosal functions.

Abnormalities of the above mentioned characteristic innervation of the gastric mucosa are considered to play an important role in impairments of mucosal microcirculation and epithelial cell functions, leading to ulcer formation.

ACKNOWLEDGMENTS

The present study was supported by the Grant-in-Aid for Scientific Research of the Ministry of Education, Science, and Culture in the year of 1983 (#58370024) and 1984 (#59370025).

REFERENCES

1. Cushing H.: Peptic ulcers and the interbrain. Surg Gynecol Obstet, 55:1–34, 1932
2. Bergamann G.: Das spasmogene Ulcus Pepticum. Münch. Med. Wochenschr., 60:169–174, 1913
3. Sun D.C.H.: Etiology and pathology of peptic ulcer, In: Gastroenterology Vol 1 Edited by H.C. Bockus, Ed. W.B. Saunders Co, Philadelphia, pp 579–610, 1974
4. Tsuchiya M., Oda M., Nakamura M., Watanabe N. and Ohya Y.: Gastric mucosal microcirculation and its disturbances—with special reference to gastric ulcerogenesis; In: Defence Mechanism of Gastrointestinal Mucosa. Mucosal Blood Flow. Proceedings of the 2nd Symposium Defence Mechanism of Gastrointestinal Mucosa, March, 1981, Kyoto, Japan. Ed. K. Kawai. Iryokenkyushinsha, Kyoto, pp 93–99, 1981
5. Syay H.: Stress and gastric secretion. Gastroenterology, 26:316–319, 1954
6. Hollander F.: The two-component mucous barrier. Its activity in protecting the gastroduodenal mucosa against peptic ulceration. Arch Intern Med, 93:107–120, 1954
7. Oda M., Nakamura M., Watanabe N., Nagata H. and Tsuchiya M.: Microcirculatory changes in the restraint-induced gastric ulcer formation of the rat—a vital and electron microscopic study. In: Advances in Experimental Ulcer. Proceedings of the 4th International Conference for Experimental Ulcer, October 18–19, 1980, Tokyo, Japan. Eds. S. Umehara and H. Ito. Tokyo Medical College, Tokyo, pp 226–236, 1982
8. Davenport H.W.: Gastric mucosal injury by fatty and acetylsalicylic acids. Gastroenterology, 46:245–253, 1964
9. Lanciault G. and Jacobson E.D.: Progress in gastroenterology. Gastroenterology, 71:851–873, 1976
10. Nakamura M., Watanabe N., Tsukada N., Oda M. and Tsuchiya M.: Demonstration of the adrenergic nerves in the rat gastric mucosa—a histofluorescence and electron microscopic study in comparison with the distribution of the cholinergic nerves. Okajima's Folia Anat Jpn, 59:65–86, 1982
11. Van-Driel C. and Drukker J.: A contribution study of the architecture of the autonomic nervous system of the digestive tract of the rat. J Neural Trans, 34:301–320, 1973
12. Gabella G.: Innervation of the gastrointestinal tract. Int Rev Cytol, 59:129–193, 1979
13. Llewellyn-Smith I.J., Furness J.B., Wilson A.J. and Costa M.: Organization and fine structure of enteric ganglia. In: Autonomic Ganglia. Ed. L-G. Elvin. John Wiley & Sons, Chinchester, pp 145–182, 1983
14. Kyösola K., Veijola L. and Rechardt L.: Cholinergic innervation of the gastric wall of the cat. Histochemistry, 44:23–30, 1975
15. Costa M. and Gabella G.: Adrenergic innervation of the alimentary canal. Z. Zellforsch., 122:357–377, 1971
16 Pearse A.G.E. and Polak J.M.: Immunocytochemical localization of substance P in mammalian intestine. Histochem., 41:373–375, 1975
17. Lundberg J.M., Hökfelt T., Schultzberg M., Uvnas-Wallensten K., Kohler C. and Said S.I.: Occurrence of vasoactive intestinal polypeptide (VIP)-like immunoreactivity in certain cholinergic neurons of the cat: evidence from combined immunohistochemistry and acetylcholinesterase staining. Neuroscience, 4:1539–1559, 1979
18. Lundberg J.M.: Evidence for coexistence of vasoactive intestinal polypeptide (VIP) and acetylcholine in neurons of cat exocrine glands: Morphological, biochemical and functional study. Acta Physiol Scand (suppl), 496:1–57, 1981
19. Iwanaga T.: Gastrin-releasing peptide (GRP)/bombesin-like immunoreactivity in the neurons and paraneurons of the gut and lung. Biomed Res 4:93–104, 1983
20. Lundberg J.M. and Hökfelt T.: Coexistence of peptides and classical neurotransmitters. Trends in Neurosci., 6:325–333, 1983
21. Panula P., Kaartinen M., Macklin M. and Costa E.: Histamine-containing peripheral neuronal and endocrine systems. J Histochem Cytochem, 33:933–941, 1985
22. Gershon M.D., Sherman D., Erde S.M. and Rothman T.P.: Serotonergic neurons and mammalian gut, In: Functional Disorders of the Digestive Tract, Ed. W.Y. Chey. Raven Press, New York, pp 59–77, 1983
23. Lackovic Z. and Relja M.: Evidence of a widely distributed peripheral dopaminergic system. Fed Proc., 42:3000–3004, 1983
24. Burnstock G.: Purinergic nerves. Pharmacol Rev, 24:509–581, 1972
25. Bell C.: Fine structural localization of acetylcholinesterase at a cholinergic vasodilator nerve-arterial smooth muscle synapse. Circ. Res., 24:61–70, 1969
26. Karnovsky M.J. and Roots L.: A direct coloring thiocholine method for cholinesterases. J Histochem Cytochem, 12:219–221, 1964
27. Nakamura M.: Studies of the cholinergic innervation in the rat fundic mucosa—with special reference to the gastric mucosal microcirculation. Keio Igaku, 63:13–28, 1986 (in Japanese)
28. Nakamura M., Watanabe N., Oda M., and Tsuchiya M.: Histochemical, fluorescence and electron microscopic studies on the distribution of autonomic nerve endings in the gastric mucosa. The Autonomic Nervous System, 17:338–345, 1980 (in Japanese)
29. Bunge R., Johnson M. and Rosse C.D.: Nature and nurture of the autonomic neuron. Science, 199:1409–1416, 1978
30. Nakamura M., Oda M., Yonei Y., Komatsu H., Tsukada N., Watanabe N. and Tsuchiya M.: Histochemical and electron microscopic cytochemical studies on the autonomic innervation of the gastric mucosa in

rats—embryological differentiation of the parietal cell and acetylcholinesterase activity. The Autonomic Nervous System, 21:386–398, 1984 (in Japanese)

31. Chamley J.H. and Campbell G.R.: Trophic influence of sympathetic and cyclic AMP on differentiation and proliferation of isolated smooth muscle cell in culture. Cell Tissue Res., 208:1–19, 1980

32. Nakamura M., Oda M., Watanabe N., Ohya Y., Sekizuka E., Tsukada N., Yonei Y., Komatsu H. and Tsuchiya M.: Dynamic aspects of the gastric mucosal microcirculation in the healthy and stress condition—with special reference to the autonomic nervous control, in: Intravital Observation of Organ Microcirculation. Proceedings of the Tokyo Symposium, June 18, 1983. Eds. Tsuchiya M., Wayland H., Oda M. and Okazaki I.. Excerpta Medica, Amsterdam pp 65–97, 1983

33. Oda M., Nakamura M., Watanabe N., Tsukada N., Yonei Y., Komatsu H., Ohya Y., Sekizuka E. and Tsuchiya M.: Dual action of the parasympathetic nerve in the gastric mucosa—significance of its overactivity in the pathogenesis of gastric ulcer, In: Gastrointestinal Function. Regulation and Disturbances of Gastrointestinal Function, September 18, 1982, Tokyo, Japan. Eds. Kasuya Y., Tsuchiya M., Nagao F. and Matsuo Y. Amsterdam Excerpta Medica, pp 145–173, 1983

34. Oda M., Nakamura M., Watanabe N., Tsukada N., Ohya Y., Sekizuka E. and Tsuchiya M.: Autonomic nerve regulation of gastric mucosal microcirculation—with special reference to the pathogenesis of stress-induced ulcer, In: Basic Aspects of Microcirculation. Proceedings of Tokyo International Symposium on Microcirculation, July 26, 1981, Tokyo, Japan. Eds. Tsuchiya M., Oda M., and Asano M. Amsterdam Excerpta Medica, pp 209–229, 1982

35. Nagata T., Nawa T. and Yokota S.: A new technique for electron microscopic drymounting radioautography of soluble compounds. Histochemie, 18:241–249, 1969

36. Nakamura M., Oda M., Yonei Y., Tsukada N., Watanabe N., Komatsu H. and Tsuchiya M.: Demonstration of the localization of muscarinic acetylcholine receptors in the gastric mucosa—light and electron microscopic autoradiographic studies using ^{3}H-quinuclidinyl benzilate. Acta Histochem Cytochem, 17:297–309, 1984

37. Nakamura M., Oda M., Yonei Y., Tsukada N., Komatsu H. and Tsuchiya M.: Muscarinic acetylcholine receptors in rat gastric mucosa—a radioautographic study using a potent muscarinic antagonist, ^{3}H-pirenzepine. Histochemistry, 83:479–487, 1985

38. Holm-Rutili L. and Öbrink K.J.: Rat gastric mucosal microcirculation in vivo. Am J Physiol, 248:G741–746, 1985

39. Guth P.H. and Smith E.: Neural control of gastric mucosal blood flow in the rat. Gastroenterology, 69:935–940, 1975

40. Ajelis V., Björklund A., Falck B., Lindvall O., Loren J. and Walles B.: Application of the aluminium formaldehyde (ALFA) histofluorescence method for demonstration of peripheral stores of catecholamines and indolamines in freeze-dried paraffin-embedded tissue, cryostat sections and whole-mounts. Histochemistry, 65:1–15, 1979

41. Falck B. and Hillarp N.: Fluorescence of catecholamine and related compounds condensed with formaldehyde. Histochem Cytochem, 10:348–354, 1973

42. Furness J.B.: The adrenergic innervation of the vessels supplying and draining the gastrointestinal tract. Z. Zellforsch., 113:67–82, 1971

43. Read J. and Burnstock G.: Competitive histochemical studies of adrenergic nerves in the enteric plexuses of vertebrate large intestine. Comp. Biochem. Physiol., 27:505–517, 1968

44. Nakamura M., Ohya Y., Morishita T. and Oda M.: The structure of the gastric mucosal microcirculatory system and its regulatory mechanism—with special reference to autonomic nervous function. J Japanese College of Angiology, 24:11–18, 1984

45. Bell C., Lang W.J. and Laska F.: Dopamine-cotaining axons supplying the arteriovenous anastomosis of the canine paw pad. J Neurochem, 31:1329–1333, 1978

46. Hase T. and Moss B.J.: Microvascular changes of gastric mucosa in the development of stress ulcer in rats. Gastroenterology, 65:224–234, 1973

47. Kitajima M., Wolfe R.R., Trelftadt R.L., Allsop J.R. and Burk J.F.: Gastric mucosal lesion after burn injury: Relationship to H^+-back diffusion and the microcirculation. J Trauma, 18:644–650, 1978

48. Guth P.H. and Rosenberg A.: In vivo microscopy of the gastric microcirculation. Am J Dig Dis, 17:391–398, 1972

49. Guth P.H.: In vivo microscopy of the gastric microcirculation: anatomical and physiological findings, In: Basic Aspects of Microcirculation. Proceedings of Tokyo International Symposium on Microcirculation, July 26, 1981, Tokyo, Japan. Eds. M Tsuchiya, Oda M. and Asano M. Excerpta Medica, Amsterdam pp 209–229, 1982

50. Szurszewski J.H. and Weems W.A.: A study of peripheral input to and its control by postganglionic neurones of the inferior mesenteric ganglion. J Physiol, 256:541–556, 1976

51. Schwartz J.C., Pollard H. and Quach T.T.: Histamine as a neurotransmitter in mammalian brain. J Neurochem, 35:26–33, 1980

52. Ash A.S. and Schild H.O.: Receptors mediating some actions of histamine. Br J Pharmacol Chemother, 27:427–439, 1966

53. Blach J.W., Duncan W.A.M., Durant C.J., Ganellin C.R. and Parsons E.M.: Definition and antagonism of histamine H_2-receptors. Nature, 236:385–390, 1972

54. Soll A.H.: The interaction of histamine with gastrin and carbamylcholine on oxygen uptake by isolated mammalian parietal cells. J Clin Invest, 61:381–389, 1978

55. Guth P.H., Smith E. and Moler T.: H_1 and H_2 receptors in rat gastric submucosal arterioles. Microvasc Res, 19:320–328, 1980

56. Curwain B.P., Holton P. and Spencer J.: Evidence that the inhibitory effect of burimamide on gastric secretion is not due to decreased gastric mucosal blood flow. J Physiol, 230:33p–34p, 1973

57. Nakamura M., Oda M., Yonei Y., Kaneko K., Komatsu H., Tsukada N., Tsuchiya M. and Fujishiro Y.: Radioautographic demonstration of localization of histamine H_1 and H_2 receptors in the gastric mucosa. In: Annual report 1985 Japanese Society for Microcirculation. Eds. Tsuchiya M., Asano M., Oda M. and Okazaki I. Amsterdam Excerpta Medica, pp 217–223, 1985

58. Mortillaro N.A., Granger D.N. and Kvietys P.R.: Effects of histamine and histamine antagonists on intestinal capillary permeability. Am J Physiol 240:381–386, 1981

5

Non-Hodgkin's Lymphomas of the
Gastrointestinal Tract:
A Review with Special Reference to the
Gut-associated Lymphoid Tissue

P. van der Valk M.D, Ph.D
J. Lindeman M.D, Ph.D
C.J.L.M. Meijer M.D, Ph.D

Non-Hodgkin's lymphomas (NHL) are intriguing tumors for several reasons. First, they show a marked variety of histological pictures. Second, though most common in the lymphoid tissues, they can be found in any tissue or organ of the body; and third, they are related to the immune system, as lymphocytes are the cells composing that system. Our knowledge concerning NHL has increased enormously in the last 20 years, due largely to technical advances, such as immunohistochemistry with monoclonal antibodies and electron microscopy. Basic to our present insights is the realization that normal lymphocyte physiology can be seen mirrored in NHL. Malignant lymphoid cells resemble normal lymphocytes in some state of their development, both morphologically and functionally. As lymphocytes are engaged in reactions in the immune response and malignant lymphoid cells mimic normal lymphocytes in morphology and behavior, NHL can be regarded as neoplastic counterparts of the immune reactions. This concept[1,2,3,4] is the basis of proper understanding of NHL and is re-

flected in the classification schemes according to Lukes & Collins[2] and Kiel.[3]

This concept is based largely on knowledge of NHL of the (peripheral) lymph nodes. The lymphoid tissue, however, is not confined to the lymph nodes: accumulations are found as watchdogs against antigenic attacks along the epithelia of the gut (gut-associated lymphoid tissue (GALT)) with concentrations in the terminal ileum and appendix,[5] of the bronchi (bronchus-associated lymphoid tissue or BALT),[6] of the genital tract,[7] and some foregut-related appendages, such as thyroid[8] and salivary glands.[9] As these systems have features in common, morphologically[6] and functionally,[10] the term mucosa-associated lymphoid tissue (MALT) was introduced.[11] Here we shall stick to the term GALT as we are concerned with gastrointestinal lymphoid tissue only.

The GALT and the peripheral lymph nodes differ in some essential points. Most important of these is that the GALT acts to prevent extensive reactions against antigens and generally has a dampening influence immunologically,[12] whereas in the lymph nodes, reactions against antigens are meant to augment immune responses. The goal of this "tolerance" for some antigens is to prevent undue reactions against molecules in the gastrointestinal lumen. This is partly achieved by covering these molecules with IgA.[13]

This difference in function between GALT and peripheral lymph nodes is achieved, among others, through a difference in homing of lymphocyte subsets to GALT. Thus, B-cells preferentially home to the GALT, whereas T-lymphocytes tend to favor the peripheral lymph nodes.[14] Of the B-cells, IgA carrying lymphocytes are found in much higher numbers in the GALT compared to the peripheral nodes. In the T-lymphocytes there appear to be subsets preferentially localizing in the GALT,[15] which of course may cause differences in function.[16] The peculiar distribution of suppressor T-cells and helper T-cells found in the GALT, with intraepithelial lymphocytes being of suppressor/cytotoxic phenotype and lamina propria lymphocytes mainly of helper/inducer phenotype[12,17] may explain the tendency towards tolerance innate to the GALT.

Thus, the GALT has its own cellular pool and physiology. In short, cells are brought in contact with antigen in the bowel wall. Here, the epithelium may play a role as GALT localizations are covered by a specialized epithelium containing cells with microfolds on their luminal surface, the so-called M-cells.[5] After antigenic contact B-cells migrate to the mesenteric lymph nodes and via the thoracic duct and the peripheral blood, back to the GALT. During this journey they differentiate towards plasma cells. These plasma cells, finally, are found in the GALT in the lamina propria, while most of their precursors are not, at least under normal conditions. These precursors (e.g., the follicle center cell phase) can be found in other (earlier) locations such as the mesenteric lymph nodes or that part of the bowel wall where contact with the antigen takes place.[5]

Since NHL from peripheral lymph nodes mimic the normal behavior of peripheral lymph node cells, NHL arising in the GALT can be expected to do the same. Therefore, in discussing gastrointestinal NHL, the concept of the GALT has to be considered. Not all GI-tract NHL arise in the GALT, however. According to the GALT concept, the following subdivision can be made:

I. *Primary GI-NHL.* They arise in the GALT and may be confined to the GALT and regional lymph nodes (Ia) or show dissemination beyond the regional lymph nodes (Ib).
II. *Secondary GI-NHL,* in which the GI tract involvement is secondary to wide dissemination.

Approximately 40% would fall into category Ia, primary GI-NHL restricted to GALT,[18] whereas a similar percentage is reported for primary GI-NHL with dissemination beyond the GALT.[19]

Involvement of the GI tract secondary to a "peripheral" NHL is recognized in ± 20% of all NHL,[19] but at autopsy higher percentages are found, ranging from 45–70%.[18,19]

In the next paragraphs we will discuss incidence and localization of GI-NHL. In the part on pathology the significant NHL categories are considered. The importance of marker studies in diagnosis and classification is stressed. Next, prognosis, prognostic factors and implications for staging procedures and treatment are discussed, and finally some remarks on therapy will be made. Where possible reference shall be made to the above-mentioned categories (Ia and b and II).

INCIDENCE

Extranodal NHL are not uncommon: 20–40% arise outside the lymph nodes.[20,21] From these primary extranodal localizations, the GI tract is involved most frequently, followed by Waldeyer's ring, skin, the oribital region, salivary glands, bone, and lungs.[20] Of all NHL 4–10% are primarily located somewhere along the gastrointestinal tract,[20,22,23] while 1–4% of all GI tumors are NHL. That involvement of the GI tract in NHL, regardless of the initial localization, is fairly common was mentioned before (20% of all NHL recognized during life and 45–70% at autopsy).

CLINICAL DATA

GI tract NHL show no clear age predilection and are found twice more often in men than in women. They usually cause symptoms, such as abdominal pain or discomfort, bleeding with hematemesis or melena, obstruction, intussusception, perforation with or without peritonitis, and/or general symptoms such as fever, weakness, weight loss, etc.[18] Obstruction is seen most frequently in small intestine localizations. Intussusceptions are especially frequent in ileocecal localizations and are thus seen most frequently in children.[22,24] Perforation is a dreaded complication; it is reported in 1–28% of all cases.[22]

LOCALIZATION

Though accounts tend to vary, the majority of studies show the stomach to be involved most often. Small intestine follows closely. Some studies list the ileocecal region separately. It is involved in approximately 10% of the cases, as is the large intestine. Table 5-1 lists the data of several studies from the literature, as well as the data from our material.

In children most GI tract NHL are located in the ileocecal region.[22] Most studies mentioned concern primary GI-NHL, which makes it likely that these tumors originated in the GALT. However, distinguishing between a GALT lymphoma with extensive dissemination (Ib) and a nodal NHL with involvement of the GI tract (II) is not always possible. Though likely, it is not absolutely certain that GALT-NHL (group I) follow the pattern of localization outlined above. Reports on six GALT-NHL mention the stomach (5×) and the small intestine (1×) as localizations.[25,26,27]

TABLE 5-1

Localization of NHL in GI Tract (in percentages).

Reference	n	Stomach	SI	ICR	LI
Lewin et al.[22]	117	41	32	12	9
Isaacson et al.[34]	66	36	49	12	3
Saraga et al.[28]	66	55	30	NS	15
Weingrad et al.[23]	104	73	14	NS	13
Filippa et al., 1983[31]	60	75	7	NS	18
Grody et al.[30]	25	68	20	NS	12
Our material	51	27	17	NS	7

n = number of patients   SI = small intestine
LI = large intestine   ICR = ileocecal region
NS = not stated

PATHOLOGY

Macroscopy

There are no specific macroscopic features. Ulceration is fairly common,[22] but is seen in nonmalignant lesions as well.[28] A diffuse thickening of the bowel wall is found in roughly a quarter of the cases and is very suspicious for lymphoma. More commonly, however, lymphomas produce a discrete mass, in some cases polypoid.[28]

Microscopy

Microscopically, most GI tract-NHL are large-cell lymphomas; there is a predominance of diffuse over follicular NHL.[19,22,28–30] Here we will discuss several categories of NHL separately:

B-cell NHL: Follicle Center Cell Lymphomas (FCC)

True follicular NHL in the GI tract are less common, with percentages reported varying from 2.7–10%.[18,19,28–30]

Among all diffuse GI-NHL, there is a predominance of FCC.[23,30–33] Isaacson et al[34] report an FCC origin for all their lymphoid GI-

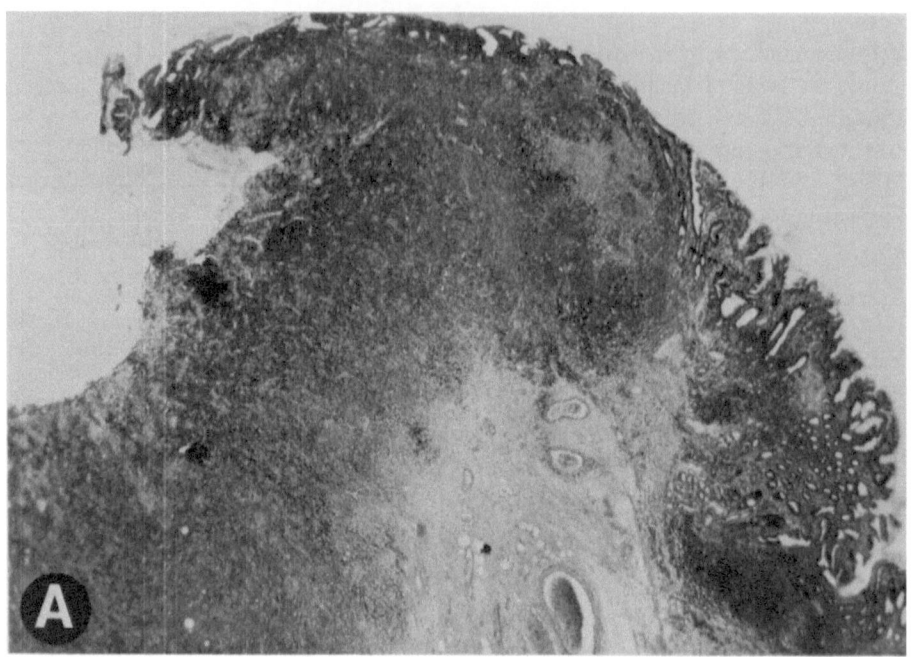

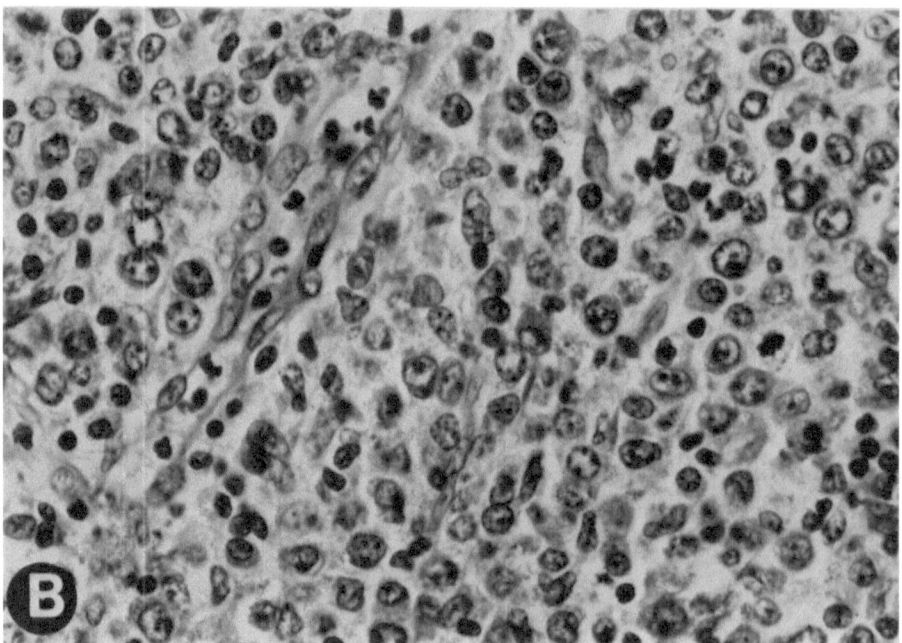

Fig. 5-1. Centroblastic lymphoma localized in the antrum of the stomach. (a) Low power view of the tumor. (HE stain ×25). (b) Detail of the tumor cells. (HE stain ×400). (c) Nearly all neoplastic cells stain with a monoclonal antibody against κ light chain immunoglobulin.

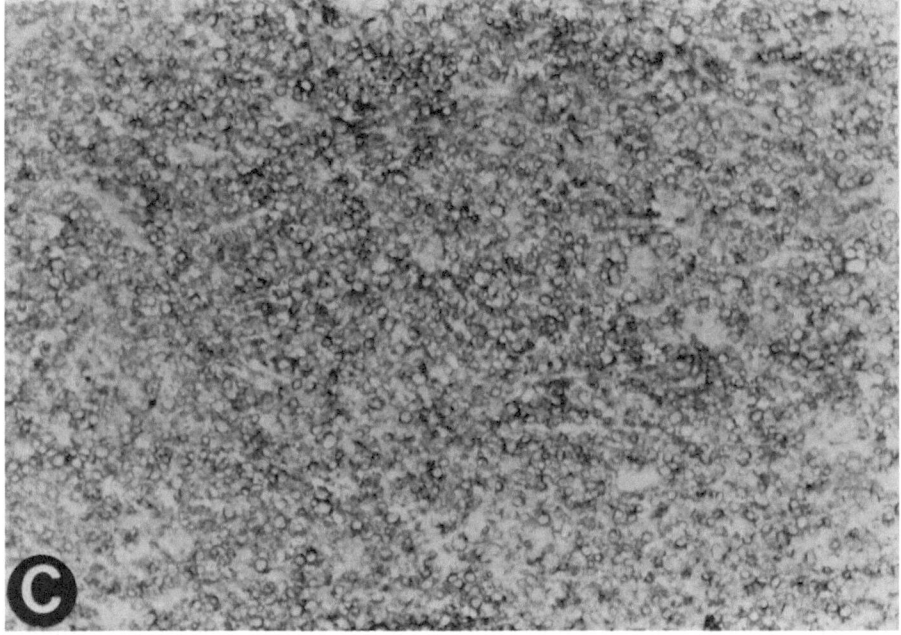

Fig. 5-1. *(continued)*

NHL. Most common are the *large non-cleaved* or *centroblastic NHL* (Fig. 5-1). They consist predominantly of large cells with large, vesicular nuclei, 1–3 marginal nucleoli, and little cytoplasm. Usually there is some mixture with cells having single and central nucleoli and ample cytoplasm. (i.e., immunoblast-like cells). If this admixture is pronounced and the number of immunoblasts does not exceed the number of centroblasts, the term polymorphic centroblastic lymphoma is used.

Futhermore, there are always large cells with cleaved nuclei present. Small, dark, and angular/cleaved cells or centrocytes can be seen in varying numbers, usually scant. In centroblastic NHL, macrophages are usually present in high numbers (10–15%).[35] Occasionally, these large cell FCC can resemble carcinomas.

Centroblastic/centrocytic lymphomas are often diffuse, though it is not uncommon to find follicular areas. These areas are difficult to differentiate from lymphoid hyperplasia,[28,36] even when applying strict morphological criteria. In resection specimens the diffuse areas will provide the important clue to diagnosis of malignancy, but in a small biopsy specimen these areas may be missing. Marker studies, especially demonstration of monoclonality by immunoglobulin light chain typing, are essential here, as they are in all NHL diagnostics.

Centrocytic lymphomas are diffuse. They can be present in a very typical way: as multiple polypoid lesions along large parts of the GI tract.[24] These NHL consist entirely of small cells with angular or cleaved nuclei with moderately dense chromatin and scanty cytoplasm. They show a relative high tendency to become leukemic.

B-cell NHL: B-immunoblastic NHL (B-IB)

B-IB are found somewhat less frequently than centroblastic NHL, but this may vary per localization: Otto et al.[37] report a predominance of B-IB in their *intestinal* large-cell lymphomas. B-IB tends to involve the entire bowel wall. It destroys the muscularis, producing fissures that explain the high rate of perforation in these tumors.[24] The microscopic picture of this NHL is typical. The cells are large, with large nuclei. There is usually one large (para)central nucleolus, though more nucleoli are occasionally seen. The cytoplasm is ample and basophilic. There is some differentiation to plasma cell morphology. Admixed small cells have round nuclei. Macrophages can be numerous.

B-Cell NHL: (Lympho)plasmacytoid NHL

Plasmacytomas show no preference for a certain site,[22,38,39] but lymphoplasmacytoid NHL are somewhat more prevalent in the small intestine.[28,37] Plasmacytomas are usually easily recognized, however, atypical cases occur. Plasmacytomas where the cells have signet ring cell morphology have been described.[27,40] We have seen a plasmacytoma where the nuclei were deformed by immunoglobulin-containing vacuoles in the cytoplasm. The nuclei were angular and/or dented and the cells did not resemble plasma cells at all. Such cases can cause diagnostic problems and immunohistochemistry is necessary.

Lymphoplasmacytoid NHL consists of lymphocytes with moderate amounts of cytoplasm, and round to slightly irregular nuclei that show a tendency to a spoke-wheel pattern of chromatin. Plasma cells can be seen, and sometimes a few immunoblasts can be found. In this context mention must be made of the so called *"Mediterranean lymphoma,"* or *immunoproliferative small intestine disease (IPSID)* as it has come to be called. This is a clinicopathologic entity; clinical features are chronic diarrhea, weight loss, and abdominal pain.[41,42] Furthermore, a number of these patients have an abnormal IgA molecule in their serum, which can also be found in the cells of the concomitant mucosal infiltrate in the small intestine,[43] and that has led to the name α-chain disease. However, not all patients with IPSID have α-chain disease.[44] Pathologically there are two variants of IPSID. One is the classical diffuse (lympho)plasmacytoid infiltration of the duodenal and/or jejunal mucosa, associated with α-chain disease.

Transformation of this variant into B-immunoblastic lymphomas is frequently found in this setting. In the other there is a follicular lymphoid hyperplasia. Lymphomas developing in this setting are frequently of the undifferentiated type (Rappaport classification).[45] These two types are probably both a reflection of GALT physiology. There is an initial phase (FCC reaction, not necessarily taking place at the site of the lymphoplasmacytoid infiltrate), and a terminal lymphoplasmacytoid phase that develops in the end phase of plasmacytic differentiation. Both phases can take place in separate portions of the gut, but not necessarily so. Under sufficient antigenic pressure, follicles (the initial phase of the reaction) can arise anywhere in the GI tract. Support for this theory is found in marker studies. They have identified an identical immunophenotype on cells of both phases (initial FCC phase, and terminal lymphoplasmacytoid phase) of a lymphoma in a single patient.[46] Thus, IPSID appears to be an example of a GALT-NHL. Classification of a lymphoma with both phases represented in the histology is sometimes difficult. They can best be classified as a pleomorphic immunocytoma. An FCC origin for these lymphomas in the lymph nodes (similar to the GALT situation), was suggested earlier.[35,47]

B-Cell: B Lymphoblastic NHL (Burkitt or Non-Burkitt Type)

These lymphomas show a characteristic clinicopathologic picture. They are most frequent in children, with boys predominating (M:F = 2:1). The patients often have an acute obstruction, due to intussusception in the ileocecal region where these lymphomas are found most frequently, though not exclusively.[22,37] In fact a clinical presentation like that in a child is highly suggestive for lymphoblastic NHL. Microscopically, the tumor seems to spare the muscularis even when it is disseminated beyond the bowel. Another striking feature is the reluctance to invade the regional lymph nodes. Lymph nodes can be seen, completely encased by tumor, but without infiltration of the lymph node itself.[24] Besides their locally invasive character that leads to fixation of the bowel to adjacent structures, there is a clear tendency to dissemination[48] involving extranodal localizations such as the kidney, the gut, pleura, and central nervous system.[24,48]

The histology of these NHL is monotonous (Fig. 5-2). It is a uniform proliferation of medium-sized cells, with little cytoplasm and some degree of nuclear polymorphism. In cytology the vacuolated aspect of the cytoplasm is especially well appreciated. In many, especially Burkitt-type cases, the abundance of admixed macrophages causes the so-called "starry sky" pattern. It is striking, but not specific (centroblastic lymphomas can also show a starry sky pattern) and not invariably present in our experience.

Occasionally we have seen lymphoblastic NHL where the cells resembled small centroblasts, with 2–3 marginal, though less conspicuous nucleoli, but with the grayish, finely dispersed chromatin characteristic of lymphoblasts. The clinical course of these cases does not appear to be different from other lymphoblastic NHL, Burkitt, or non-Burkitt type.

T-Cell Lymphomas

Lymphomas of T-lymphocytes in the GI tract are very rare by all accounts, probably reflecting the preference of these cells for the peripheral lymph nodes over the GALT.[14] Grody et al.[30] reported two T-cell lymphomas among their 25 patients (8%), which is the highest number we found in the literature. Classification of T-cell lymphomas is still troublesome, even in the peripheral lymph nodes and with the scarcity of cases, this makes any statement on GI-T-cell lymphomas difficult. Of interest is the report on a T-cell NHL in the gut showing marked epitheliotropism,[49] not unlike the epidermotropism seen in mycosis fungoides. Interestingly, the tumor cells were Leu2a positive (i.e., of suppressor/cytotoxic phenotype). Since intraepithelial lymphocytes have a similar phenotype, this case underlines the similarity between normal and malignant lymphocytes. But

many more cases will have to be studied in order to obtain a clear picture of T-cell lymphomas in the GI tract.

Histiocytic Sarcomas or True Histiocytic Lymphomas

Though as an entity histiocytic sarcoma is established, its frequency among NHL is controversial. The controversy was sparked off by Isaacson et al.[34] who drew attention to this tumor in the gut and reported a frequency of 50% in their 66 primary GI-NHL. Other investigators did not find such high percentages; some even questioned the existence of histiocytic sarcoma as a primary GI-NHL.[30] Other percentages mentioned were 18 (lysozyme positive),[29] 18.4 (lysozyme and/or α_1-antitrypsin positive),[50] and 9.[51] In our experience the incidence of histiocytic sarcoma in the GI tract is not essentially different from that of the whole group of histiocytic sarcomas, (i.e. 5–10%).[52,53]

Many of these histiocytic sarcomas were associated with malabsorption states, such as celiac disease.[54,55]

After starting this controversy on incidence, Isaacson and colleagues recently published data indicating a T-cell origin for four cases previously diagnosed as malignant histiocytosis of intestine,[56] suggesting that most celiac disease-associated lymphomas are actually of T-cell origin. The reason for this sudden change was the presence of the 3A1 pan-T-cell antigen on the tumor cells and the finding of lymphoid tumors that were α_1-antitrypsin positive,[57] while α_1-antitrypsin was considered the most important marker criterion for histiocytic tumors by Isaacson et al.[34] This clearly illustrates that markers alone are not the solution to the problem. Apart from the presence of 3A1 antigen in all four neoplasms the tumor cells of three cases also showed rearrangements of genes for the β-chain of the T-cell antigen receptor. Questions concerning the specificity of this finding, however, can also arise. Little or nothing is known about gene rearrangements in macrophages/histiocytes and gene rearrangements are not 100% lineage-specific, as T-cell lym-

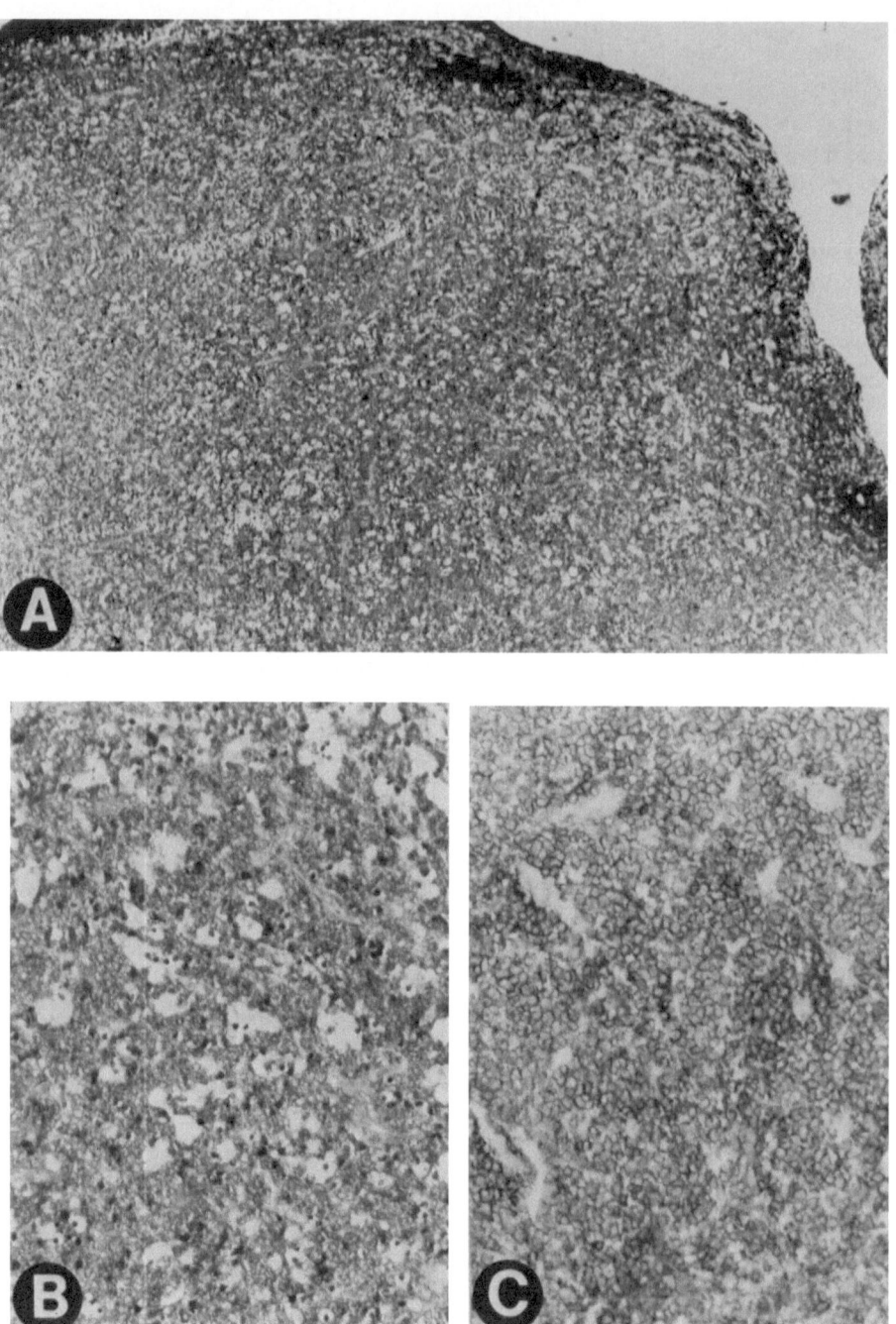

Fig. 5-2. Primary localization of lymphoblastic lymphoma, Burkitt type in the ileocoecal region of a 7 year old boy. (a) Low magnification; note starry sky appearance. (HE stain, paraffin embedding. ×25) (b) Higher magnification. Optical empty spaces are filled by nuclei of macrophages with often brushed, very pale staining cytoplasm. (×100). (c) Demonstration of the B cell nature by the pan B cell monoclonal antibody Leu 14. (d) High power view of the lymphoblastic cells. (HE stain ×400).

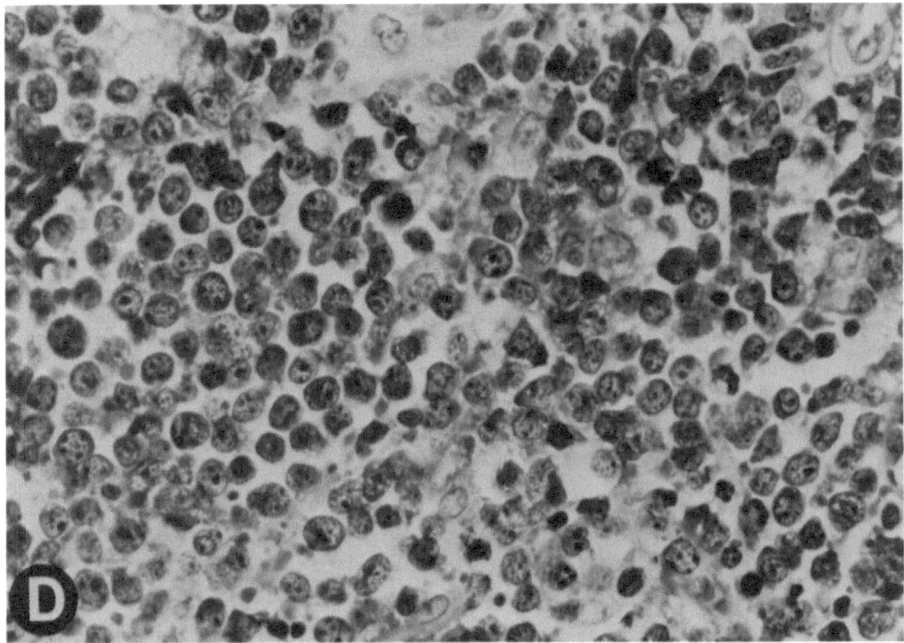

Fig. 5-2. *(continued)*

phomas have been described with immuno-globulin gene rearrangements.[58]

Though the findings of Isaacson et al.[56] are certainly suggestive, we feel that this matter is not yet settled and consistent, and that extensive marker studies (including, when possible, gene rearrangement studies) are of vital importance. As an illustration of the diversity in this field, we cite the report of Otto et al.,[37] who claim a B-cell nature for their celiac disease-associated lymphomas, since these NHL show monoclonal cytoplasmic immunoglobulins. It is not unlikely that all three possibilities (for celiac disease-associated NHL) can occur: B-cell, T-cell, and histiocytic origin.

The histology of histiocytic sarcoma has been amply described.[53] The cells are large, with large and mostly (very) irregular nuclei with conspicuous nucleoli and nuclear membranes (Fig. 5-3). Cytoplasm is ample and the cells show signs of phagocytosis. Multinucleated giant cells are virtually always present. Immunologically, lysozyme, α_1-antitrypsin and/or α_1-antichymotrypsin and nonspecific esterase and acid phosphatase can be dem-

onstrated in the cytoplasm. Furthermore, the tumor cells react with monoclonal antibodies against monocytes/histiocytes[53] and lack T-(Leu4, Leu5, 3A1,) and B-cell (Leu14, B1) markers.

THE IMPORTANCE OF MARKER STUDIES

From several of the above-mentioned facts, the crucial importance of marker studies emerges. Their role in diagnosis cannot be overestimated: the diagnosis of NHL can hinge on the use of markers.

There are some basic rules that have to be maintained in using markers:[60]

The material should be handled optimally.

Never rely on a single marker. Always use a small panel to avoid confusion because of cross-reactions.

Use markers as an *additional* technique to morphology.

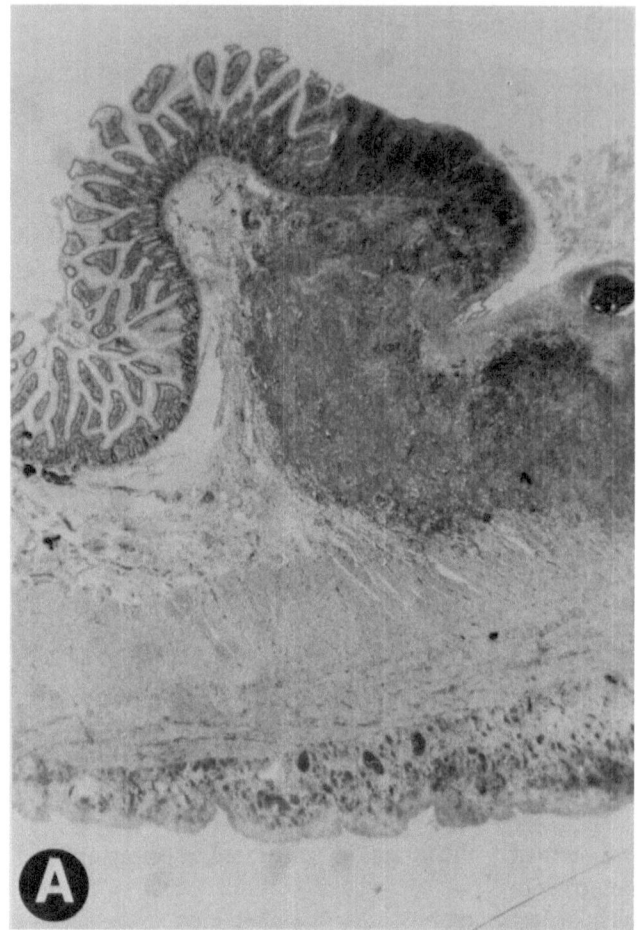

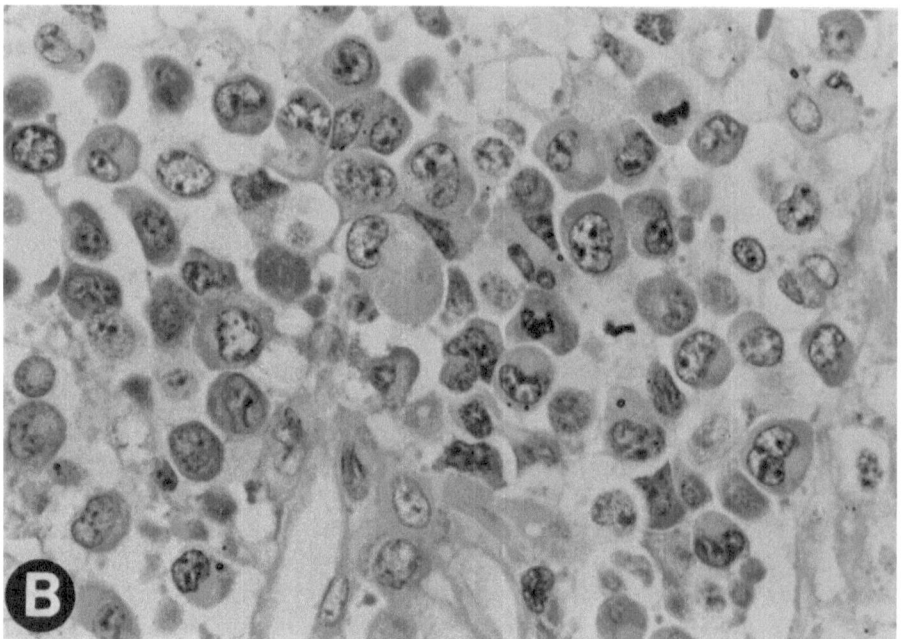

Fig. 5-3. True histiocytic lymphoma of the small intestine. (a) Low power view of the tumor. (HE stain ×25). (b)Higher power view of the neoplastic cells. Note the irregular nuclear contour and the ample cytoplasm. (Giemsa staining, glycol methacrylate embedding, ×400)

Lymphoma versus Carcinoma

Cases of gastrointestinal tumors where a differential diagnosis of carcinoma and lymphoma was considered may not be frequent, but they are by no means rare. Whether this is because carcinoma cells can look like transformed lymphocytes (especially lymphoblasts and centroblasts) or lymphocytes take on (e.g.) a signet ring cell appearance (mentioned above) is irrelevant. In some cases the distinction is impossible on clinical and morphologic grounds. Here markers are a necessity and it has been shown that a small panel of monoclonal antibodies, (i.e., 115D8 directed against the MAM6 antigen, cytokeratins; vimentin; NKI-C3, a melanoma-associated antigen and leucocyte common antigen), can effectively distinguish among carcinoma, lymphoma, sarcoma, and melanoma in cases of undifferentiated tumors.[59-61]

Lymphoma vs. Pseudolymphoma

Also mentioned above was the difficulty in distinguishing lymphomas from reactive lymphoid lesions. Though criteria have been mentioned to distinguish between benign (pseudolymphomas) and malignant lesions (NHL) in the GALT,[28,36,62] and the BALT,[63] there are an increasing number of reports stating that it is often difficult and sometimes even impossible to diagnose a lesion properly without immunological markers.[28,33,64-66] In practice distinguishing between lymphoma and pseudolymphoma is limited to follicular lesions. If monoclonality for light chain immunoglobulins is demonstrated the lesion is malignant and a lymphoma; if not the lesion is a pseudolymphoma or lymphoid hyperplasia, a term we prefer as it is more apt and less confusing than pseudolymphoma. The clinical relevance of the demonstration of monoclonality has been stressed.[67] Marker studies also are imporant for pathologists with less experience in this difficult field.

Marker studies can and should also be applied to material removed for staging procedures, as staging is very important; especially when on morphological grounds distinction between benign versus malignant processes in lymph nodes removed during staging procedures and showing multiple monotonous follicles cannot be made. Demonstration of monoclonality is crucial here.

Immunophenotyping of Lymphoma

Additionally, there is the role of markers in diagnosing the type of lymphoma (i.e., B-cell, T-cell, histiocytic). In contrast to node-based NHL, this appears to have limited prognostic value for GI-NHL (see Prognostic Factors). There are, however, only a limited number of large series of GI-NHL classified after really extensive marker studies and the relevance of such typing has yet to emerge fully. Considering the debate generated by the question of the incidence of histiocytic tumors in the GI-tract, marker studies are here to stay.

A marker panel should consist of pan-B-cell markers (B1 and/or Leu14), and anti-light chain antisera to demonstrate monotypic surface and intracytoplasmic immunoglobulin staining and pan-T-cell markers, even if T-cell lymphomas are rare in the GI-tract (e.g., monoclonal antibodies Leu4/OKT3, Leu5/OKT11 and 3A1). Thus a lymphoid origin can be established. If these markers are negative and morphology suggests a histiocytic origin, with histiocytic markers such as lysozyme, α_1-antitrypsin, and/or α_1-antichymotrypsin the revealed diagnosis is histiocytic sarcoma.

PROGNOSTIC FACTORS

Overall survival of primary (Group I) GI-NHL is reported to be 44% in two large series.[22,23] Secondary involvement of GI-tract by lymphoma (Group II) usually spells doom for the patient. The median survival is reported to be 9.1 months.[19] There are, however, several factors that influence the prognosis:

Size of the tumor. Several investigators report the size to be a prognostically important factor.[31] However, it is probably closely related to other factors, such as stage of disease and infiltration of adjacent structures.[33,68]

Histology and immunophenotype of the NHL. Surprisingly this has only limited bearing on prognosis. Follicular lymphomas tend to do better than diffuse ones.[18,68] Lymphoplasmacytoid NHL are reported to have a slightly better prognosis[23,31] perhaps because these cells, reflecting normal GALT physiology, tend to home back to the GALT and thus remain localized there. The group of NHL studied by Evans[69] shows some examples of such cases. Most studies, however, clearly state that histology is not a prognostic factor.[22,24,28]

The marker profile of the neoplastic cells is also of limited importance, but as mentioned above, more data are needed. Nevertheless, absence of immunoglobulin staining on B-cell NHL appears to correlate with an unfavorable prognosis.[28,29]

Site. Taken as a group, lymphomas in the stomach do better than small intestinal lymphomas, which do better than NHL from the large intestine.[18,33] This is irrespective of type of NHL. Ileocecal lymphomas are often lymphoblastic; they have a poor prognosis.

Perforation. This is an ominous sign,[7] reported with a varying incidence of 1–28%.[22]

Staging. Most studies agree that staging is the most important factor prognostically. As with perforation, infiltration of adjacent structures by NHL is a bad sign.[18] It should be looked for. The most important factor, however, is whether the NHL has spread beyond the GALT or not.[18,22,23,28,33] Whether involvement of regional lymph nodes is prognostically unfavorable is controversial, but most authors agree it is not.[22,23,28] These viewpoints have led to alternative staging schemes.[18,70,71] These schemes resemble staging according to the TNM staging scheme for carcinomas, stressing that the histology of NHL is of relatively little relevance for prognosis.

With prognosis dependent on whether or not the NHL is restricted to the confines of the GALT system (including the regional lymph nodes) staging procedures become very important. However, there is no consensus concerning the methods of staging, whether abdominal CT scan with or without lymphangiography is sufficient, or if laparotomy is always indicated. This is more or less dependent on the choice of therapy. If a patient will receive radiation therapy, a radiation field can be chosen to treat potentially involved lymph nodes, an operation can be avoided, and CT scanning will suffice.

Unfortunately no studies are available comparing treatment results in patients receiving radiation therapy and patients who have undergone extensive staging (laparotomy) with surgical treatment plus possibly chemotherapy and/or radiotherapy. Studies like that are needed to settle the question of which staging method (and which therapeutic modality) to choose. In any case special care must be taken to document spread beyond the GALT. Abdominal CT scan/laparotomy and, if indicated, investigation on laparotomy of paraaortic or more distant lymph nodes, with bone marrow aspiration and/or biopsy and, on indication, liver biopsy are important. It must be kept in mind that the lymph nodes can show numerous monotonous follicles, suggestive of NHL. In these cases demonstration of monoclonality by markers (κ or λ light chains) brings the definitive answer.

THERAPY

As GI-NHL are not very frequent, experience with different therapeutic regimens is limited. As was stated before, no studies are available comparing survival of patients treated with radiotherapy alone to that of patients treated with surgery with or without additional radiotherapy. In practice most people are treated surgically with or without additional chemo- and/or radiotherapy. While awaiting the results of such a comparative study, the current data from the literature are as follows: For group I patients (GI-NHL restricted to GALT) resection of the stomach or bowel specimen with regional lymph nodes is usually effective.[18,23,24,33] Additional radiotherapy does not appear to influence survival,[18,23] though Herrmann et al.[19] do find a beneficial effect on relapse-free survival time.

"Complete" resection, (i.e., bowel and nodal disease and invaded adjacent structures), gives superior results compared to incomplete removal.[18] Investigation by frozen sections of the resection edges can give important information on radicality of the resection. Though complete resection is the obvious goal, it is best not to be tempted to perform heroic surgery such as thoraco-abdominal explorations since they have high risk at operation. Moreover, in lymphomas, absolute certainty about "completeness" of a resection is never obtained, given the fact that lymphoma cells recirculate. Thus for GALT-restricted NHL a laparotomy with removal of the affected part of the bowel and sampling of regional lymph nodes as well as non-contiguous lymph nodes, investigated if possible with marker studies, is indicated for both proper staging (prognosis) and therapy. (Of course staging will also have to include bone marrow biopsy, palpation, and investigation of peripheral lymph nodes, if necessary).[33]

For the group Ib and II patients, systemic therapy seems to be indicated. Resection may still play a part as many patients develop local complications (12 of 31 patients (39%!) reported by Herrmann et al.)[19] Otherwise, radiotherapy may be helpful, especially in patients where an operation is unattractive (older and/or debilitated patients). Maybe for some patients from group Ib, especially those with not too extensive a spread of lymphoma, radiation therapy alone will give satisfactory results, but as stated before, this awaits prospective studies.

CONCLUSIONS

GI-NHL are mostly derived from the GALT.

Approximately 10% of all NHL are located primarily in the GI-tract. The most common type of lymphoma is the diffuse large-cell

NHL, with those of FCC origin predominating. The majority of GI-NHL are of B-cell origin. Histiocytic sarcomas occur, but their incidence is uncertain. T-cell lymphomas are rare.

Immunophenotyping is important for: (a) distinguishing pseudolymphoma from NHL; and (b) distinguishing between lymphoid and nonlymphoid lesions. And, to a lesser degree, it has prognostic implications. Nearly half of the patients with GI-NHL have regional lymph node involvement at diagnosis.

Prognosis depends more on the extent of the disease than on the histology of the neoplasm. NHL restricted to the GALT (including the regional lymph nodes) have a much better prognosis than those NHL that have disseminated beyond the confines of the GALT, or those in which GI tract involvement is part of a widely disseminated "nodal" NHL.

Staging procedures are important and should include investigation for peripheral lymphadenopathy and splenomegaly, bone marrow aspiration and/or biopsy, and either abdominal CT-scan or laparotomy. This last point is not yet settled. If there are enlarged nonregional nodes, histologic and immunologic investigation is indicated.

REFERENCES

1. Lennert K.: Follicular lymphoma. A tumor of the germinal centers. Malignant Disease of the Hematopoietic System. GANN monograph on Cancer Research, vol 15. University of Tokyo Press, Tokyo, pp. 217–231, 1973
2. Lukes R.J., Collins R.D.: A functional approach to the classification of malignant lymphoma. Recent Results Cancer Res. **46**:18–30, 1974
3. Lennert K: Malignant lymphomas, other than Hodgkin's disease. Handbuch der speziellen pathologischen Anatomie und Histologie. Band I, Teil 3B, Springer-Verlag 1978
4. Mann R.B., Jaffe E.S., Berard C.W.: Malignant lymphomas: A conceptual understanding of morphologic diversity. Am J Pathol **94**:104–191, 1979
5. Parrott D.M.V.: The gut as a lymphoid organ. Clin. Gastroenterol. 5:211–228, 1976
6. Bienenstock J., Johnston N., Perey D.Y.E.: Bronchial lymphoid tissue I. Morphologic characteristics. Lab Invest 28:686–698, 1973
7. Morris H., Edwards J., Tiltman A., Emms M.: Endometrial lymphoid tissue: An immunohistological study. J Clin Pathol 38:644–652, 1985

8. Anscombe A.A., Wright D.H.: Primary lymphoma of the thyroid, a tumour of mucosa-associated lymphoid tissue: Review of seventy-six cases. Histopathology 9:81–97, 1985

9. Segatto O., Giacomini P., Santoro L., Perrino A., Natali P.G.: Lymphoid stroma of Warthin's tumour: Phenotypic analogies with gut-associated lymphoid tissue. Clin Immunol Immunopathol 34:39–47, 1985

10. MacDermott M.R., Bienenstock J.: Evidence for a common mucosal immunologic system. I. Migration of B-immunoblasts into intestinal, respiratory, and genital tissues. J Immunol 122:1892–1898, 1979

11. Bienenstock J., Befus A.D., McDermott M.: Mucosal immunity. From: Monographs in Allergy, vol 16: Essays on the anatomy and physiology of lymphoid tissues. Karger S.: Basel pp 1–18, 1980

12. Brown W.R.: Immunology. Chapter 7 from the Gastro-enterology Annual/2 eds., Kermÿn F., Blum A.L.: Elsevier, Amsterdam, pp. 190–213, 1984

13. Thompson R.A.: Immunological mechanisms. From: Immunology of the gastrointestinal tract. Ed: P. Asquith. Churchill Livingstone, Edinburgh, pp 14–22, 1979

14. Stevens S.K., Weissman I.L., Butcher E.C.: Differences in the migration of B and T lymphocytes: Organ-selective localization in vivo and the role of lymphocyte-endothelial cell recognition. J Immunol 128:844–851, 1982

15. Cahill R.N.P., Poskitt D.C., Frost H., Trnka Z.: Two distinct pools of recirculating T lymphocytes: Migratory characteristics of nodal and intestinal T lymphocytes. J Exp Med 145:420–428, 1977

16. Elson C.O., Heck J.A., Strober W.: T-cell regulation of murine IgA synthesis. J Exp Med 149:632–643, 1979

17. Selby W.S., Janossy G., Bofill M., Jewell D.P.: Intestinal lymphocyte subpopulations in inflammatory bowel disease: an analysis by immunohistological and cell isolation techniques. Gut 25:32–40, 1984

18. Blackledge G., Bush H., Dodge O.G., Crowthers D.: A study of gastrointestinal lymphoma. Clin Oncol 5:209–219, 1979

19. Herrmann R., Panahon A.M., Barcos M.P., Walsh D., Stutzman L.: Gastrointestinal involvement in non-Hodgkin's lymphoma. Cancer 46:215–222, 1980

20. Freeman C., Berg J.W., Cutler S.J.: Occurrence and prognosis of extranodal lymphomas. Cancer 29:252–260, 1972

21. Haak H.L., Kluin Ph.M, Meijer C.J.L.M., Otter R., Steijnen Th.: Population-based registration of non-Hodgkin's lymphoma in the region covered by the Comprehensive Cancer Centre West. Neth. J. Med. 29:105–110, 1987

22. Lewin K.J., Ranchod M., Dorfman R.F.: Lymphomas of the gastrointestinal tract. A study of 117 cases presenting with gastrointestinal disease. Cancer 42:693–707, 1978

23. Weingrad D.N., DeCosse J.J., Sherlock P., Straus D., Lieberman P.H., Filippa D.A.: Primary gastrointestinal lymphoma: A 30-year review. Cancer 49:1258–1265, 1982

24. Blackshaw A.J.: Non-Hodgkin's lymphomas of the gut. Recent Advances in Gastrointestinal Pathology. Wright R. (Ed). Philadelphia, Wm. Saunders 1980 pp 213–240

25. Isaacson P. Wright D.H.: Malignant lymphoma of mucosa-associated lymphoid tissue. A distinctive type of B-cell lymphoma. Cancer 52:1410–1416, 1983

26. Isaacson P. Wright D.H.: Extranodal malignant lymphoma arising from mucosa-associated lymphoid tissue. Cancer 53:2515–2524, 1984

27. Hernandez J.A., Sheehan W.W.: Lymphomas of the mucosa-associated lymphoid tissue. Signet ring cell lymphomas presenting in mucosal lymphoid organs. Cancer 55:592–597, 1985

28. Saraga P., Hurlimann J., Ozzello L.: Lymphomas and pseudolymphomas of the alimentary tract. An immunohistochemical study with clinicopathologic correlations. Hum Path 12:713–723, 1981

29. Seo I.S., Binkley W.B., Warnez T.F.C.S., Warfel K.A.: 442 A combined morphologic and immunologic approach to the diagnosis of gastrointestinal lymphomas: I Malignant lymphoma of the stomach (22 cases). Cancer 49:493–501, 1982

30. Grody W.W., Magidson J.G., Weiss L.A., Hu E., Warnke R.A., Lewin K.J.: Gastrointestinal lymphomas. Immunohistochemical studies on the cell of origin. Am J Surg Pathol 9:328–337, 1985

31. Filippa D.A., DeCosse J.J., Lieberman P.H., Bretsky S.S., Weingrad D.N.: Primary lymphomas of the gastrointestinal tract. Analysis of prognostic factors with emphasis on histological type. Am J Surg Pathol 7:363–372, 1983

32. Wright D.H., Isaacson P.G.: Extranodal malignant lymphomas. From: Biopsy Pathology of the Lymphoreticular System. Chapman & Hall, London, pp 267–309, 1983

33. Appelman H.D., Schnitzer B., Hirsch S.D., Loon W.W.: Clinicopathologic overview of gastrointestinal lymphomas. Am J Surg Pathol 9:71–83, 1985

34. Isaacson P. Wright D.H., Judd M.A., Mepham B.L.: Primary gastrointestinal lymphomas. A classification of 66 cases. Cancer 43:1805–1819, 1979

35. Valk P. van der, Jansen J., Daha M.R., Meijer C.J.L.M.: Characterization of B-cell Non-Hodgkin's lymphomas. Virchows Arch. A 401:289–305, 1983.

36. Ranchod M., Lewin K.J., Dorfman R.F.: Lymphoid hyperplasia of the gastrointestinal tract. A study of 26 cases and review of the literature. Am J Surg Pathol 2:383–400, 1978

37. Otto H.F., Bettman I., Weltzien J.V., Gebbers J.O.: Primary intestinal lymphoma. Virchows Arch A 391:9–31, 1981

38. Kotner L.M., Wang C.C.: Plasmacytoma of the upper air and food passages. Cancer 30:414–418, 1972

39. Asselah F., Crow J., Slavin G., Sheldon C., Asselah H.: Solitary plasmacytoma of the intestine. Histopathology 6:631–645, 1982

40. Tweel J.G. van der, Taylor C.R., Parker J.W., Lukes R.J.: Immunoglobulin inclusions in non-Hodgkin's lymphomas. Am J Clin Pathol 69:306–313, 1978

41. Rappaport H., Ramot B., Hulu N., Part J.K.: The pathology of the so-called Mediterranean abdominal lymphoma with malabsorption. Cancer 29:1502–1511, 1972

42. Khojasteh A., Haghshenass M., Haghighi P.: Immunoproliferative small intestinal disease. A "Third-World lesion." N Eng J Med 308:1401–1405, 1983

43. Isaacson P.: Middle-East lymphoma and α-chain disease. An immunohistochemical study. Am J Surg. Pathol. 3:431–441, 1979

44. Gilinsky N.H., Mee A.S., Beatty D.W., Novis B.H., Young G., Price S., Purves L.R., Marks I.L.: Plasmacell infiltration of the small bowel: Lack of evidence for a non-secretory form of alpha-heavy chain disease. Gut 26:928–934, 1985

45. Nassar V.H., Salem P.A., Shadid M.J., Alami S.Y., Balikian J.B., Salem A.A., Nasrallah S.M.: Mediter-

ranean abdominal lymphoma" or immunoproliferative small intestinal disease. Part II. Pathological aspects. Cancer 41:1340–1354, 1978

46. Isaacson P., Price S.K.: Light chains in Mediterranean lymphoma, J Clin Pathol 38:601–677, 1978

47. Wright D.H.: The identification and classification of non-Hodgkin's lymphomas: A review. Diagn Histopathol 5:73–111, 1982

48. Banks A.M., Arseneau J.C., Gralnick H.R., Canellos G.P., De Vita V.T., Berard C.W.: American Burkitt's lymphoma: A clinicopathologic study of 30 cases. II Pathologic correlations. Am J Med 58:322–329, 1975

49. Foucar K., Foucar E., Mitros F., Clamon G., Goeken J., Crossett J.: Epitheliotropic lymphoma of the small bowel. Report of a fatal case with cytotoxic/suppressor T-cell immunotypes. Cancer 54:54–60, 1984

50. Mir R., Kahn L.B.: Immunohistochemistry of primary gastrointestinal lymphomas: A study of 38 cases. Lab Invest 48:59A, 1983

51. MacLennan K.A., Bennett M.H., Tu A.: The pathology of primary gastrointestinal lymphoma (report no. 10). Clin Radiol 32:513–518, 1982

52. Valk P. van der, Meijer C.J.L.M., Willemze R., Oosterom A.T. van, Spaander P.J., Velde T. te: Histiocytic sarcoma (true histiocytic lymphoma): A clinicopathological study of 20 cases. Histopathology 8:105–123, 1984

53. Valk P. van der, Meijer C.J.L.M: Histiocytic sarcoma. Clinical picture, morphology, markers, differential diagnosis. Pathol Annu 20(Part 2):1–28, 1985

54. Isaacson P., Wright D.H.: Malignant histiocytosis of the intestine. Its relationship to malabsorption and ulcerative jejunitis. Hum Pathol 9:661–677, 1978

55. Isaacson P., Wright D.H., Jones D.B.: Malignant lymphoma of true histiocytic (monocytic/macrophage) origin. Cancer 51:80–91, 1983

56. Isaacson P.G., O'Connor N.T.J., Spencer J., Bevan D.H., Conolly C.E., Kirkham H., Pollock D.J., Wainscoat J.S., Stein H., Mason D.Y.: Malignant histiocytosis of the intestine: A T-cell lymphoma. Lancet 2:688–691, 1985

57. Stein H., Lennert K., Feller A.C., Mason D.Y.: Immunohistological analysis of human lymphoma: Correlation of histological and immunological categories. Adv. Cancer. Res. 42:67–73, 1984

58. Knowles II D.M., Dodson L., Burke J.S., Ming Wang J., Bonetti F., Pelicci P.G., Flug F., Favera R., Wang C.Y.: SIg -, E - ("null-cell") non-Hodgkin's lymphomas. Multiparametric determination of their B- or T-cell lineage. Am J Pathol 120:356–370, 1985

59. Meijer C.J.L.M., Willemze R., Henzen-Logmans S.C., ván der Valk P.: Monoclonal antibodies in the histopathological diagnosis of non-Hodgkins's lymphomas. Neth J Med 20:138–141, 1985

60. Meijer C.J. L.M., ván der Valk P., Poppema S.: Markers of malignant lymphomas. Diagnostic implications. In: Tumor Immunology—Mechanisms, Diagnosis, Therapy. Eds. Wolen Otter, E. J. Ruiteabey, Elseviers Science Publ Chap 12, pp, 187–226, 1987

61. Meijer C.J.L.M., Mulliak M., Hearen-Rogmans S.C.: Practical application of monoclonal antibodies to diagnostic tumor pathology and sòme future perspectives. In: Application of monoclonal antibodies in tumor pathology. Eds D. J. Raiter et. al. Martinus Nyhoff Publ Chap 17, pp 299–318, 1987

62. Faris T.D., Saltzstein S.L.: Gastric lymphoid hyperplasia: A lesion confused with lymphosarcoma. Cancer 17:207–212, 1964

63. Saltzstein S.L.: Pulmonary malignant lymphomas and pseudolymphomas. Classification, therapy, and prognosis. Cancer 16:928–955, 1963

64. Greenberg S.D., Heisler J.G., Gyorkey F., Jenkins D.E.: Pulmonary lymphoma versus pseudolymphoma: A perplexing problem. South Med J 65:775–784, 1972

65. Julsrudd P.R., Brown L.R., Li G-Y., Rosenow III E.C., Crowe J.K.: Pulmonary processes of mature-appearing lymphocytes: Pseudolymphoma, well differentiated lymphocytic lymphoma, and lymphocytic interstial pneumonitis. Radiology 127:289–296, 1978

66. Lerman-Sagie T., Zio Y., Rubin M., More C., Dintsman M.: Gastric lymphoma versus pseudolymphoma: The importance of immunological differentiation. Am J Gastroenterol 80:763–707, 1978

67. Vimadalal S.D., Said J.W., Voyles III H.: Gastric lymphoreticular neoplasms: An immunologic study of 36 cases. Am J Clin Pathol 80:792–799, 1983

68. Brooks J.J., Enterline H.T.: Primary gastric lymphomas: A clinicopathologic study of 58 cases with long-term follow-up and literature review. Cancer 51:701–711, 1983

69. Evans H.L.: Extranodal small lymphocytic proliferation: A clinicopathologic and immunocytochemical study. Cancer 49:84–96, 1982

70. Lim F.E., Hartman A.S., Tan E.G.C., Cody B., Meissner W.A.: Factors in the prognosis of gastric lymphomas. Cancer 39:1715–1720, 1977

71. Musshoff K.: Klinische Stadieneinteilung der Nicht-HodgkinLymphome. Strahlentherapie 153:218–221, 1977

6

Endocrine Tumors of the Gastrointestinal Tract: Classification, Function and Biological Behavior

Eiichi Tahara, M.D.

The gastrointestinal (GI) tract, which has many different types of hormones and peptides, is the largest endocrine organ of the body. GI hormones and peptides are present in both endocrine cells and nerves and act as endocrines, paracrines, and neurocrines in regulating digestion, absorption, motility, and growth of the GI tract.

The representative tumor related to GI peptides is carcinoid, but its concept or definition has been altered with the identification of 18 distinct endocrine cells of the GI tract.[1] Moreover, confusion has arisen from the needless abuse of the term carcinoid, and furthermore, the classification of endocrine tumors of the gut varies remarkably by authors.

On the other hand, endocrine cells are well known to occur in ordinary carcinoma of the GI tract, aside from classical carcinoid. The frequency of endocrine cells differs according to the localization, histologic type, and infiltrative growth of GI carcinoma.[2-5] Carcinoma with numerous argentaffin or argyrophil cells diffusely presenting in the tissue is referred to variously in reports as "diffuse argentaffinoma,"[3] "argentaffin cell adenocarcinoma,"[6] "atypical carcinoid,"[7] and "argyrophil cell carcinoma."[4] More recently, the term "neuroendocrine carcinoma" has been proposed by Gould et al.[8-10]

BASIC DEFINITION AND NEW CLASSIFICATION

Endocrine tumor of the GI tract is a general term for neoplasms in that the vast majority of tumor cells arising in the GI tract show endocrine differentiation. It does not, however, imply that the endocrine tumors are derived from endocrine cells.

GI endocrine tumors, from the standpoint of their microscopic characteristics, functional differentiation, and biologic behavior can be divided into three histological types. The first is classical, "typical" carcinoid, corresponding to A or B type of Soga's carcinoid classification.[11] The second is mucocarcinoid,[12] involving tumors described under the term goblet-cell carcinoid and mucinous carcinoid. The third is endocrine cell carcinoma, which is regarded as a malignant epithelial tumor consisting predominantly of neoplastic endocrine cells with cellular pleomorphism, atypism, and numerous mitoses. Depending on the amount of stromal connective tissue, endocrine cell carcinoma is subdivided into medullary type and scirrhous type. The author's classification is shown in Table 6-1, in comparison with the WHO classification[12] of tumors of the diffuse endocrine system and Soga's carcinoid classification.[11]

TABLE 6-1
Classification of Gastrointestinal Endocrine Tumors

Author's Classification	WHO Classification (1980)[12]	Soga's Carcinoid Classification (1971)[11]
I Carcinoid	I Carcinoid	A type
	A. Enterochromaffin cell (EC-cell) carcinoid	
	B. G-cell tumor (G-cell carcinoid)	B type
	C. Other carcinoid	
II Mucocarcinoid	II Mucocarcinoid	C type
III Endocrine cell carcinoma		
A. Medullary type		
1. Well differentiated		
2. Poorly differentiated	III Mixed carcinoid-adenocarcinoma	D type
3. Undifferentiated		
B. Scirrhous type		

Carcinoid

Morphology

Carcinoid frequently shows a pattern of submucosal tumor, as tumor cells usually arise from the deep mucosa of the GI tract and from an early stage they infiltrate into the submucosa. It may be yellowish or grey and solid on the cut surface. Multiple tumors are not rare. Gastric and rectal carcinoids occupy over 60% of GI carcinoids in Japanese patients,[13] whereas appendicular carcinoids occupy about 40% in European and American patients.

Histologically, the term should be limited only to tumors composed of uniform endocrine cells that form a pattern of solid nests or trabecular, ribbon, or lobular patterns (Fig. 6-1a,b). Nuclear pleomorphism and mitotic figures are almost never seen. Ultrastructurally, endocrine granules of a variety of shapes and sizes are present in the cells' cytoplasm. The stroma is abundant in blood vessels and fibrous tissue. Most of the cells are positive with the argyrophil reaction regardless of the site of the tumor (Fig. 6-2a). EC-cell carcinoids, which are strongly positive with argentaffin stain, usually occur in the small intestine, appendix and right side of the colon.

Function

Carcinoid is well known to produce serotonin, histamine, and catecholamine. However, the incidence of carcinoid syndrome is from 2% to 5% of GI carcinoids. When metastasis occurs, it may be associated with the carcinoid syndrome. Gastric carcinoids may on occasion produce histamine and 5-HT (5-hydroxytryptamine) synchronously, the patient showing a skin flush due to hyperhistaminemia. The gastric tumors originating from ECL (enterochromaffin-like cells) usually occur in atrophic fundic glands of chronic atrophic gastritis, achylia gastrica, or pernicious anemia.[14,15] The patients show hypergastrinemia via a negative feedback mechanism.

On the other hand, these tumors produce numerous hormones and peptides, such as gastrin, CCK (cholecystokinin), somatostatin, glucagon, insulin, glicentin, motilin, substance P, neurotensin, enkephalin, endorphin, PP (pancreatic polypeptide), PYY (polypeptide YY), ACTH, calcitonin, NPY (neuropeptide Y), and GRP (gastrin-releasing peptide).[15-21] Among GI carcinoids, more than 40% show multiple peptide-immunoreactivities. Moreover, the tumors occasionally produce both peptides and amines. Carcinoids producing only one peptide are rare.

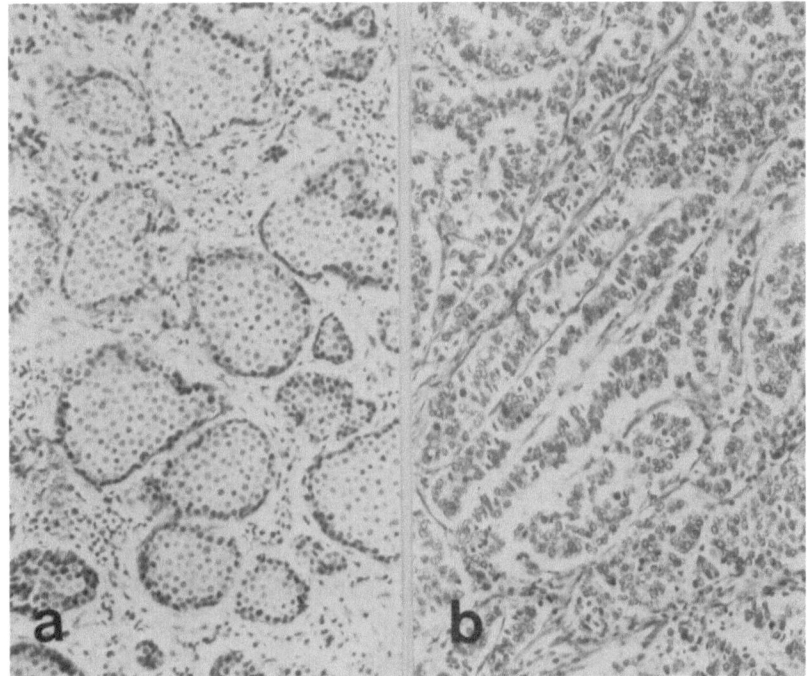

Fig. 6-1 a and b. (a) Appendicular carcinoid showing solid nests. (b) Gastric carcinoid showing trabecular or ribbon patterns. H&E, × 300.

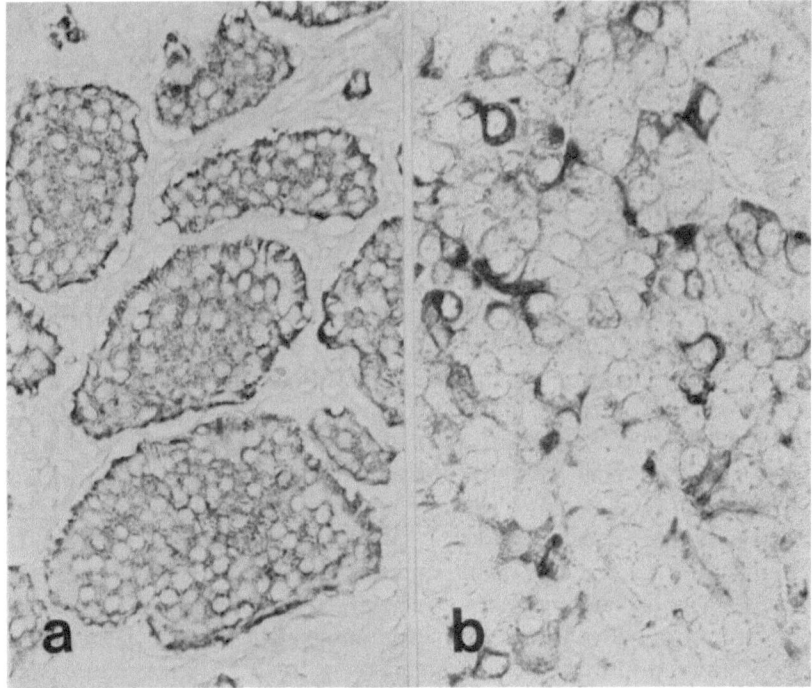

Fig. 6-2 a and b. The same tumor as in Fig. 1a. (a) Tumor cells are strongly positive with argyrophil reaction. Grimelius stain, ×420. (b) Some tumor cells show CEA immunoreactivity, PAP stain, ×600.

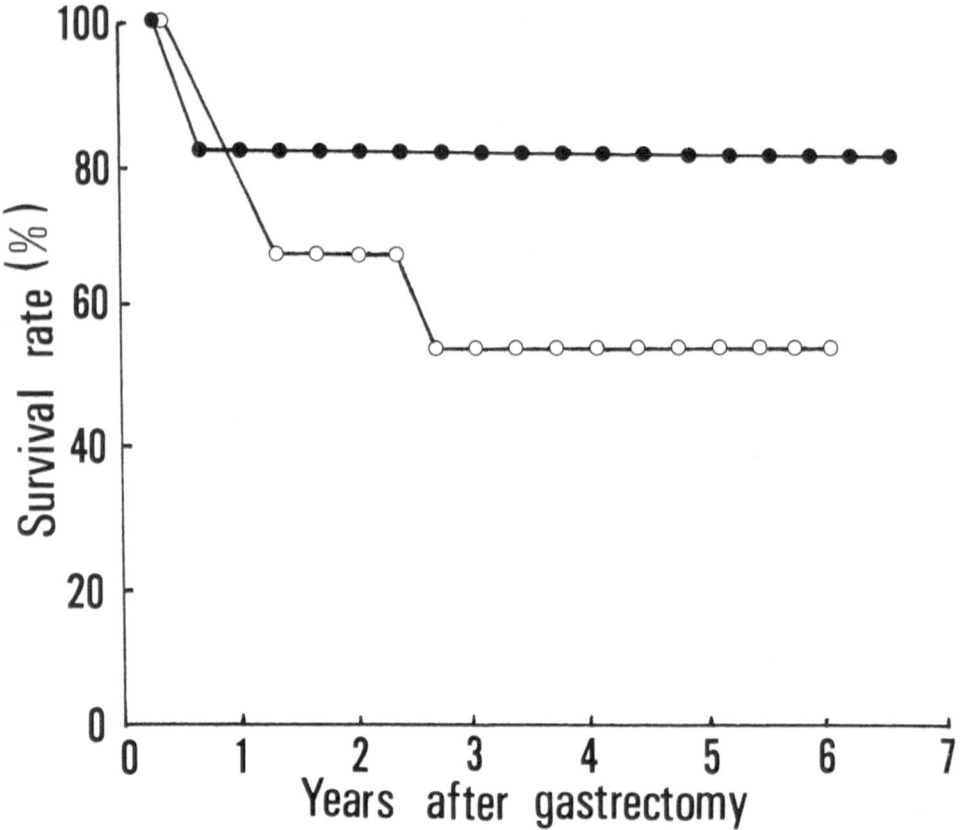

Fig. 6-3. Comparison of 7-year cumulative survival rates between gastric carcinoid and colon-rectum carcinoid.
Open circle: 9 cases of gastric carcinoid (mean age, 67.1 yr). Closed circle: 15 cases of colon-rectum carcinoid (mean age, 60.4 yr).

With regard to the relation between peptide production and tumor site, gastrin and CCK are seen occasionally in gastric and duodenal carcinoids, but glucagon or glicentin, PP, and PYY are rather frequently observed in colonic and rectal carcinoids. The expression of these peptides within the tumor is similar to the normal distribution of GI endocrine cells.

Paraendocrine syndrome due to peptides produced by tumor cells does not usually occur. The reason for this seems to be as follows: (1) The amount of peptides within the tumor is low; (2) peptides produced by tumor cells are in inactive form or prohormone; (3) extracellular secretion of peptide from tumor cells is small, especially into the blood vessels; and (4) simultaneous production of multiple peptides shows mutual competition. Gastri-

noma consisting of gastrin-producing cells may on occasion occur in the duodenum, the patients showing Zollinger-Ellison syndrome.[22] Both duodenal and pancreatic gastrinomas may occur as part of MEN (multiple endocrine neoplasia) type I. ACTH producing tumor associated with Cushing syndrome[23] is very rare.

Except for amines and peptides, GI carcinoids produce a variety of glycoproteins and enzymes together with amines or peptides.[24,25] Immunohistochemically, CEA related antigens (Fig. 6-2b), SC (secretory component) and hCG (human chorionic gonadotropin) within the tumor are seen in about 60%, 15%, and 13% of all GI carcinoids, respectively. NSE (neuron specific enolase) occurs in 33% of the gastric tumors and in 66% of intestinal

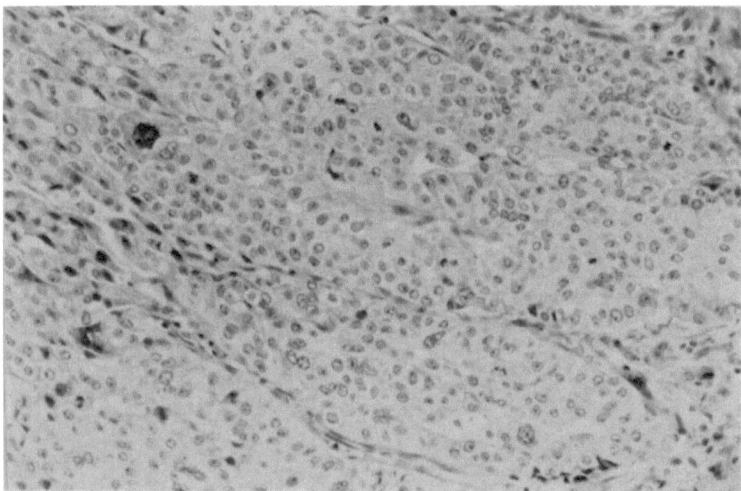

Fig. 6-4. *Well differentiated type* of medullary ECC of the stomach. Tumor cells have numerous mitoses and pleomorphism. H&E, ×300.

carcinoids. Expression of S-100 protein, however, is less common than that of NSE, and its incidence is about 25% of all GI carcinoids. Alpha$_1$-antitrypsin (AAT)-immunoreactivity is also noted, its incidence being 15% of all GI carcinoids.

Biological Behavior

All GI carcinoids are regarded as malignant tumors on pathologic and biologic grounds, but their malignancy is generally of a low grade. More than 70% of gastric carcinoids, however, show metastases to local lymph nodes and liver. Figure 6-3 shows a comparison of the 7-year cumulative survival rates between gastric carcinoid and colon-rectum carcinoid. For gastric carcinoid, the 7-year cumulative survival rate is about 50%, while that for colon-rectum carcinoid is about 80%. The prognosis for gastric carcinoid thus is worse than that for colon-rectum carcinoid.

Endocrine Cell Carcinoma

Carcinoma fulfilling the following two criteria should be diagnosed as endocrine cell carcinoma (ECC): (1) The vast majority of tumor cells are endocrine cells with atypia,

pleomorphism, and many mitoses, and (2) these endocrine cells are present with diffuse distribution throughout the tumor tissue. ECC can be divided into medullary type and scirrhous type according to the amount of stromal connective tissue. Moreover, according to the cellular and structural atypicality of tumor cells, medullary ECC is subdivided into well differentiated, poorly differentiated, and undifferentiated types. Most of the ECC cells show a positive reaction to Grimelius' stain.

Subclassification of ECC

1. Medullary ECC
   a. Well Differentiated Type
      Medullary ECC of well differentiated type frequently occurs in the stomach, being especially more common in the fundus than in the antrum. Macroscopically, gastric tumors usually show polypoid carcinomatous growth corresponding to Borrmann's type 1. By light microscopy these tumors have solid islands or trabecular patterns, resembling carcinoid but remarkable mitoses and pleomorphism are often seen (Fig. 6-4).

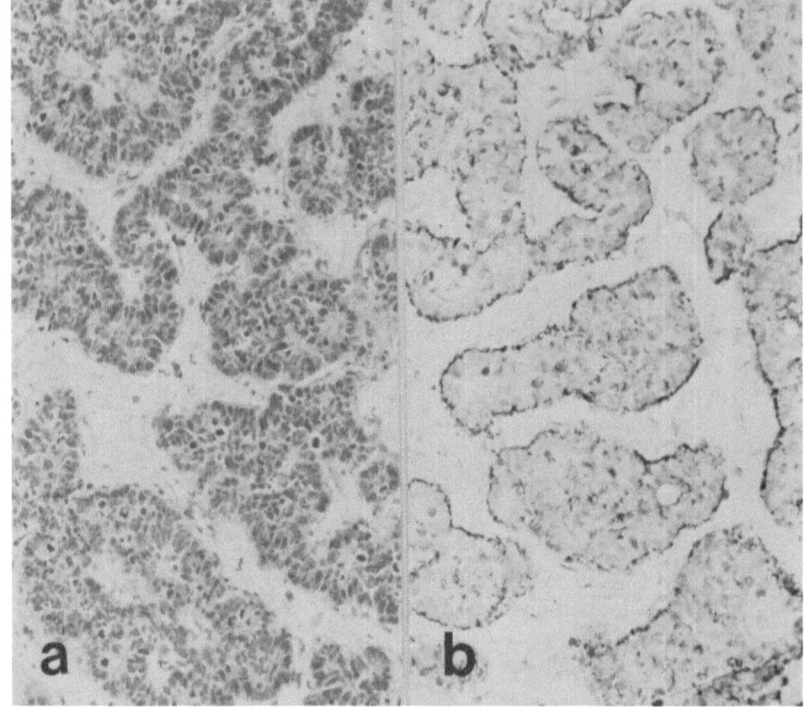

Fig. 6-5 a and b. *Poorly differentiated type* of medullary ECC of the stomach. (a) Tumor cells with remarkable mitoses form tubular structures, resembling adenocarcinoma. H&E, ×300. (b) Tumor cells are diffusely positive with argyrophil reaction. Grimelius stain, ×300.

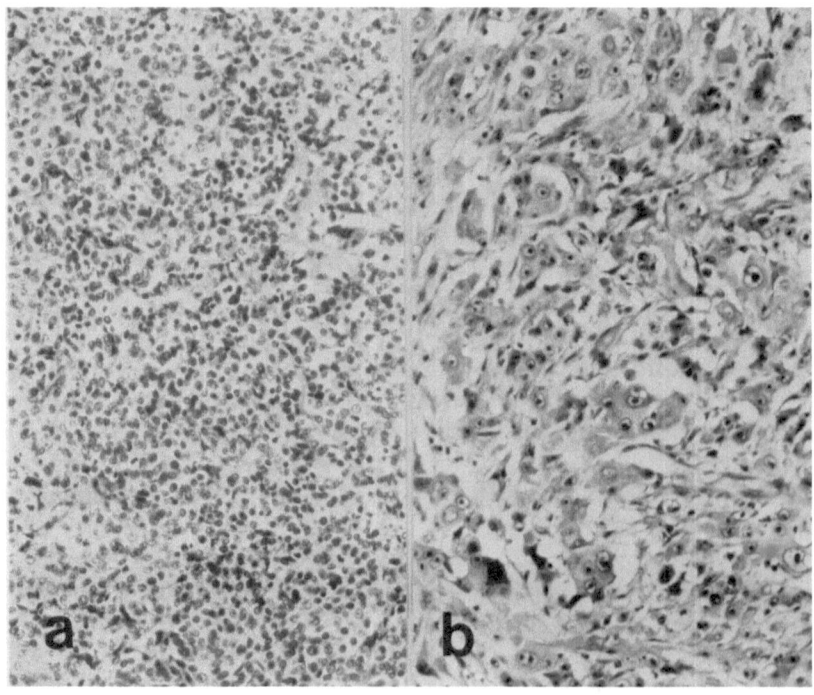

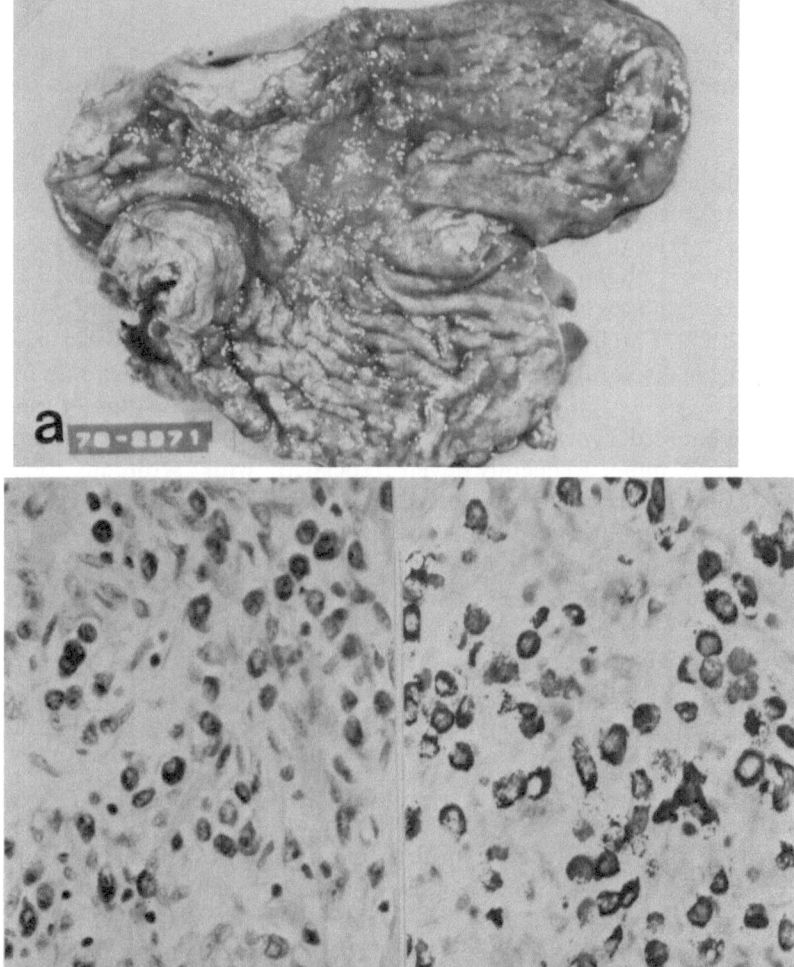

Fig. 6-7 a, b and c. *Scirrhous ECC* of the stomach from a 44-year-old woman, showing diffusely infiltrative carcinoma or Borrmann's type 4 carcinoma (a). (b) The tumor has abundant fibrosis. H&E, ×500. (c) Tumor cells with fine eosinophilic granules are diffusely positive with Grimelius stain. ×500.

←————————————————————————————

Fig. 6-6 a and b. *Undifferentiated type* of medullary ECC of the esophagus (a) and the colon (b). (a) Tumor cells are of small cell type. (b) Tumor cells are of giant cell type with prominent nucleoli. H&E, ×300.

b. Poorly Differentiated Type

This type of medullary ECC frequently occurs in the colon and rectum. The tumor usually cannot be distinguished from ordinary carcinoma macroscopically. By light microscopy the tumor cells form glandular or tubular structures, resembling ordinary adenocarcinoma (Fig. 6-5a,b). Carcinoid pattern may be occasionally seen in a part of the tumor.

c. Undifferentiated Type

This type of tumor frequently develops in the esophagus and stomach and shows the same macroscopic appearance as in ordinary solid carcinoma. The tumor cells vary in size, including such varieties as small cell or oat cell type, intermediate cell type, and large cell type (Fig. 6-6a,b). The tumor may show very rapid growth and remarkable vascular invasion.

2. Scirrhous ECC

Scirrhous ECC usually occurs in the stomach, especially in the fundus, and often grossly manifests as a diffusely infiltrative carcinoma or Borrmann's type 4 carcinoma (Fig. 6-7a). It may be rarely seen in the rectum. Microscopically, the tumor resembles poorly differentiated adenocarcinoma with abundant fibrosis (Fig. 6-7b,c). Many tumor cells have fine or strongly stained eosinophilic granules in the cytoplasm. Signet ring cells may be rarely noted.

Function

ECC as well as carcinoid produce serotonin, and its incidence is about 75% of scirrhous ECC. Moreover, the number of serotonin-immunoreactive cells is greater in ECC than in carcinoid (Fig. 6-8a,b,c,d,e). Vanillylmandelic acid, 5-hydroxy-3-indoleacetic acid and catecholamine also are biochemically detected within the tumor.[8] It is yet unknown, however, whether ECC produces histamine.

On one hand, ECC shows a broad array of peptide-immunoreactivity, such as gastrin, CCK, somatostatin, glucagon, glicentin, PP, ACTH, calcitonin, β-endorphin, and GRP. Synchronous production of these peptides is not a rare phenomenon and is frequently associated with serotonin. Particularly, in young patients under the age of 30 scirrhous ECC of the stomach has a tendency to produce multiple peptides synchronously (Fig.6-9a,b,c,d). The number or distribution density of peptide-immunoreactive cells is greater in ECC than in carcinoid (Fig. 6-10a,b). Ultrastructurally, various endocrine granules are usually seen in the tumor cells (Fig. 6-11a,b,c).[4]

Medullary ECC of the esophagus may on occasion produce ACTH and calcitonin.[10] Gastrin, PP, calcitonin, and glicentin-immunoreactive cells are detected in from 25% to 50% of gastric scirrhous ECC.[4,26] ECC of the colon may have a fair number of gastrin-immunoreactive cells.[27] Compared with carcinoid, ECC appears capable of producing a broader spectrum of peptide hormones. The incidence of peptide-immunoreactivity in ECC examined by the author is summarized in Table 6-2.

Endocrine disturbance due to hyperproduction of peptide hormones in ECC as well as in carcinoid is not usually seen. Hypergastrinemia may on occasion occur in gastric scirrhous ECC.[4]

A variable number of glycoproteins and enzymes is also detected in ECC and the inci-

→

Fig. 6-8 a, b, c, d and e. *Scirrhous ECC* of the stomach from a 31-year-old man. (a) Ulcerative lesion (arrow) in the intermediate zone (b, cut section of the ulcer). Diffuse fibrosis is seen around the deep ulcer. (c) The tumor shows productive fibrosis. H&E, ×150. (d) Many tumor cells have positive immunoreactivity for serotonin. ABC stain, ×150. (e) They are also positive with argentaffin reaction. Masson-Fontana stain, ×150.

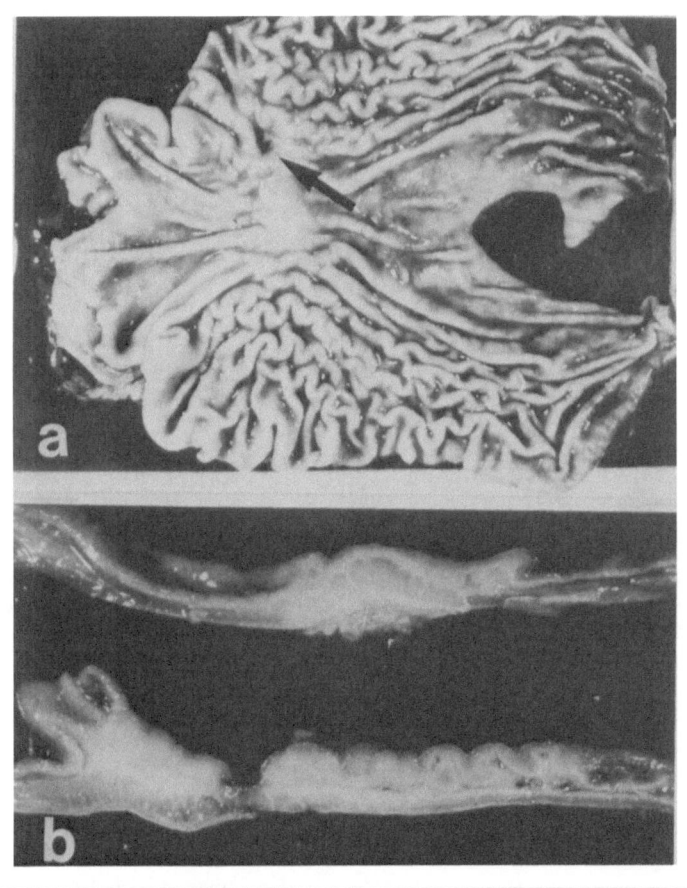

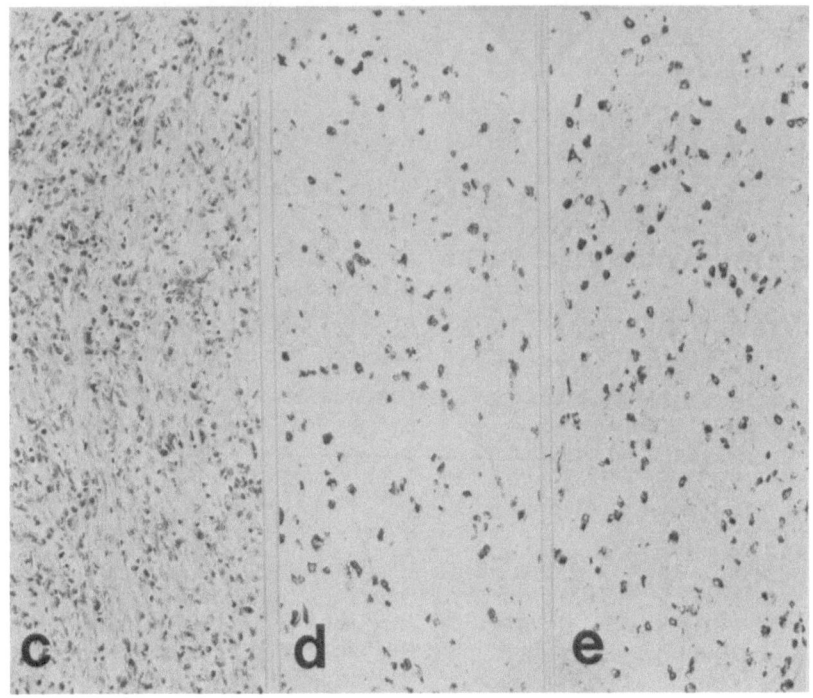

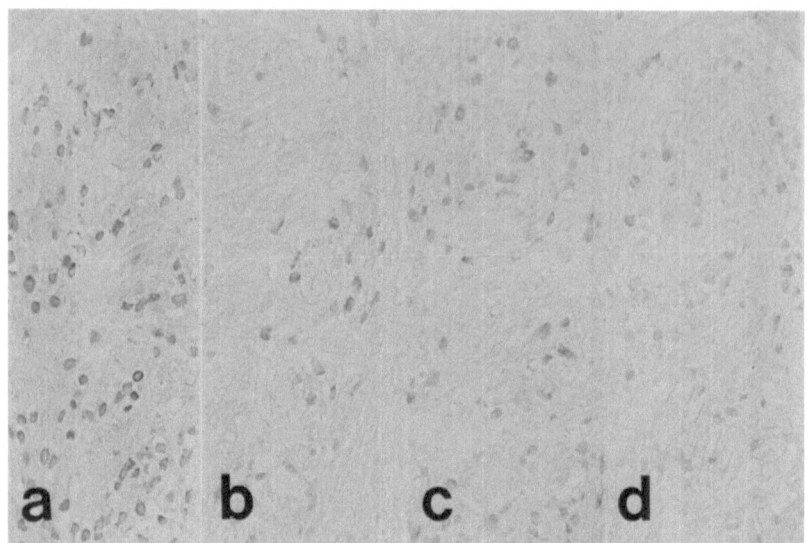

Fig. 6-9 a, b, c and d. *Scirrhous* ECC of the stomach from a 29-year-old man, with synchronous production of six polypeptides, CEA, SC and lysozyme. Tumor cells showed gastrin- (a), glicentin- (b), glucagon (c), calcitonin- (d), somatostatin- and pancreatic polypeptide-immunoreactivity synchronously. PAP stain, ×160.

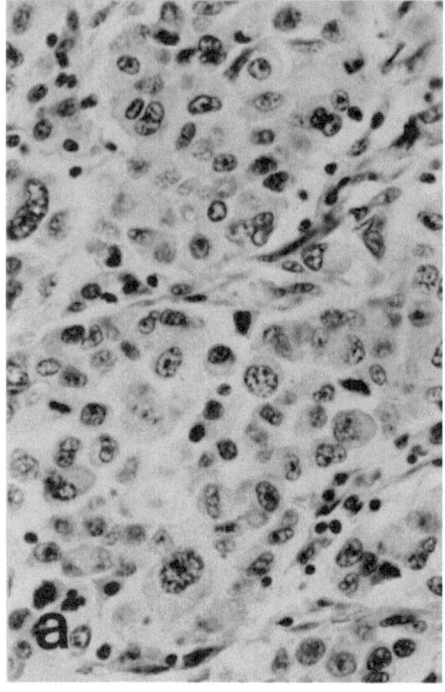

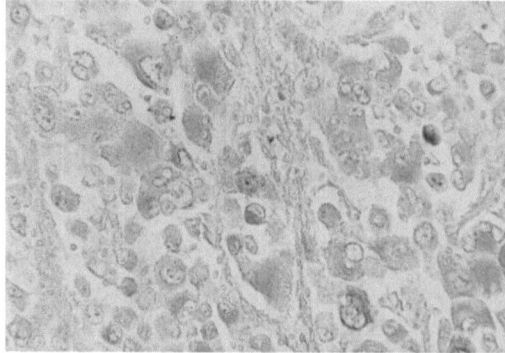

Fig. 6-10 a and b. *Medullary* ECC (*undifferentiated type*) of the stomach. (a) Tumor cells are of large cell type. H&E stain, ×600. (b, color) Most of the tumor cells show strong immunoreactivity for glicentin. PAP stain, ×500.

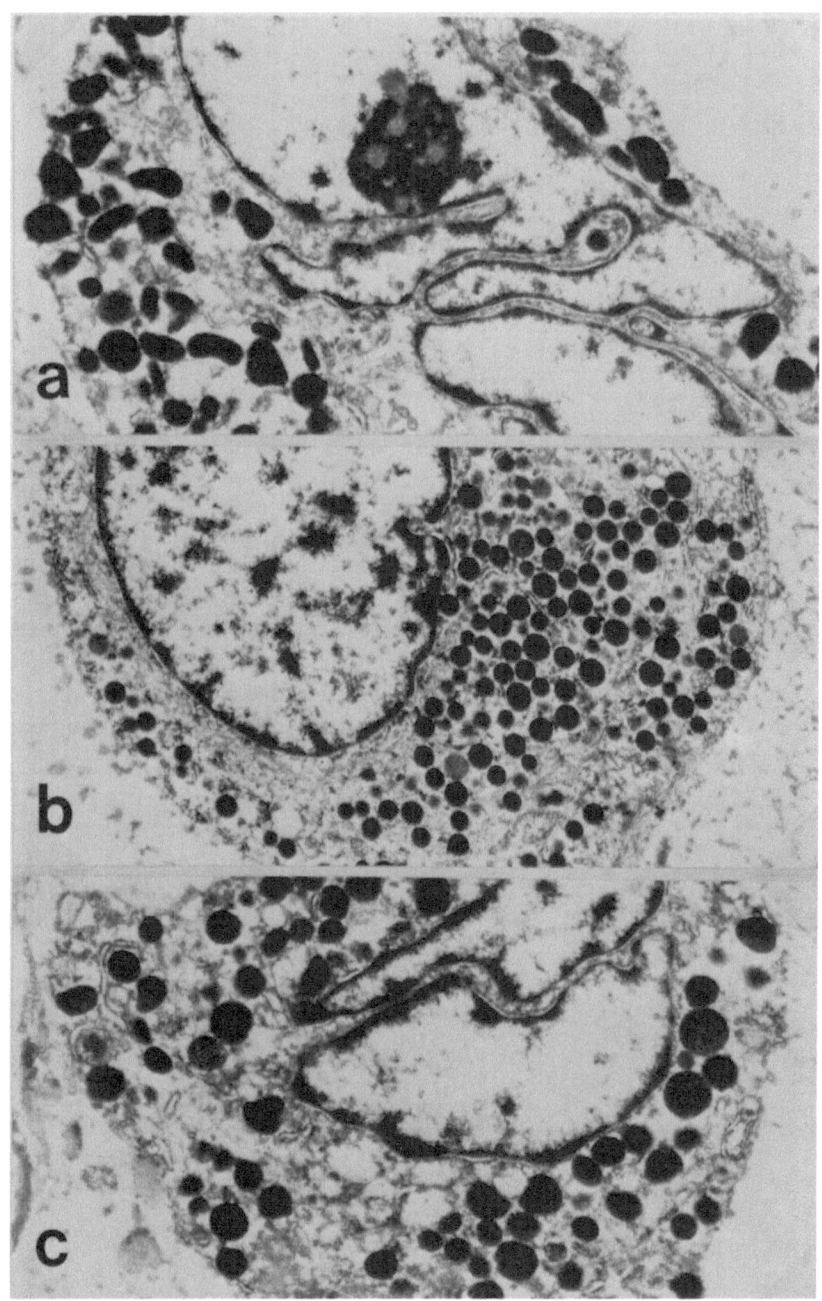

Fig. 6-11 a, b and c. Ultrastructure of the same tumor as in Fig. 7. Tumor cells have three types of secretory granules. (a) Pleomorphic and highly osmophilic granules (400-480 nm). ×11,000. (b) Round and electron dense granules (240-320 nm). ×11,000. (c) Round and large granules (440-480 nm). ×11,000.

TABLE 6-2
Peptide-Immunoreactivity in ECC of the Gastrointestinal Tract

Localization	Subclassification	Number of Cases	Peptide-immunoreactivity[a]							Serotonin-immunoreactivity
			G	S	Glu	Gli	PP	Ca	ACTH	
Esophagus	Medullary	2	0	0	0	0	0	0	0	0
Stomach	Medullary	16	1	1	0	3	0	0	0	6
	Scirrhous	14	4	5	2	5	2	4	0	9
Colon	Medullary	4	1	0	0	0	2	1	0	1

[a] G, gastrin; S, somatostatin; Glu, glucagon; Gli, glicentin; PP, pancreatic polypeptide; Ca, calcitonin; ACTH, adreno-corticotropic hormone.

dence of these markers is greater than in carcinoid. CEA-related antigen and SC are seen in the majority of ECC (Fig. 6-12a,b). hCG is found in from 6% to 43% of gastric and colonic ECC. S-100 protein and NSE expression does not differ between ECC and carcinoid (Fig. 6-13a,b). Over 60% of gastric ECC have lysozyme-immunoreactivity (Fig. 6-14a). AAT expression in ECC is greater than that in carcinoid and over 50% of gastric medullary ECC are characterized by AAT expression (Fig. 6-14b). Table 6-3 shows the incidence of glycoprotein and enzyme-immunoreactivity in ECC.

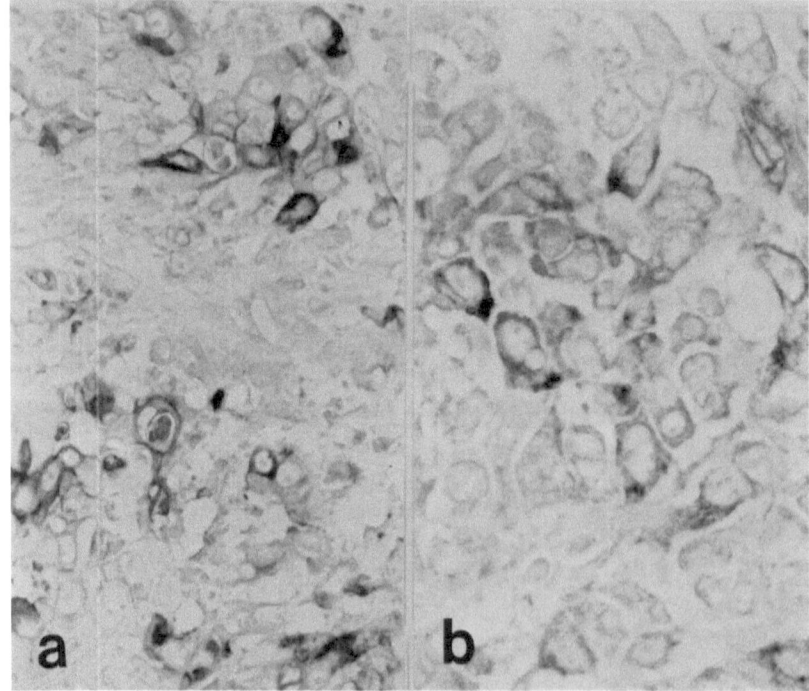

Fig. 6-12 a and b. (a) The same tumor as in Fig. 6b. Tumor cells are partially positive with CEA. PAP stain, ×600. (b) The same tumor as in Fig. 10. Tumor cells show SC-immunoreactivity. ABC stain, ×600.

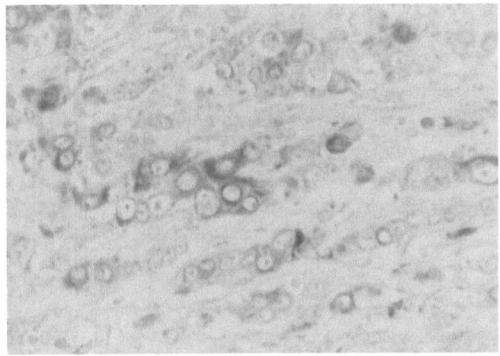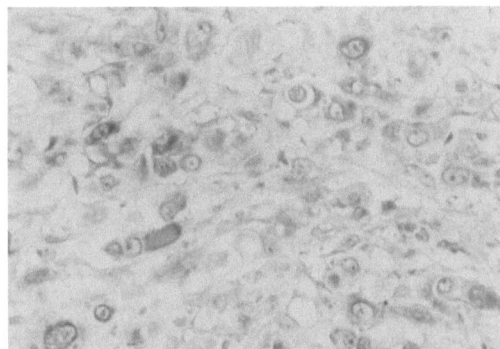

Fig. 6-13 a and b. The same tumor as in Fig. 6b. Many tumor cells are diffusely positive with S-100 protein (a, color) and NSE (b, color). ABC stain, ×600.

Biological Behavior

The incidence of ECC among gastrointestinal cancers is about 1% among esophageal tumors and 0.2% of colonic tumors. Gastric medullary ECC occurs in 0.1% of all gastric cancer. Gastric scirrhous ECC is seen in about 30% of gastric scirrhous carcinomas that correspond to Borrmann's type 4 carcinoma.

ECC of the esophagus and colon frequently occurs in 50–60 year old patients without a sex difference in its incidence. In gastric ECC, however, the ratio of male to female is 1.6 to 1 in the medullary type, but in the scirrhous type it is 1 to 1.3 (Table 6-4). Moreover, gastric scirrhous ECC evidently occurs in younger patients (30–40 years old) compared to those with gastric medullary ECC (50–60

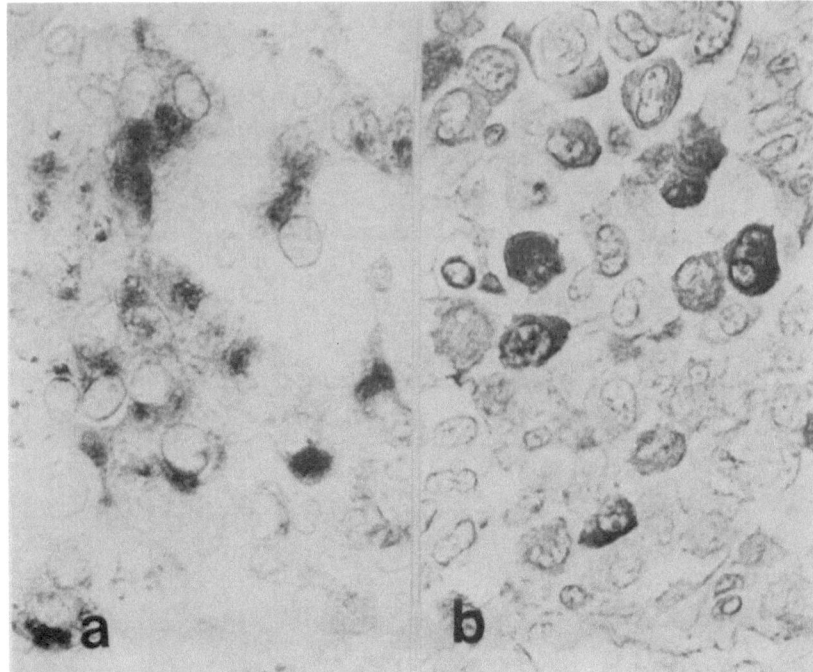

Fig. 6-14 a and b. The same tumor as in Fig. 10. Tumor cells show lysozyme- (a) and AAT- (b) immunoreactivity. ABC stain, ×600.

TABLE 6-3

Glycoprotein- and Enzyme-Immunoreactivity in ECC of the Gastrointestinal Tract

Localization	Subclassification	Number of Cases	Glycoprotein- and Enzyme-immunoreactivity[a]						
			CEA	S-100	NSE	hCG	Ly	AAT	SC
Esophagus	Medullary	2	2	0	0	0	0	0	0
Stomach	Medullary	16	13	1	6	1	9	9	8
	Scirrhous	14	14	3	4	6	10	3	11
Colon	Medullary	4	4	1	0	2	1	1	1

[a] CEA, carcinoembryonic antigen; S-100, S-100 protein; NSE, neuron specific enolase; hCG, human chorionic gonadotropin; Ly, lysozyme; AAT, α_1-antitrypsin.

years old) (Table 6-4). In addition, the mean age of the patients with gastric ECC is lower than that of the patients with gastric carcinoid.

Figure 6-15 shows a comparison of 5-year cumulative survival rates between ECC and carcinoid of the stomach. For gastric ECC the 5-year survival rate is under 40%, whereas that for gastric carcinoid is about 50%. Gastric ECC biologically shows a higher grade of malignancy than gastric carcinoid.

Mucocarcinoid

The tumors are composed of mucus-producing cells and endocrine cells. The former resemble goblet cells and form acinar or duc-

tal structures surrounded by a small number of endocrine cells (Fig. 6-16a). The endocrine cells usually show serotonin immunoreactivity (Fig. 6-16b). Mucocarcinoids frequently develop in the appendix.

Mucocarcinoids can be regarded as adenocarcinomas showing differentiation to both mucus-producing cells and endocrine cells and may correspond to the tumors described under the term "goblet-cell carcinoid"[28] or "mucinous carcinoid."[29]

Tumors with Endocrine Cells

Except for carcinoid and ECC, argyrophil cells or endocrine cells frequently occur in ordinary adenocarcinomas, adenomas and po-

TABLE 6-4

Sex and Age of Patients with Endocrine Tumors of the Gastrointestinal Tract

Site of Tumor	Classification of Tumor	Number of Cases	Female	Male	Mean Age, Years
Stomach	Carcinoid	9	3	6	67.1 ± 10.8[a]
	ECC				
	medullary	16	6	10	60.5 ± 8.7
	scirrhous	14	8	6	40.8 ± 8.3
Colon	Carcinoid	12	8	4	60.8 ± 15.8
	ECC, medullary	4	2	2	60.5 ± 8.6

[a] Mean age ± S.D.

→

Fig. 6-16 a and b. Mucocarcinoid of the appendix. (a) Tumor cells resembling goblet cells form acinar and tubular patterns. H&E, ×300. (b) The same tumor as in Fig. 16a. Serotonin-positive cells surround goblet tumor cells. ABC stain, ×500.

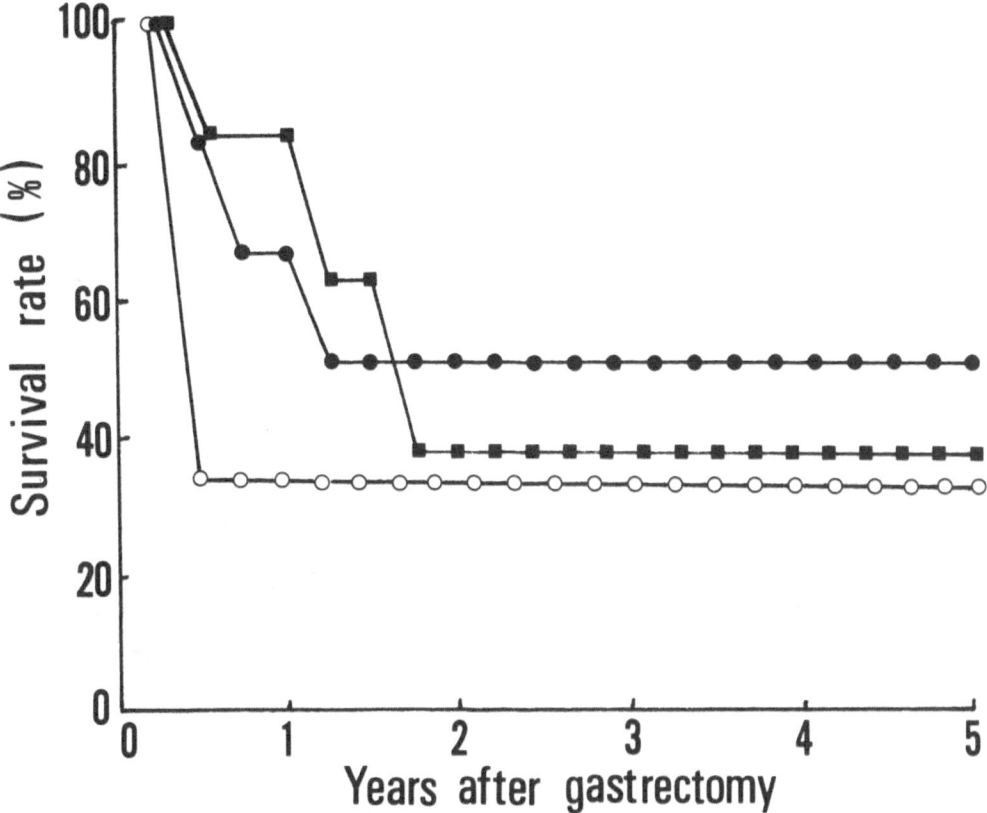

Fig. 6-15. Comparison of 5-year cumulative survival rates between ECC (Stages III and IV) and carcinoids of the stomach. Open circle: 3 cases of scirrhous ECC. Closed square: 6 cases of medullary ECC. Closed circle: 6 cases of carcinoid.

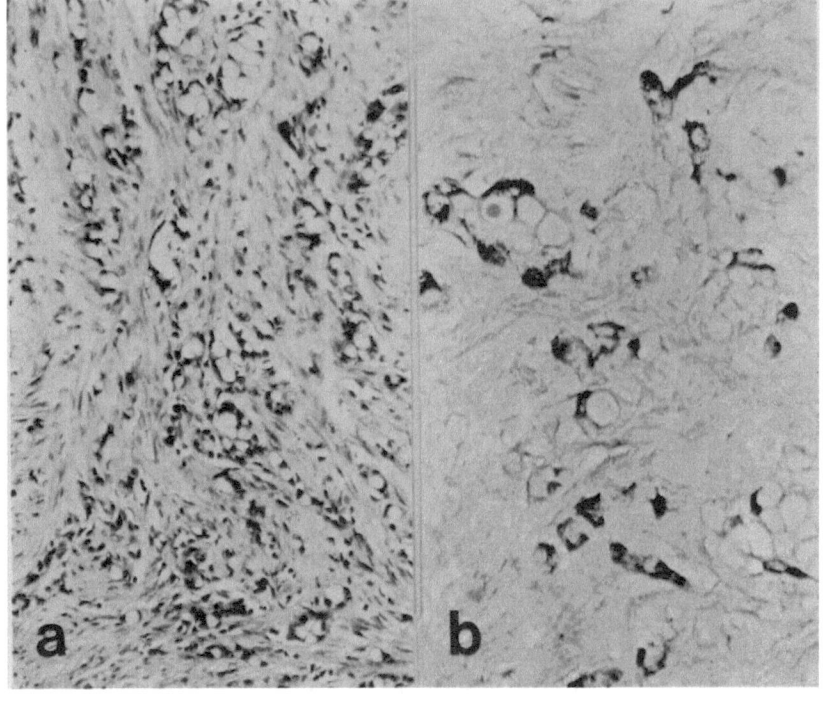

TABLE 6-5
Endocrine Cells in Adenocarcinoma of the Stomach

Stage	Histological Type[a]	Number of Cases	Peptide-Immunoreactivity				Argyrophil Cells
			Gastrin	Somat[b]	Glicentin	Calcitonin	
Early Cancer	Well	44	8(18.2)[c]	8(18.2)	3(6.8)	0	10(22.7)
	Poor	21	3(14.3)	2(9.5)	1(4.8)	0	4(19.0)
Advanced Cancer	Well	58	10(17.2)	10(17.2)	7(12.1)	0	12(26.7)[d]
	Poor	94	12(12.7)	19(20.2)	9(9.6)	12(12.7)	39(48.1)[d]

[a] Well: well differentiated adenocarcinoma; Poor: poorly differentiated adenocarcinoma.

[b] Somat: somatostatin.

[c] Values in parentheses represent incidence of cases with peptide-immunoreactivity or argyrophil cells (percentages).

[d] Significantly different ($P < 0.01$).

lyps of the GI tract. In ordinary adenocarcinomas, however, endocrine cells are present in a small number in the neoplastic glands, so that they constitute only a small portion of the tumor. The occurrence of endocrine cells differs by site, histological type, and depth of invasion of ordinary adenocarcinomas. In adenomas the number and distribution of endocrine cells are usually greater than those in ordinary adenocarcinomas.

Adenocarcinoma of the Stomach

The frequency of endocrine cells in gastric adenocarcinomas varies considerably in individual studies, but it may range from 20% to 30% of all gastric adenocarcinomas. Table 6-5 shows the incidence of endocrine cells in early and advanced adenocarcinoma of the stomach. In early gastric cancer, there is no significant difference in the incidence of endocrine cells between well differentiated adenocarcinoma and poorly differentiated adenocarcinoma, but in advanced cancer the incidence of argyrophil cells is higher in the poorly differentiated type (48%) than in the well differentiated type (26.7%), the difference being significant ($P < 0.01$).

By immunohistochemistry, the incidence of gastrin- and somatostatin-immunoreactivity in well differentiated adenocarcinoma is identical in early cancer (18.2%) and in advanced cancer (17.2%), and the ratio of gastrin to somatostatin is 1 to 1. This may correspond to the ratio of the number of gastrin-producing (G) cells to somatostatin producing (D) cells in human fetal antral mucosa at the end of gestation (Fig. 6-17.) On the other hand, in advanced poorly differentiated adenocarcinoma, gastrin- and somatostatin-positive tumor cells are detected in 13% and 20%, respectively, and the ratio is 1 to 1.5. The ratio in the tumor may correspond to that of the number of G cells to D cells in human fetal antral mucosa at six or seven months of gestation (Fig. 6-17). Glicentin-immunoreactive tumor cells are seen more frequently in the well differentiated type than in the poorly differentiated type, its incidence being from 7% to 12%. The occurrence of glicentin in gastric adenocarcinoma can be regarded as an expression of intestinal or fetal type endocrine cells. Glicentin is normally localized in adult small intestine and also in fetal fundic stomach. Calcitonin-immunoreactivity is seen only in advanced poorly differentiated adenocarcinoma, its incidence being about 13%. Calcitonin is present in normal antral mucosa and is immunohistochemically detected within G cells.[30]

Expression of peptide hormones in gastric adenocarcinoma is more closely related to patient age rather than to site of the tumor. When the frequency of peptides in poorly differentiated adenocarcinoma is compared between young patients (under 30 years old,

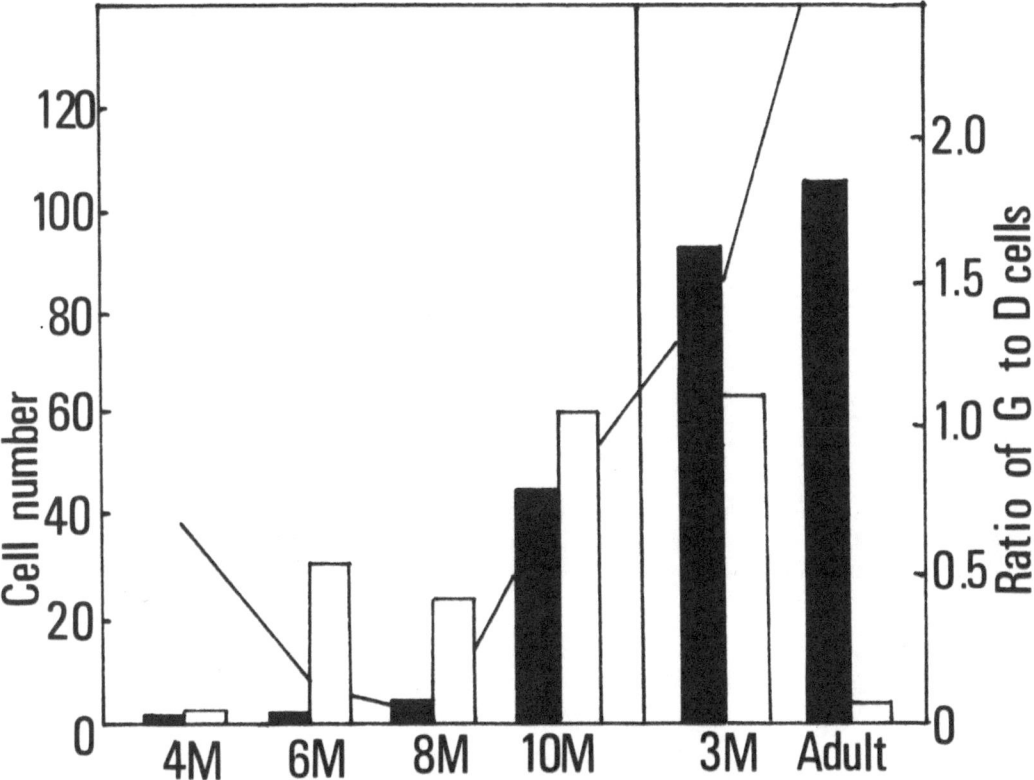

Fig. 6-17. The number of G cells and D cells in human fetal and newborn antral mucosa. Open column: The number of D cells among 1000 cells. Closed column: The number of G cells among 1000 cells. Diagonal line: The ratio of the number of G cells to D cells.

mean age 27.1 years, female 10 cases, male 18 cases) and older patients (over 70 years old, mean age 75.8, female 11 cases, male 13 cases), the frequency of somatostatin is significantly higher in aged patients than in young patients, whereas that of gastrin, glicentin and calcitonin is evidently higher in young patients (Table 6-6).

ECC was observed in five (17.9%) of the young patients, but only in one (4.2%) of the aged patients. Moreover, the simultaneous production of over two peptides is seen in six

TABLE 6-6
Comparison of the Incidence of Endocrine Cells in Poorly Differentiated Gastric Adenocarcinoma
Between Young Patients and Older Patients

Age	Number of Cases	Peptide-immunoreactivity				Argyrophil Cells	ECC
		Gastrin	Somat[a]	Glicentin	Calcitonin		
Young Patients (under 30 years old)	28	4(14.3)[b]	5(17.9)[c]	6(21.4)	5(17.9)	18(64.3)[c]	5(17.9)
Older Patients (over 70 years old)	24	1(4.2)	9(37.5)[c]	2(8.3)	1(4.2)	7(29.2)[c]	1(4.2)

[a] Somat: somatostatin.

[b] Values in parentheses represent incidence of cases with peptide-immunoreactivity, argyrophil cells and ECC (percentages).

[c] Significantly different (P<0.05).

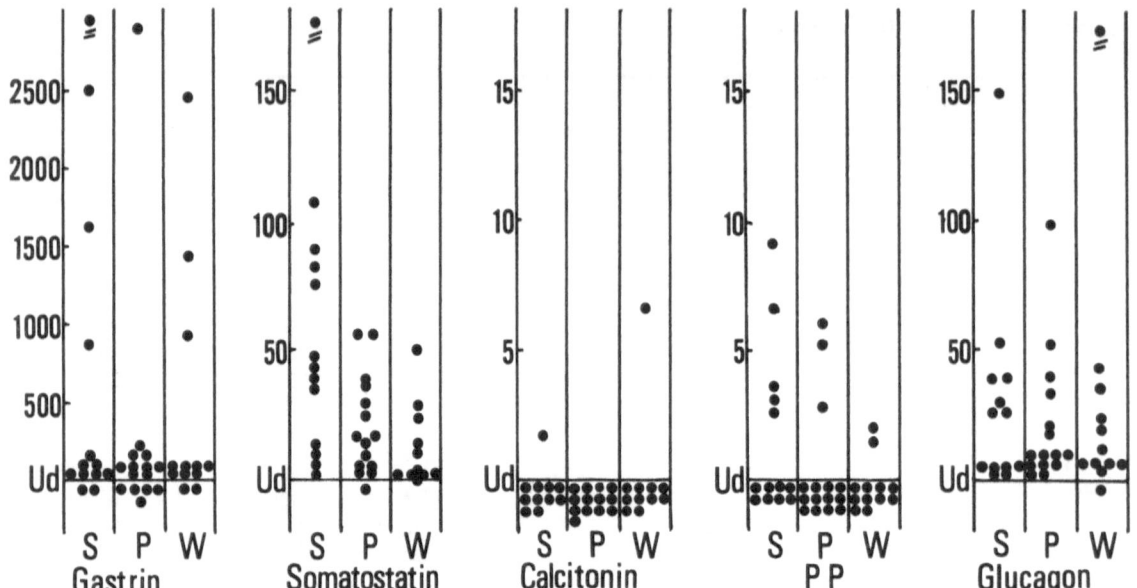

Fig. 6-18. Content of peptide hormones in gastric adenocarcinoma by radioimmunoassay.
Values are represented by ng/g wet weight. Ud: Undetectable. S: Scirrhous type. P: Poorly differentiated type. W: Well differentiated type.

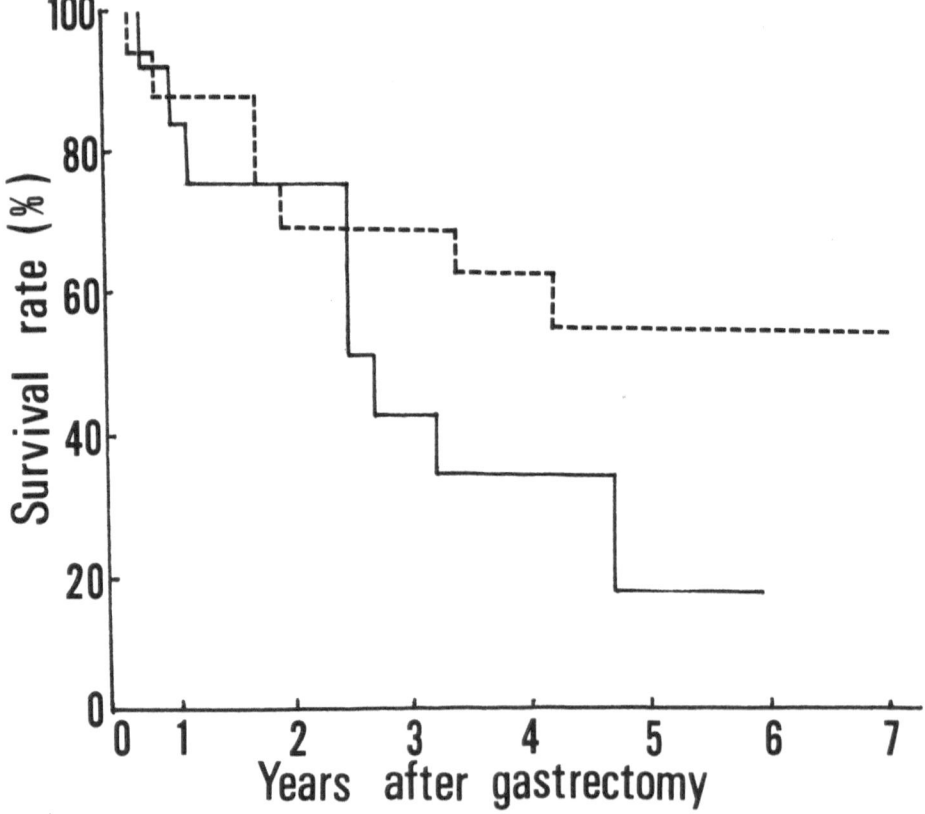

Fig. 6-19. Comparison of 7-year survival rates of Stages II and III gastric adenocarcinoma (poorly differentiated type) between patients with peptides and without peptides.
Continuous lines: 13 cases with peptide-producing cells (mean age, 69.1 yr). Dotted line: 17 cases without peptide-producing cells (mean age, 64.5 yr).

TABLE 6-7
Endocrine Cells in Adenocarcinoma of the Colon and Rectum

Localization	Number of Cases	Peptide-immunoreactivity[a]					Serotonin-immunoreactivity	Argyrophil Cells
		G	S	Glicentin	PP	Ca		
Right Colon	8	0	0	1(12.5%)	0	0	1(12.5%)	2(25.0%)
Trans. Colon[b]	15	0	0	2(13.3%)	0	0	0	5(33.3%)
Sigmoid Colon	27	0	0	0	0	0	1(3.7%)	5(18.5%)
Rectum	28	0	0	2(7.1%)	0	0	2(7.1%)	21(75.0%)
Total	78			5(6.4%)			4(5.1%)	33(42.3%)

[a] G: gastrin; S: somatostatin; PP: pancreatic polypeptide; Ca: calcitonin.

[b] Trans. colon: transverse colon.

(21.4%) of the young patients, but in only two (8.3%) of the older patients (Table 6-5). These findings suggest the possibility that rapid growth of gastric carcinoma in young patients is in part correlated with peptide expression within the tumor. By radioimmunoassay, various hormones such as gastrin, somatostatin, calcitonin, PP, and glucagon are detected. Gastrin and somatostatin content is higher in scirrhous carcinoma than in other histological types (Fig. 6-18).

When the 7-year survival rates of stages II and III advanced carcinomas (excluding scirrhous carcinomas) are compared for patients with peptide-positive and those negative for peptide hormones, the survival rate is 20% for the former, while that for latter is 50% (Fig. 6-19). Patients with peptide hormones evidently have a significantly poorer prognosis than those without peptide hormones (P < 0.05).

Adenocarcinoma of the Colon and Rectum

Colorectal adenocarcinomas as well as gastric adenocarcinomas have a variable number of endocrine cells.[31,32] The incidence of argyrophil cells is about 40% among all colorectal cancer.

Endocrine cell incidence is higher in rectal carcinoma than in colonic carcinoma and is also higher in well differentiated adenocarcinoma than in poorly differentiated adenocarcinoma.

Immunohistochemically, glicentin- and serotonin-positive tumor cells are found in 6.4% and 5.1%, respectively (Table 6-7). There is a case report of an ACTH-producing colon cancer.

No evident correlation exists between peptide expression within the tumor and prognosis of the patients.

Adenoma of the Stomach

Gastric tubular adenoma also has a marked heterogeneity, comprising SC producing epithelial cells, lysozyme-containing cells, CEA-producing cells, and endocrine cells. The incidence and distribution density of endocrine cells in gastric tubular adenoma are higher than those in gastric adenocarcinoma.

Serotonin-positive EC cells, often showing hyperplasia, occur most frequently (73.5%) throughout the tubular adenoma, followed by glicentin-(67.3%), somatostatin-(30.6%), motilin-(14.3%) and gastrin-(12.2%) positive tumor cells (Table 6-8). Glucagon-positive tumor cells are not seen in the gastric tubular adenoma. Most of these endocrine cells are located in deeper adenomatous glands. The number of endocrine cells markedly decreases with increase in the degree of atypicality of tubular adenomas, and there are no endocrine cells in the foci of carcinoma within some tu-

TABLE 6-8

Relationship between Histological Grade and Distribution Density of Endocrine Cells in Tubular
Adenomas

Histological Grade	Number of Cases	Cases with Endocrine Cell (%) Distribution Density of Endocrine Cells				
		EC-cell[a]	L-cell	D-cell	Mo-cell	G-cell
Mild	18	15(83.3%)	15(83.3%)	7(38.9%)	5(27.8%)	6(33.3%)
Atypia		222.6 ± 88.1[b,c]	97.3 ± 28.8	16.6 ± 13.9	7.4 ± 4.3	0.5 ± 0.2
Moderate	24	19(79.2%)	15(62.5%)	6(24.0%)	2(8.3%)	0
Atypia		101.7 ± 40.6	78.3 ± 33.7	7.3 ± 6.3	0.1 ± 0.01	
Severe	7	2(28.6%)	2(28.6%)	2(28.6%)	0	0
Atypia		2.7 ± 2.3	12.0 ± 6.7	2.3 ± 1.7		
Total	49	36(73.5%)	33(67.3%)	15(30.6%)	7(14.3%)	6(12.2%)

[a] EC-cell: serotonin-containing cell; L-cell: glicentin-containing cell; D-cell: somatostatin-containing cell; Mo-cell: motilin-containing cell; G-cell: gastrin-containing cell.

[b] Distribution density of each endocrine cell was obtained as follows: Total number of endocrine cells in tubular adenoma × 5 mm/diameter of adenoma (mm).

[c] Results are expressed as mean ± S.E.

bular adenomas. Similar changes are seen in lysozyme- and SC-positive cells as well.

Glicentin-containing L cells, which are not present in normal gastric mucosa, but preferentially appear in intestinal metaplasia, first occur in the gastric mucosa of the transitional area between metaplastic and intact gastric glands. They frequently show hyperplasia or micronoduli in the budding area of the deeper metaplastic glands (Fig. 6-20a,b,c),[26] but in completely intestinalized mucosa these endocrine cells decrease remarkably. In view of the localization of glicentin-positive cells in tubular adenoma and the physiological function of glicentin, which has a trophic action on intestinal epithelia and inhibits gastric acid secretion, the selective increase of glicentin-containing L cells in intestinal metaplasia may be correlated with the development of gastric tubular adenoma.

Adenoma of the Colon and Rectum

Colorectal adenoma also has a good number of endocrine cells, of which glicentin- and serotonin-positive cells are dominant, as in gastric adenoma. PYY producing cells are present in the colorectal mucosa and PYY and PP-immunoreactivity is also detected within L cells. There is a possibility that colorectal adenoma has PYY- or PP-positive cells. The occurrence of endocrine cells has the tendency to increase in adenomas of the lower large intestine rather than in those of the upper large intestine. Malignant changes in colorectal adenoma induce a decrease in the number of endocrine cells within the tumor.

Hyperplasia of Endocrine Cells

Hyperplasia of G cells is seen in the antrum of patients with Zollinger-Ellison syndrome type I or duodenal ulcer showing hypergastrinemia.

Micronoduli, which are composed of 4 to 5 endocrine cells, frequently occur not only in chronic atrophic gastritis, but also in the gastric mucosa adjacent to gastric ulcer, carcinoma, and adenoma. Endocrine cell types of micronoduli include G cells, EC cells, and L cells. Hyperplasia of D cells is not seen and D

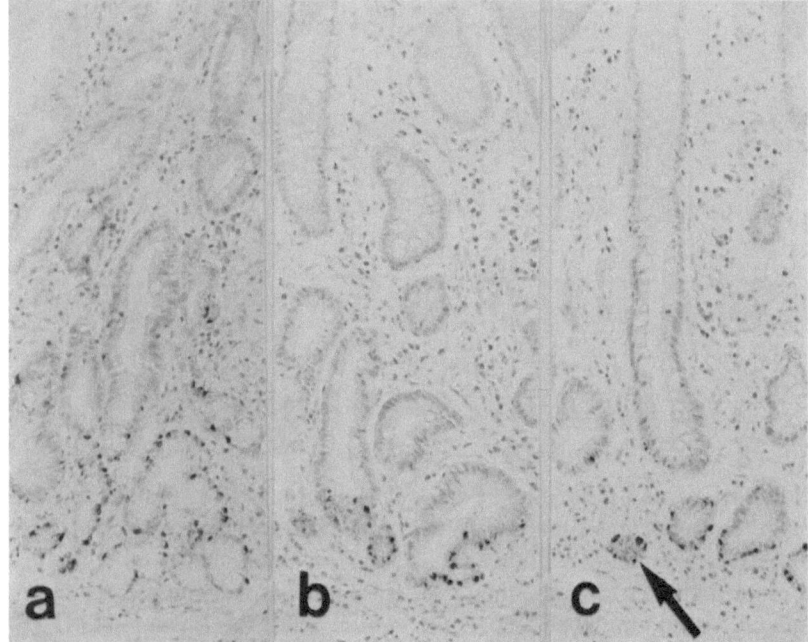

Fig. 6-20 a, b and c. (a) and (b) significant numbers of glicentin-immunoreactive cells are found in the deeper portion of intestinal metaplasia, showing budding, PAP stain, ×160. (c) Micronodule composed of glicentin-positive cells (arrow). PAP stain, ×160.

cells rapidly decrease with extension of intestinal metaplasia. In pernicious anemia and severe atrophic gastritis associated with hypergastrinemia, multifocal hyperplasia of ECL cells frequently occurs and may on occasion develop into carcinoid.[15,33] Micronoduli of endocrine cells are derived not from "neuroendocrine cells"[34] or "stromal endocrine cells"[35] in the lamina propria mucosae, but from endocrine cells of gastric glands.

In the colorectal mucosa, micronoduli of endocrine cells are rare, compared with those in gastric mucosa. In familial polyposis, multiple micronoduli of endocrine cells and microcarcinoid may on occasion occur.

HISTOGENESIS OF ENDOCRINE TUMORS

The relationship between endocrine cells in the GI tract and endocrine or other tumors can be analyzed as follows: (1) classical carcinoids of endocrine cell origin, (2) ECC, and (3) endocrine cell clones scattered in the tumor (Fig. 6-21).[36,37] As for its origin ECC has several possibilities, such as epithelial stem cells, endocrine cells, carcinoid, and endocrine cell clones within adenocarcinoma. In view of the morphological and functional heterogeneity of ECC, totipotent stem cells and endocrine cell clones in adenocarcinoma may be the most closely related to the development of ECC. Endocrine cell clones in the tumor may not originate from endocrine cells, but may be based on differentiation of some tumor cells into endocrine cells. There is an interesting theory of "cell hybridization," which postulates that hybridization of tumor cells with endocrine cells will progress into a tumor with mixed cell populations.[5]

Production processes of peptide hormones by tumor cells essentially seem to be the same as those of normal endocrine cells but larger molecule types of hormones or fragments are detected more frequently in the tumors than

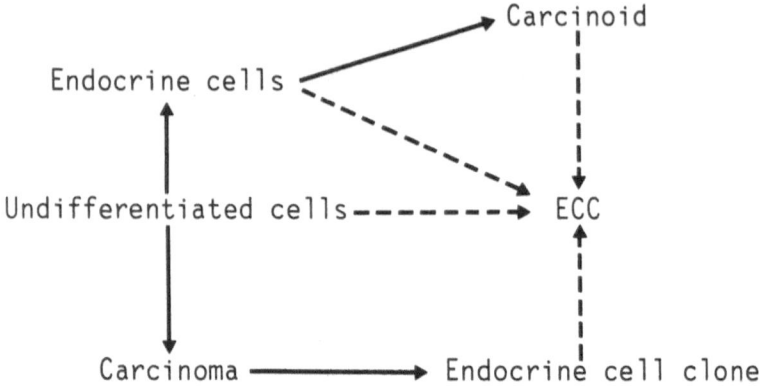

Fig. 6-21. Relation between GI endocrine cells and tumors.

in normal endocrine tissue.[38] This may be accounted for by the abnormal processing of prohormone after translation, involving a deficiency of processing enzymes or enhancement of processing within tumor cells. The differences in regulatory gene expression between peptide hormone-producing tumors and normal endocrine tissues should be elucidated in the future.

PEPTIDE HORMONES, GROWTH FACTORS AND ONCOGENE PRODUCTS

Gut hormones as well as growth factors regulate the growth and differentiation of GI epithelial cells through endocrine and paracrine mechanisms. Gastrin, CCK, glicentin, and glucagon have growth-trophic actions on target cells specifically and they can be regarded as "growth factors." These peptides also stimulate the growth of tumor cells of GI carcinomas both in vitro and in vivo.[39–42] The growth of human gastric carcinoma cell line TMK-1, which shows parietal cell differentiation (Fig. 6-22), is promoted by gastrin in a dose-dependent manner (Fig. 6-23).[42] These data suggest that some of the GI carcinomas have peptide hormone receptors and that their growth is stimulated by peptides derived from tumor cells themselves through endocrine, paracrine or autocrine secretion in vivo.

Many biological events caused by peptide hormones are linked to cAMP metabolism. cAMP production and cAMP-dependent protein kinase are responsible for the growth-promoting effect of gastrin on TMK-1 and xenotransplantable human gastric carcinoma SC-6-JCK.[40,42] cAMP-dependent protein kinase is classified into type I and type II isoenzymes according to differences in the molecular form of the regulatory subunits. Type I isoenzyme is involved in cell growth and transformation, while type II isoenzyme is involved in differentiation and inhibition of cell growth. The proportion of type I isoenzyme is significantly elevated in human gastric carcinoma in comparison with normal gastric mucosa (Table 6-9).[43] Moreover, type I cAMP-dependent protein kinase can play an important role in the enhanced effect of gastrin on rat stomach carcinogenesis induced by N-methyl-N′-nitro-N-nitrosoguanidine.[44] cAMP-dependent protein kinase and oncogenic tyrosine kinase comprise a single divergent gene family, owing to the homology of amino acid sequences.[45] In addition, G protein regulating cAMP metabolism shares a limited sequence homology with *ras* oncogene product p21.[46]

On one hand, gastrin and the transforming protein (middle T-antigen) of polyoma virus may have evolved from a common ancestor because of their highly homologous amino acid sequences.[47] Furthermore, epidermal growth factor (EGF) receptor has a close se-

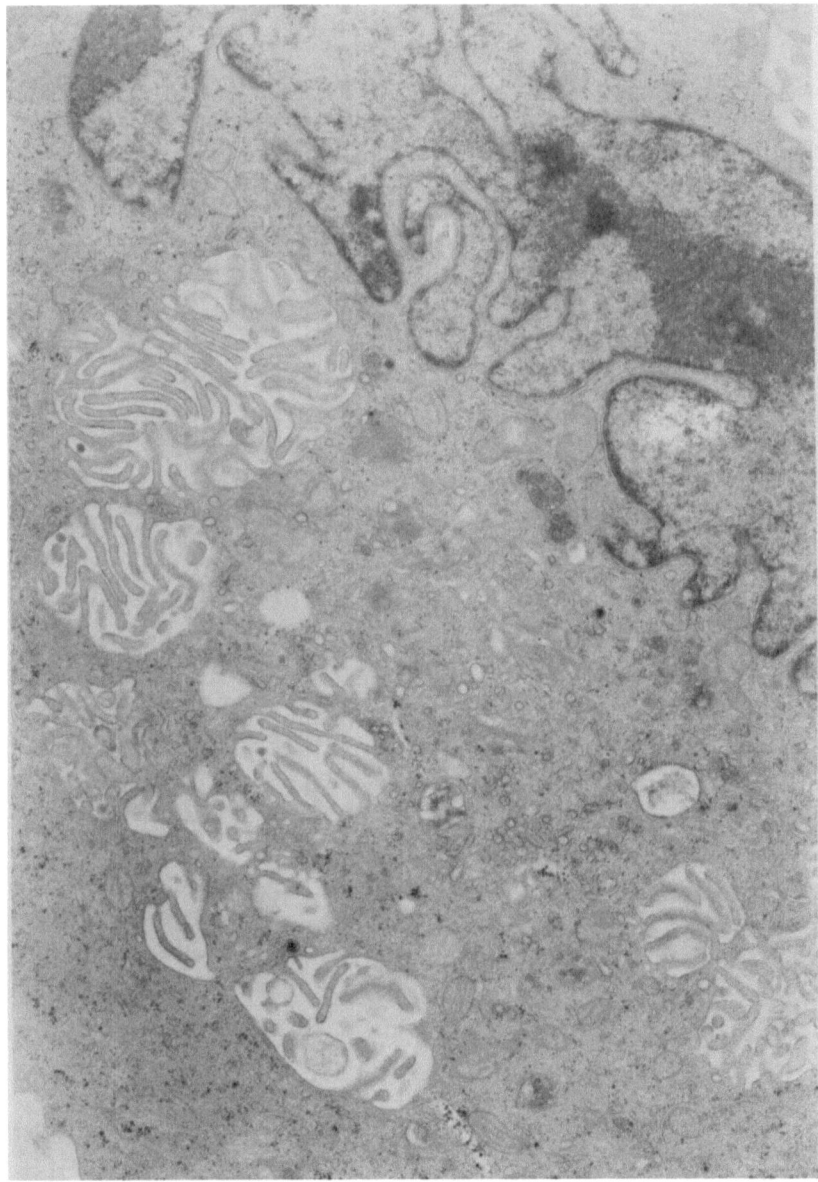

Fig. 6-22. Ultrastructure of TMK-1 cells. The tumor cell shows parietal cell differentiation characterized by abundant mitochondria, tubulovesicles and intracellular canaliculi filled with numerous microvilli. ×20,000.

quence homology with erythroblastosis virus oncogene protein (*erb*-B). The relation between "growth factors" or their receptors and oncogenes or oncogene products provides a clue in clarifying "autocrine secretion" for self-stimulation, whereby a tumor cell secretes peptides for which the tumor cell itself has peptide receptors.

Endocrine tumors of the GI tract as well as ordinary carcinomas produce human EGF (Fig. 6-24a).[49] It is detected in 11% of gastric carcinoid and in 21% of gastric scirrhous ECC (Table 6-10). The incidence of human EGF expression in gastric carcinoid is clearly lower than that in advanced gastric carcinomas. Transforming growth factor (TGF)α, which

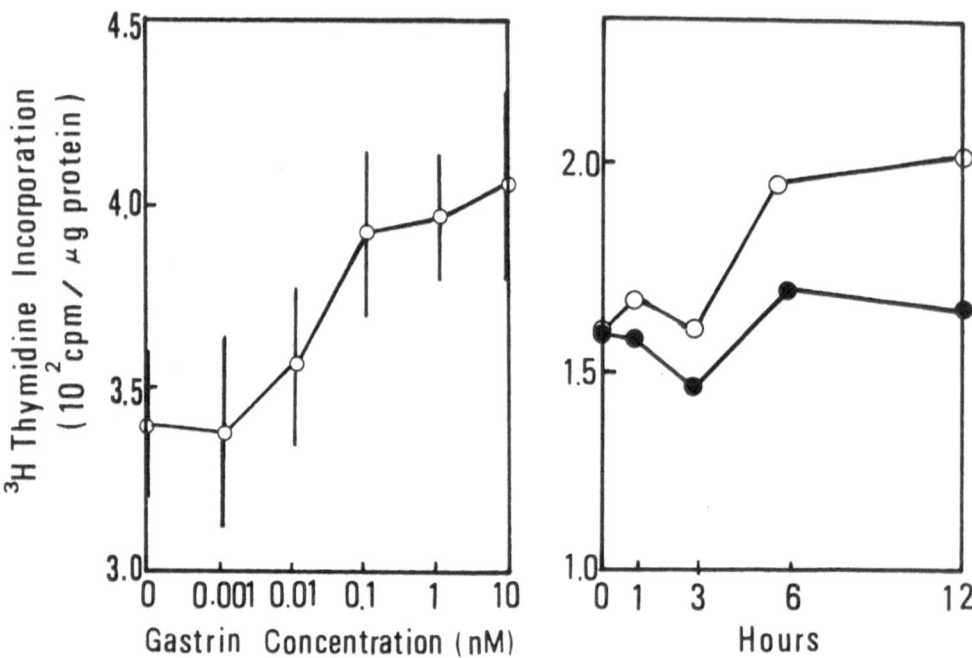

Fig. 6-23. Gastrin stimulated DNA synthesis of TMK-1 cells.[42] (Left) Gastrin dose-dependent curve. Points: Mean of 3 experiments. Bars: S.D. (Right) Time course of gastrin stimulated DNA synthesis. Open circle: Addition of 10 nM human gastrin. Closed circle: Addition of phosphate buffered saline. Points: Mean of 3 experiments.

TABLE 6-9

The Proportion of Types I and II cAMP-Dependent Protein Kinase in Human Gastric Mucosa and Carcinoma[43]

| | Relative Activity[a](%) | | |
	Type I	Type II	Type I: Type II
Normal Mucosa	16.2 ± 1.21^b	78.5 ± 2.03	5.01 ± 0.59
Fundus	14.9	80.7	5.60
Antrum	18.2	75.2	4.13
Gastric Carcinoma			
Well[c]	24.7 ± 3.00	64.0 ± 1.57	2.75 ± 0.38
Poorly[c]	22.9 ± 1.00	70.4 ± 2.10	3.04 ± 0.17
SC-6-JCK[d]	34.0 ± 3.00^e	55.2 ± 4.83^e	1.70 ± 0.30^e
St-15[d]	30.6 ± 1.73^e	54.3 ± 3.97^e	1.81 ± 0.21^e

[a] The proportion of Types I and II in total cAMP-dependent protein kinase activity eluted from DEAE-cellulose column.

[b] Mean $\pm$ S.E. from at least 4 experiments.

[c] Well: well differentiated adenocarcinoma, Poorly: poorly differentiated adenocarcinoma.

[d] Xenotransplantable human gastric carcinomas in nude mice.

[e] Significantly different from normal gastric mucosa ($P<0.05$).

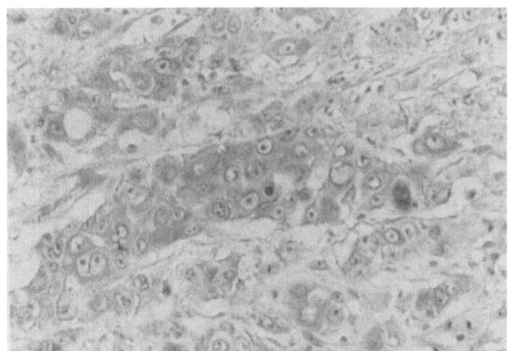
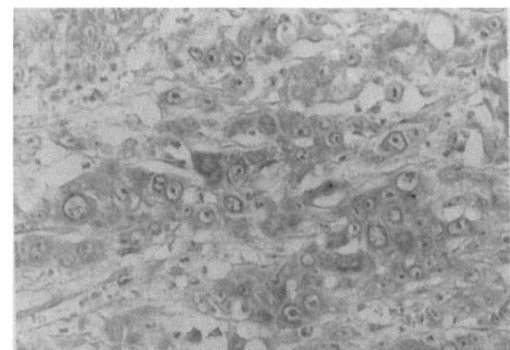
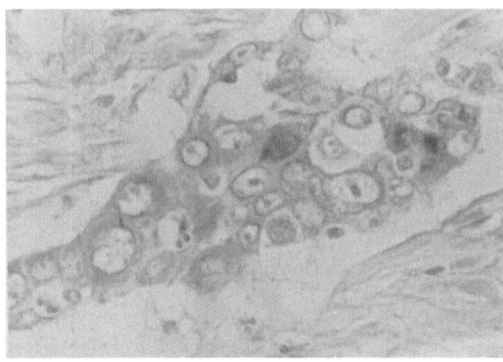

Fig. 6-24 a, b and c. The same tumor as in Fig. 6a. Tumor cells of medullary ECC show immunoreactivity for human EGF (a, color), TGFα (b, color) and Ha-*ras* p21 (c, color) synchronously. ABC stain, ×600.

TABLE 6-10

Growth Factors- and Ha-*ras* p21-Immunoreactivity in Endocrine
Tumors of the Stomach

Endocrine Tumors	Number of Cases	Immunoreactivity[a]		
		EGF	TGFα	p21
Carcinoid	9	1 (11.1%)	1 (11.1%)	1 (11.1%)
ECC				
Medullary	16	1 (6.2%)	6 (37.5%)	4 (25.0%)
Scirrhous	14	3 (21.4%)	6 (42.8%)	1 (30.6%)

[a] EGF: epidermal growth factor; TGFα: transforming growth factor α.

has sequence homology to EGF and competes with EGF for binding to the EGF receptor,[50] is detected in 11% of gastric carcinoid and in 40% of gastric ECC (Fig. 6-24b). Expression of Ha-*ras* oncogene product p21 in gastric medullary ECC (25%) is also higher than that in gastric carcinoid (11%) (Table 6-10, Fig. 6-24c). GI hormones, growth factors or their receptors and *ras* oncoprotein may be closely interrelated with growth and invasiveness of ECC. Moreover, calcium-activated, phospholipid-dependent protein kinase (protein kinase C), which is activated by many growth factors and phorbol esters, is considered to play an important role in cellular proliferation. Protein kinase C activity in the soluble fraction in human gastric carcinoma is significantly higher than that in nonneoplastic gas-

TABLE 6-11

Distribution of Protein Kinase C in Soluble and Particulate Fractions of Gastric Mucosa and Carcinoma[51]

| | Protein Kinase C Activity[a] | | | | |
| | Soluble Fraction | | Particulate Fraction | | Total Activity in Soluble Fraction (%) |
Tissue	units/g tissue	units/g protein	units/g tissue	units/g protein	
Gastric Mucosa (8)[b]	11.19 ± 1.12[c]	215.3 ± 23.5	2.40 ± 0.41	111.5 ± 15.7	81.4 ± 39.5
Fundus (4)	10.61	224.0	2.34	110.5	81.0
Antrum (4)	11.77	206.5	2.45	112.6	81.8
Gastric Cancer (8)	18.13 ± 1.92[d]	357.7 ± 57.5[e]	2.16 ± 0.52	86.7 ± 20.8	89.5 ± 19.3
Well[f] (4)	19.53	396.9	1.29	41.7	93.8
Poorly (4)	16.74	318.5	3.03	131.7	85.3

[a] Each tissue was homogenized and centrifuged. The supernatant was employed as soluble fraction and the precipitate was resuspended, sonicated and treated with Triton X-100.

[b] Numbers in parentheses are numbers of experiments.

[c] Mean ± S.E.

[d] Value is significantly higher than that in nonneoplastic mucosa ($P<0.01$).

[e] Value is significantly higher than that in nonneoplastic mucosa ($P<0.05$).

[f] Well: well differentiated adenocarcinoma; Poorly: poorly differentiated adenocarcinoma.

tric mucosa (Table 6-11).[51] Further study is necessary to clarify the interaction between protein kinase C and gut hormones in the growth of ECC.

REFERENCES

1. Solcia E., Polak J.M., Larsson L.I., et al: Update on Lausanne classification of endocrine cells, in Bloom S.R., Polak J.M. (eds): Gut Hormones. London, Churchill Livingstone, 1981, pp 96–100
2. Azzopardi J.G., Pollock J.M.: Argentaffin and argyrophil cells in gastric carcinoma. J Pathol Bacteriol 86:443, 1963.
3. Kubo T., Watanabe H.: Neoplastic argentaffin cells in gastric and intestinal carcinomas. Cancer 27:447, 1971
4. Tahara E., Ito H., Nakagami K., et al: Scirrhous argyrophil cell carcinoma of the stomach with mutliple production of polypeptide hormones, amines, CEA, lysozyme and HCG. Cancer 49:1904, 1982
5. Tahara E., Ito H., Shimamoto F., et al: Argyrophil cells in early gastric carcinoma: An immunohistochemical and ultrastructural study. J Cancer Res Clin Oncol 103:187, 1982
6. Soga J., Tazawa K., Aizawa O., et al: Argentaffin cell adenocarcinoma of the stomach. Cancer 28:999, 1971
7. Sweeney E.C., McDonnell L.: Atypical gastric carcinoids. Histopathology 4:215, 1980
8. Chejfec G., Gould V.E.: Malignant gastric neuroendocrinomas: Ultrastructural and biochemical characterization of their secretory activity. Human Pathol 8:433, 1977

9. Gould V.E., Memoli V.A., Sobel H.J., et al.: Neuroendocrine carcinomas with multiple immunoreactive peptides and melanin production. Ultrastructural Pathol 2:199, 1981
10. Reyes C.V., Chejfec G., Jao W., Gould V.E.: Neuroendocrine carcinomas of the esophagus. Ultrastructural Pathol 1:367, 1980
11. Soga J., Tazawa K.: Pathologic analysis of carcinoids: Histologic reevaluation of 62 cases. Cancer 28:990, 1971
12. Williams E.D., Siebenmann R.E., Sobin L.H.: Histological classification of tumors of the diffuse endocrine system, in Histological Typing of Endocrine Tumors No. 23. Geneva, World Health Organization, 1980
13. Soga J.: Carcinoid syndrome. Surgery (Tokyo) 45:1359, 1983
14. Capella C., Polak J.M., Frigerio B., Solcia E.: Gastric carcinoids of argyrophil ECL cells. Ultrastructural Pathol 1:411, 1980
15. Taniyama K., Tahara E., Yamamoto M., Harada T.: A case of multiple microcarcinoids of the stomach. Pathol Clin Med 3:554, 1985
16. Alumets J., Hakanson R., Ingemansson S., Sundler F.: Substance P and 5-HT in granules isolated from an intestinal argentaffin carcinoid. Histochemistry 52:217, 1977
17. Wilander E., El-Salhy M., Lundzvist M., et al: Polypeptide YY (PYY) and pancreatic polypeptide (PP) in rectal carcinoids. Virchow Arch Pathol Anat 401:67, 1983
18. Solt J., Kadas I., Polak J.M., et al.: A pancreatic polypeptide-producing tumor of the stomach. Cancer 54:1101, 1984
19. Tsutsumi Y.: Neuroendocrine and related substances. Pathol Clin Med 2:1610, 1984

20. Sano T., Hizawa K., Shimoda T.: Demonstration of peptide hormone-immunoreactive cells in classical carcinoids and allied tumors: A histological and immunohistochemical study. Pathol Clin Med 1:1315, 1983

21. Yang K., Ulich T., Cheng L., Wewin K.J.: The neuroendocrine products of intestinal carcinoids: An immunoperoxidase study of 35 carcinoid tumors stained for serotonin and eight polypeptide hormones. Cancer 51:1918, 1983

22. Creutzfeldt W., Arnold R., Creutzfeldt C., Track N.S.: Pathomorphologic, biochemical and diagnostic aspects of gastrinomas (Zollinger-Ellison syndrome). Human Pathol 6:47, 1975

23. O'Neal L.W., Kipnis D.M., Luse S.A., et al.: Secretion of various substances by ACTH-secreting tumors—gastrin, melanotropin, norepinephrine, serotonin, parathormone, vasopressin, glucagon, Cancer 21:1219, 1968

24. Hata J., Taniyama K., Tahara E., et al.: Functional differentiation of gastrointestinal carcinoids. In Proceedings 42nd Annual Meeting Japanese Cancer Association, Nagoya, Japan, p 358, 1983

25. Hata J., Ito H., Tahara E., et al.: Immunohistochemical study of human gastrointestinal carcinoid: Special reference to the distribution of NSE and S-100 protein. In Proceedings 43rd Annual Meeting Japanese Cancer Association, Fukuoka, Japan, p 381, 1984

26. Ito H., Yokozaki H., Tahara E., et al.: Glicentin-containing cells in intestinal metaplasia, adenoma and carcinoma of the stomach. Virchow Arch Pathol Anat 404:17, 1984

27. Thomas R.U., Lorna C., Henry G., et al.: A colonic adenocarcinoma with argentaffin cells: An immunoperoxidase study demonstrating the presence of numerous neuroendocrine products. Cancer 51:1483, 1983

28. Warner T.F.C.S., Seo I.S.: Goblet cell carcinoid of appendix: Ultrastructural features and histogenetic aspects. Cancer 44:1700, 1979

29. Olsson B., Ljungberg O.: Adenocarcinoid of the vermiform appendix. Virchow Arch Pathol Anat 386:201, 1980

30. Ito H., Hata J., Tahara E., et al.: Immunohistochemical localization of calcitonin in human gastric mucosa and tumor tissue. IGAKU NO AYUMI 131:315, 1984

31. Iwashita A.: Argentaffin and argyrophil cells in colonic carcinomas. Fukuoka J Med 70:370, 1979

32. Smith D.M., Haggitt R.C.: The prevalence and prognostic significance of argyrophil cells in colorectal carcinomas. Am J Surg Pathol 8:123, 1984

33. Grigioni W.F., Caletti G.C., Gabrielli M., Marrano D.: Gastric carcinoids of ECL cells: Pathological and clinical analysis of eight cases. Acta Pathol Jpn 35:361, 1985

34. Rode J., Dhillon A.P., Papadaki L., Griffiths D.: Neurosecretory cells of the lamina propria of the appendix and their possible relationship to carcinoids. Histopathology 6:69, 1982

35. Stachura J., Kause W.J., Jivey K.: Ultrastructure of endocrine-like cells in lamina propria of human gastric mucosa. Gut 22:534, 1981

36. Tahara E., Haizuka S., Kodama T., Yamada A.: The relationship of gastrointestinal endocrine cells to gastric epithelial changes with special reference to gastric cancer. Acta Pathol Jpn 25:161, 1975

37. Black W.C.: Enterochromaffin cell types and corresponding carcinoid tumors. Laboratory Invest 19:473, 1968

38. Yamaguchi K., Abe K.: Clinical and endocrinological aspects of pancreatic endocrine tumors. Pathol Clin Med 2:467, 1984

39. Kobori O., Vuillot M.T., Martin F.: Growth response of rat stomach cancer cells to gastro-entero-pancreatic hormones. Int J Cancer 30:65, 1982

40. Sumiyoshi H., Yasui W., Ochiai A., Tahara E.: Effects of gastrin on tumor growth and cyclic nucleotide metabolism in xenotransplantable human gastric and colonic carcinomas in nude mice. Cancer Res 44:4276, 1984

41. Murakami H., Masui H.: Hormonal control of human colon carcinoma cell growth in serum-free medium. Proc Natl Acad Sci USA 77:3464, 1980

42. Ochiai A., Yasui W., Tahara E.: Growth promoting effect of gastrin on human gastric carcinoma cell line TMK-1. Jpn J Cancer Res (Gann) 76:1064, 1985

43. Yasui W., Sumiyoshi H., Tahara E., et al: Type I and II cyclic adenosine 3':5'-monophosphate-dependent protein kinase in human gastric mucosa and carcinomas. Cancer Res 45:1565, 1985

44. Yasui W., Tahara E.: Effects of gastrin on gastric mucosal cyclic adenosine 3':5'-monophosphate-dependent protein kinase activity in rat stomach carcinogenesis induced by N-methyl-N'-nitro-N-nitrosoguanidine. Cancer Res 45:4767, 1985

45. Baldwin G.S.: Gastrin and the transforming protein of polyoma virus have evolved from a common ancestor. FEBS Lett 137:1, 1982

46. Hurley J.B., Simon M.I., Gilman A.G., et al.: Homologies between signal transducing G proteins and ras gene products. Science 226:860, 1984.

47. Kamps M.P., Taylor S.S., Sefton B.M.: Direct evidence that oncogenic tyrosine kinase and cyclic AMP-dependent protein kinase have homologous ATP-binding sites. Nature (London) 310:589, 1984

48. Downward J., Yarden Y., Waterfield M.D., et al: Close similarity of epidermal growth factor receptor and v-erb B oncogene protein sequences. Nature (London) 307:521, 1984

49. Tahara E., Sumiyoshi H., Sakamoto S., et al: Human epidermal growth factor in gastric carcinoma as a biologic marker of high malignancy. Jpn J Cancer Res (Gann) (in press), 1986

50. Reynolds F.H., Todaro G.J., Fryling C., Stephenson J.R.: Human transforming growth factors induce tyrosine phosphorylation of EGF receptors. Nature (London) 292:259, 1981

51. Yasui W., Sumiyoshi H., Ochiai A., Tahara E.: Calcium-activated, phospholipid-dependent protein kinase in human gastric mucosa and carcinoma. Jpn J Cancer Res (Gann) 76:1164, 1985

7

Immunohistochemical Localization of Chromogranin and Neuron Specific Enolase in Gastroenteropancreatic Tumors

Ricardo V. Lloyd M.D., Ph.D.

Chromogranin and neuron specific enolase (NSE) are present in most neuroendocrine cells and tumors of the diffuse neuroendocrine system (DNES). Silver stains such as argyrophil and argentaffin stains can be used to determine if a certain cell or tumor belongs to the DNES. However, the use of well characterized polyclonal antisera or monoclonal antibodies for the immunohistochemical study of neuroendocrine cells and tumors offers the advantages of greater specificity, reproducibility, and sensitivity intrinsic to immunohistochemical procedures. The combination of chromogranin and NSE immunostaining in examining cells and tumors for neuroendocrine features has many advantages. Among these are (1) the use of two or more markers in immunohistochemical procedures, which increases the sensitivity of the method and the reliability of a positive result, especially if both markers are positive; (2) demonstration that the intracytoplasmic target structures of chromogranin and NSE are different, so a cell may express at least one of these two markers, if not both; and (3) evidence of some gastroenteropancreatic (GEP) cells and tumors that are producing peptides and other products, which have not been characterized as

yet, so specific antisera are not available to examine these lesions. The use of chromogranin and NSE can be extremely helpful in revealing the neuroendocrine features of such lesions.

IMMUNOHISTOCHEMICAL PROCEDURES

As with most other procedures, familiarity with all aspects of the techniques is essential for correct interpretation. Knowledge about the distribution and chemical composition of the antigens used to produce the antibodies, the specificity, cross-reactivity, and other features of the antibodies are critical for proper interpretation of immunohistochemical staining.

NEURON SPECIFIC ENOLASE

Moore and his co-workers[1,2] isolated two proteins S-100 and 14-3-2 from bovine brain. Antibodies developed against 14-3-2 showed that this protein was present predominantly in neurons, while S-100 protein was found mostly in glial cells. Marangos et al[3-6] characterized the 14-3-2 protein, which was initially called neuron-specific protein. It was subsequently shown that protein 14-3-2 was localized in neuronal cells within the brain and in peripheral nervous tissue with the use of specific antisera to this protein, and neuron-specific protein was designated as neuron specific enolase (NSE).[7] Subsequent studies revealed that NSE was an isoenzyme of the glycolytic enzyme enolase.[8] Further work indicated that NSE was present in most tissues of the DNES.[9,10] There are several forms of enolase that exist in the brain and other tissues. NSE has a molecular weight of 78,000 daltons and is composed of two subunits designated as $\gamma\gamma$. This form of enolase is present in neurons, peripheral nerves and cells of the DNES.

Nonneuronal enolase (NNE) is composed of two α subunits and has a molecular weight of 87,000 daltons. It is present in glial cells in the brain and in liver cells. A hybrid enolase of molecular weight 82,500 is composed of a α and a γ subunit.[6,8] The distribution of the α isoenzyme has not been well characterized in the brain. The $\beta\beta$ isoenzyme of enolase is present predominantly in muscle tissues. Because of the overlapping subunit structures between NSE and the hybrid enolase it becomes critical to characterize anti-NSE antisera rigorously before they can be used as a specific marker for NSE.

A few commercial laboratories have produced antisera against NSE. These and other polyclonal antisera have been used by many investigators as research and as diagnostic tools. Several reports indicate that some antisera presumed to be specific for NSE reacted with many nonendocrine tissues, and this raised many questions about the specificity of NSE as a marker for the DNES.[10-15] However, well characterized antisera against NSE were used by several investigators to study neuroendocrine cells and tumors, and only occasional instances of reactivity were observed.[16-20] NSE is also a valuable serum marker for small cell carcinoma of the lung and neuroblastomas.[21-22] Patients with these

neoplasms often have elevated serum levels of NSE, especially with metastatic disease, and the serum elevation of NSE may be related to the patient's prognosis.[6]

To avoid some of the problems with the specificity of polyclonal antisera, some investigators are producing monoclonal antibodies against NSE. A recent report indicated that a highly specific monoclonal antibody that did not cross-react with NSE reacted with frozen sections of normal brain tissues and small cell carcinomas of the lung.[23] A preliminary report also suggested that a monoclonal antibody against NSE was more specific than a heterologous antiserum tested for the diagnosis of neuroendocrine and other tumors.[24] If these reports can be corroborated, monoclonal antibodies against NSE may eliminate some of the problems with cross reactivity that are sometimes encountered when immunostaining is done with polyclonal antisera against NSE.

The ultrastructural localization of NSE in rat and mouse brain has shown that this enzyme is present in neuronal perikarya and is associated with ribosomes, granular rough endoplasmic reticulum and microtubules.[25]

Chromogranin

The chromogranins, a family of acidic protein molecules, have been known to be present in the adrenal medulla for some time.[26-31] Chromogranin A comprises about 40–50% of the total soluble proteins of fractionated granules. It has a molecular weight between 68,000–81,000 daltons, depending on the species of animals and the electrophoretic system used to analyze the proteins.[28] Other chromogranin molecules of different molecular weights have also been identified.[27] Human chromogranin A has a molecular weight of 68,000 daltons. Other chromogranins with higher molecular weights have also been recently described.[31]

The ubiquitous distribution of this family of proteins in most endocrine cells with secretory granules was described recently with the development of polyclonal antisera and monoclonal antibodies against chromogranin.[32-40] A recent study suggested that chromogranin immunoreactivity is also present in lymphoid cells in the spleen, lymph node, thymus, and fetal liver of rats in addition to the cells of the DNES.[41]

The immunohistochemical localization of chromogranin in some cells of the central nervous system that forms part of the DNES varied depending on the antiserum used. While some investigators found chromogranin immunoreactivity in the CNS with the use of polyclonal antisera against bovine chromogranins,[37,38] others did not observe such immunoreactivity with other polyclonal antisera against bovine chromogranin,[33] with a polyclonal antiserum against human chromogranin,[31] or with a monoclonal antibody against human chromogranin.[34,35]

Immunoreactivity in different cells of the pituitary and the GEP axis also varied with the antibody being used.[33-36,39,42,43] Ultrastructural immunohistochemical localization of chromogranin showed that it is associated with endocrine secretory granules in the adrenal medulla,[35] pituitary,[44] and pancreas.[40] Chromogranin A has also been detected in the serum of normal patients and in patients with pheochromocytomas, so it may also be a potential serum marker for patients with neuroendocrine tumors.[45]

IMMUNOHISTOCHEMICAL LOCALIZATION OF NSE AND CHROMOGRANIN IN NORMAL GASTROENTEROPANCREATIC TISSUES

NSE has been localized in all of the normal islet cells of the pancreas (Fig. 7-1).[16,18] NSE has also been found in all currently identifiable endocrine cell types and in nerves of the gut and pancreas.[16,18,42] The simultaneous localization of NSE in both endocrine cells and nerves can thus provide a rapid way of demonstrating the relationship between these two groups of tissues (Fig. 7-2).[16] The exocrine cells of the pancreas and the nonendocrine cells in the gastrointestinal tract do not react with highly specific antisera against NSE.

The localization of chromogranin within the pancreas varies with the antibody used. O'Connor et al localized chromogranin primarily of the insulin-producing cells of the islet with the polyclonal antiserum against bovine chromogranin,[46] while Cohn et al localized chromogranin A in the somatostatin and pancreatic polypeptide-producing, but not in insulin or glucagon-producing cells of the rat pancreas with polyclonal antisera against bovine parathyroid SP-I and porcine adrenal medulla chromogranin.[39] Others found chromogranin immunoreactivity predominantly in glucagon-producing cells and only weakly in insulin-producing cells of human pancreas in formalin fixed tissues with the use of a monoclonal antibody (LK2H10) against human chromogranin (Fig.7-1B).[34,35,42] Chromogranin immunoreactivity, however, was found in insulin, glucagon, somatostatin, and pancreatic polypeptide-producing cells with the same monoclonal antibody (LK2H10) using freeze-dried tissue vapor-fixed with benzoquinone by Facer et al.[43] These latter observations indicate that fixation and processing are critical to obtain optimal immunoreactivity when using antibodies against chromogranin within the GEP axis. Chromogranin immunoreactivity was found in all GEP endocrine cells examined, including cells producing gastrin, somatostatin, gastrin inhibiting polypeptide, secretin, cholecystokinin, motilin, neurotensin, enteroglucagon, peptide YY, and serotonin (Fig. 7-3).[43] Other investigators also localized chromogranin in the enterochromaffin cells of the intestine.[34,35]

NSE AND CHROMOGRANIN LOCALIZATION IN GASTROENTEROPANCREATIC CELL HYPERPLASIA

Lloyd, et al found that both NSE and chromogranin were helpful markers in re-

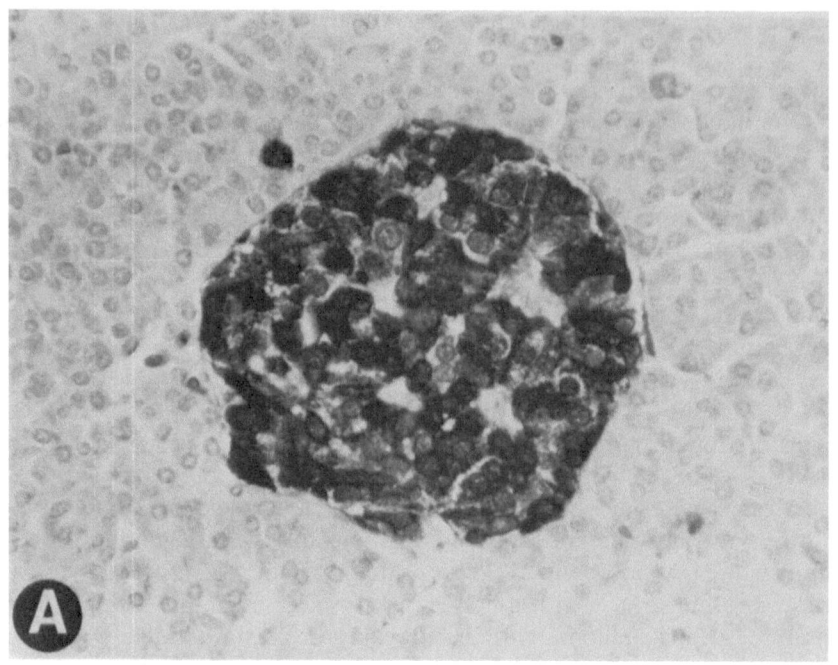

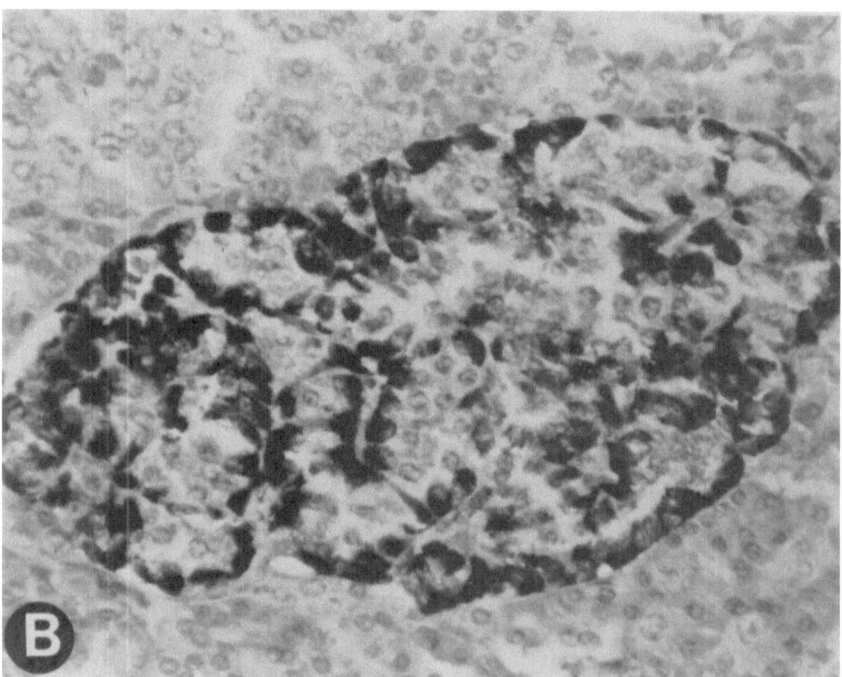

Fig. 7-1A. Pancreatic islet showing positive immunoreactivity for NSE. There is diffuse positive immunoreactivity in all of the islet cells (Immunoperoxidase ×208).
Fig. 7-1(B). Pancreatic islet showing positive immunoreactivity for chromogranin. The cells at the periphery of the islets, which are predominantly glucagon-producing cells, show the strongest immunoreactivity (Immunoperoxidase ×330).

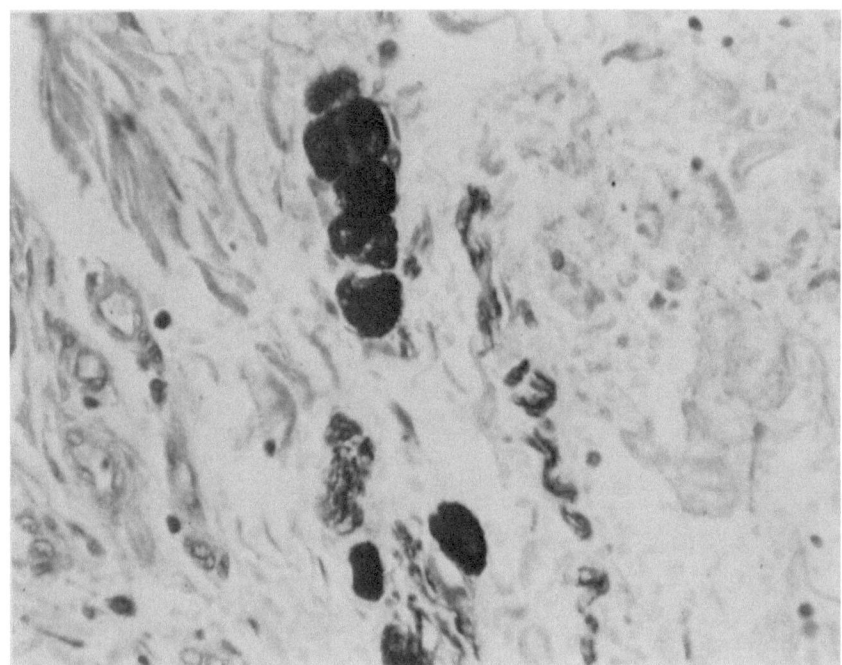

Fig. 7-2. Ganglion cells and nerve fibers from the duodenum showing positive immunoreactivity for NSE while the adjacent fibrous and vascular tissues are negative (Immunoperoxidase ×330).

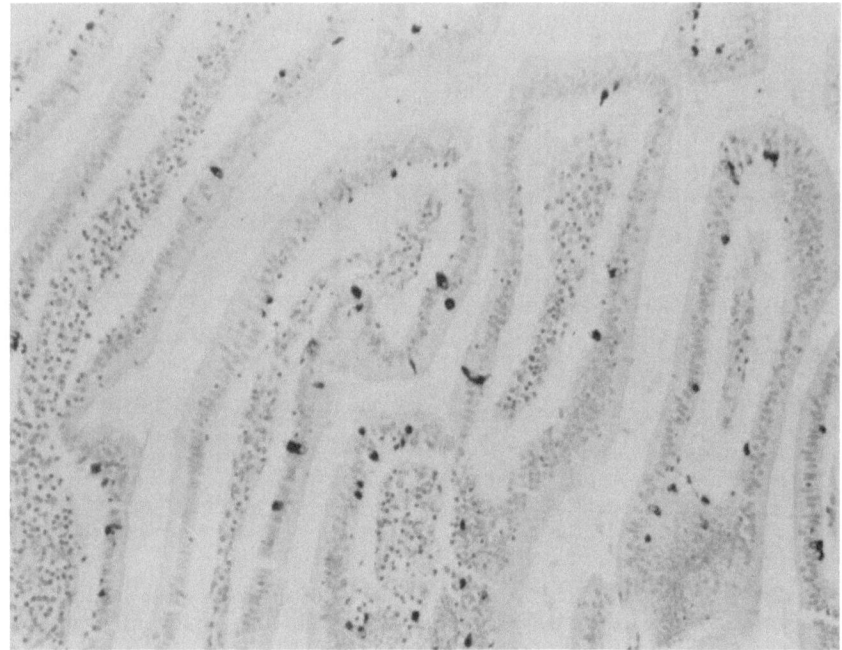

Fig. 7-3. Chromogranin immunostaining in duodenum reveals abundant endocrine cells in the villi (Immunoperoxidase ×132).

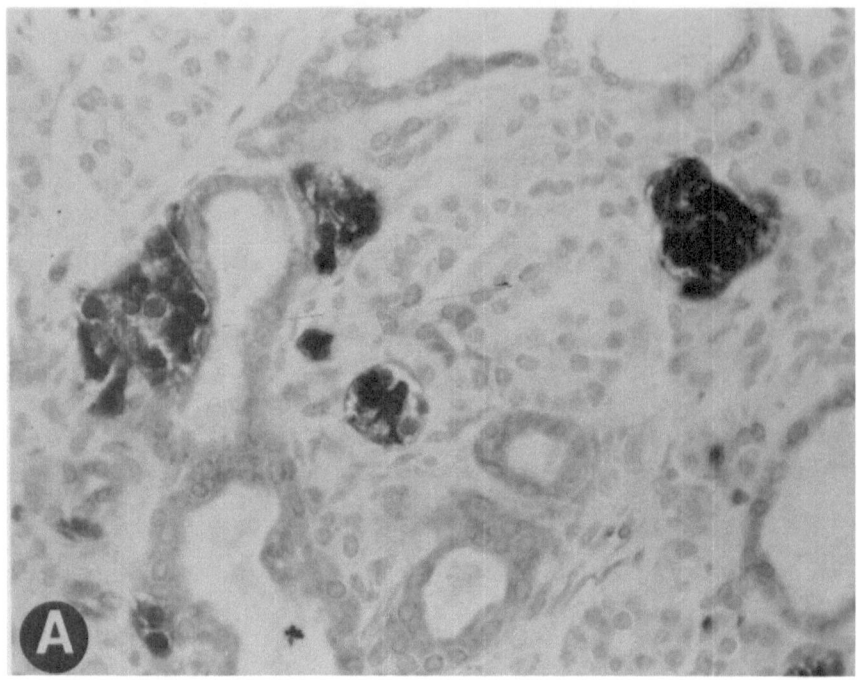

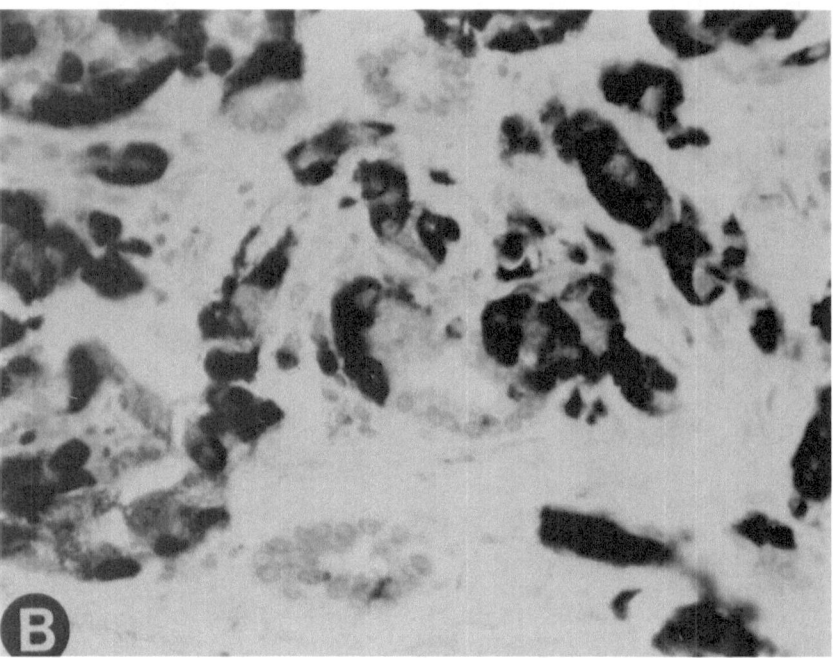

Fig. 7-4A. Pancreatic tissues showing nesidioblastosis with islet cells in close association with pancreatic ducts after immunostaining for NSE. (Immunoperoxidase ×208).

Fig. 7-4(B). Pancreatic islet tissue from a patient with multiple endocrine neoplasia type 1 showing nesidioblastosis and many small nests of islet cells after immunostaining for chromogranin. (Immunoperoxidase ×330).

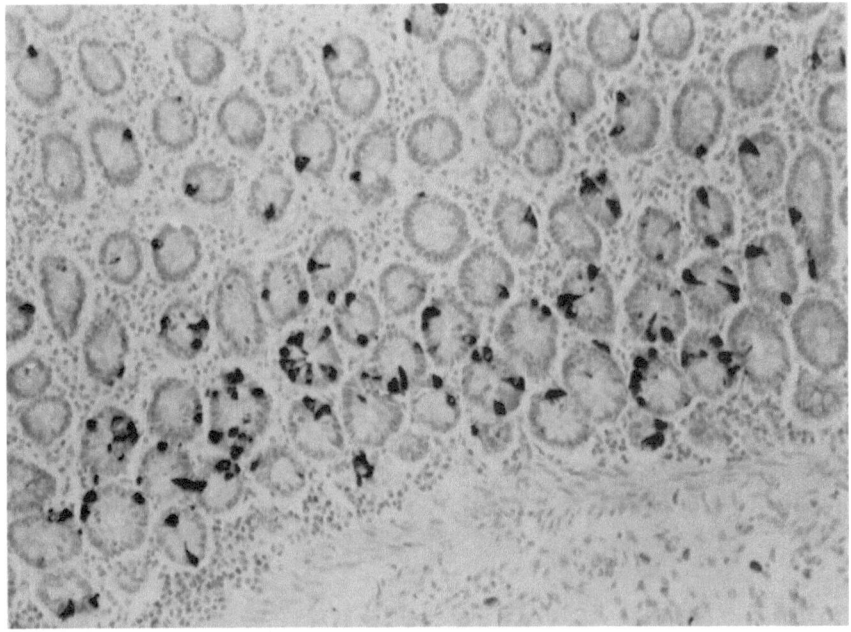

Fig. 7-5. Gastric biopsy from a patient with G-cell hyperplasia. Endocrine cells which are positive for chromogranin and for gastrin are revealed after chromogranin staining (Immunoperoxidase ×132).

vealing islet cell hyperplasia and nesidioblastosis (Figs. 7-4A and 7-4B).[42] We also observed increased staining of gastrin-producing cells in four cases of G-cell hyperplasia of the stomach with chromogranin (unpublished observations) (Fig. 7-5). NSE and chromogranin should be helpful markers in the morphometric evaluation of endocrine cell hyperplasia of the stomach and pancreas, but very little work has been done in this area to date.

NSE AND CHROMOGRANIN IN PANCREATIC ENDOCRINE TUMORS

The use of NSE and chromogranin as broad spectrum markers for pancreatic endocrine tumors is extremely helpful, especially in cases of nonfunctioning tumors that are not producing any known polypeptide hormones.[42] Since NSE stains the cytoplasm of most cells diffusely, while chromogranin

stains the secretory granules, the combined use of these markers reveals different staining patterns, and the intensity of chromogranin staining can give an estimate of the numbers of secretory granules within the tumor cells if ultrastructural studies are not available (Figs. 7-6,7-7). Glucagonomas showed intense staining in a recent study of pancreatic endocrine tumors, while insulinomas were generally negative for chromogranin.[42] Other workers detected chromogranin immunoreactivity in pancreatic endocrine tumors.[47] Walts et al recently reported on the use of chromogranin as a neuroendocrine marker for the detection of pancreatic endocrine tumors in cytologic specimens.[48] Our recent studies of normal pancreatic islets and pancreatic endocrine tumors strongly suggest that the mechanism of action of argyrophilic silver stains such as the Grimelius stain might involve binding to chromogranin.[42] This observation has also been noted by other investigators.[40]

Although the serum levels of NSE have

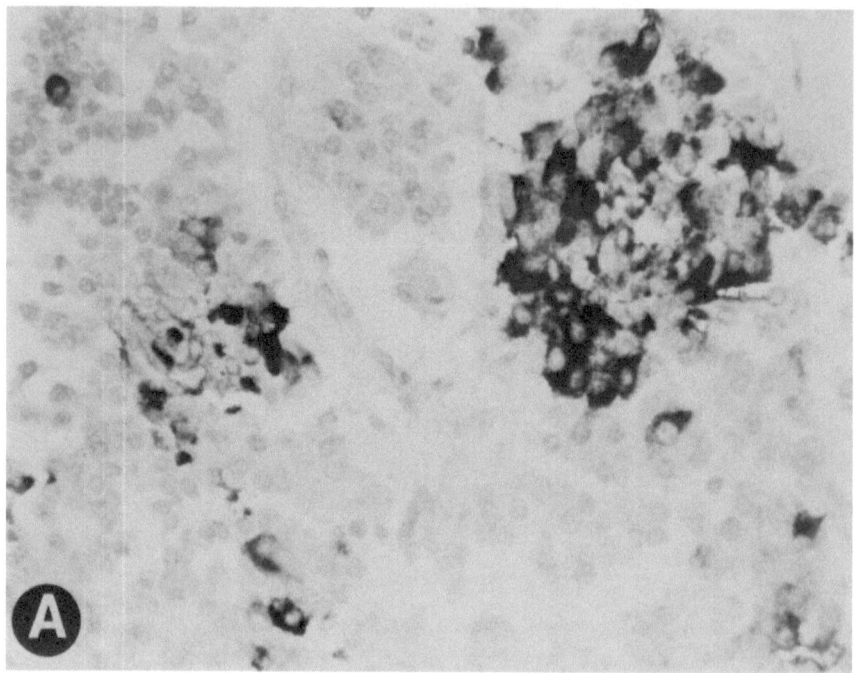

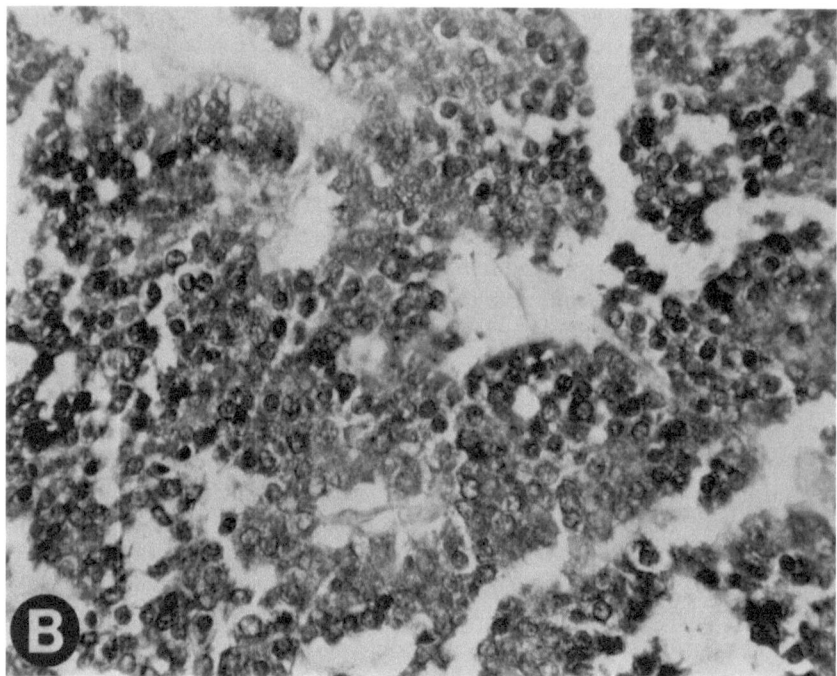

Fig. 7-6A. Pancreatic gastrinoma showing focal areas of tumor cells positive for chromogranin. These areas probably contain many endocrine granules while the chromogranin negative areas of the tumor probably contain very few endocrine granules (Immunoperoxidase ×330).

Fig. 7-6B. The same tumor as in 6A shows diffuse immunostaining for NSE. NSE immunostains the cytoplasm of endocrine cells diffusely and is not dependent on the presence of secretory granules (Immunoperoxidase ×330).

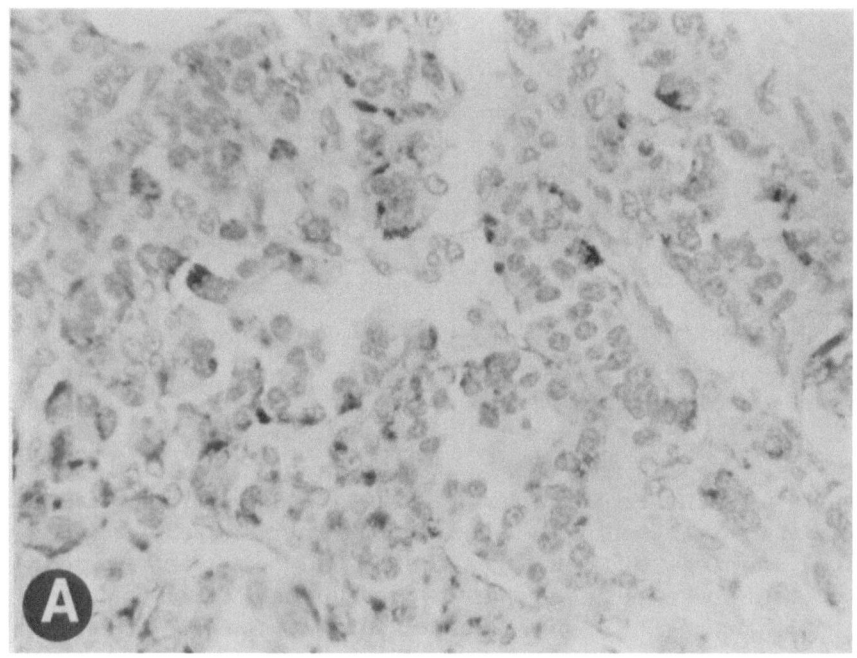

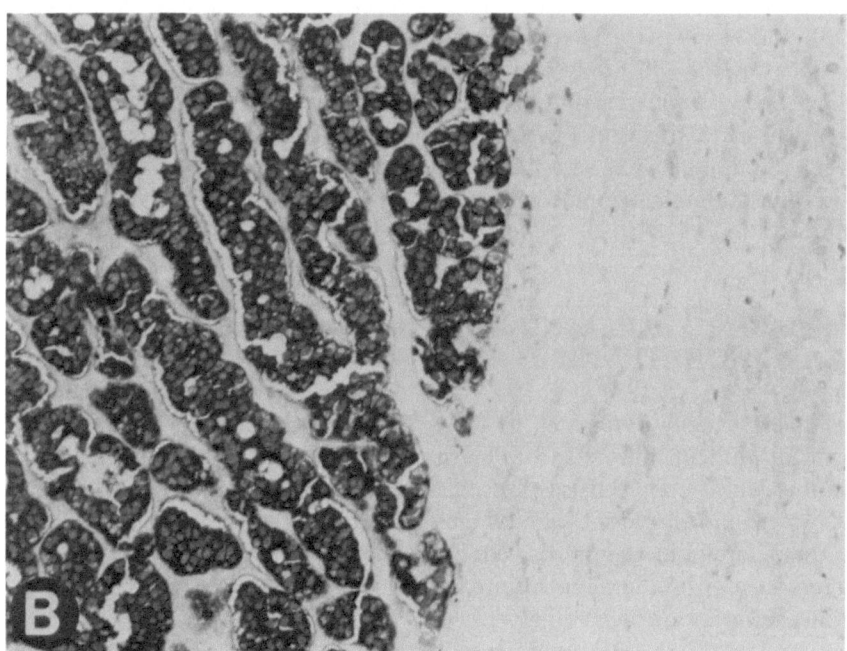

Fig. 7-7A. Metastatic pancreatic endocrine tumor to liver showing a distinct pattern of immunostaining for chromogranin in many tumor cells (Immunoperoxidase ×208).

Fig. 7-7B. The same metastatic pancreatic endocrine tumor to the liver as in 7A showing a diffuse pattern of immunostaining for NSE. (Immunoperoxidase ×132).

TABLE 7-1

Immunoreactivity for Chromogranin and Silver Staining With the Grimelius and
Fontana-Masson Stains in Gastrointestinal Carcinoid Tumors.

Tumor Location	No. of Cases	Positive Reactivity		
		Chromogranin	Grimelius	Fontana
Gastric	3	3	3	2
Small Intestine	5	5	5	5
Appendix	4	4	4	4
Colon	6	5	4	2

been examined in GEP tumors and have been found to be elevated accompanying some neoplasms,[49,50] only a few studies correlated serum levels of NSE with the immunohistochemical localization of NSE.[18] In a recent publication that examined serum levels of NSE along with immunohistochemical staining for NSE and tissue extracts analyzed by radioimmunoassay for NSE, only one of ten patients had slightly elevated serum NSE levels. This patient had a metastatic gastrinoma to the liver. The tissue levels were markedly elevated in eight of the ten patients with pancreatic tumors.[18]

NSE AND CHROMOGRANIN IN CARCINOID TUMORS

Carcinoids are usually designated as foregut, midgut, or hindgut tumors according to their anatomical location.[51] The use of specific antisera to polypeptide hormones and amines in the study of carcinoid tumors has shown that such tumors may produce a predominant polypeptide and/or amine depending on their anatomic location. Thus intestinal foregut carcinoids commonly produce somatostatin and gastrin;[52] midgut carcinoids commonly produce serotonin[52] and hindgut carcinoids often produce immunoreactive pancreatic polypeptide.[53]

The silver stains are commonly used as diagnostic tools for GEP tumors including carcinoids.[49,50] Argyrophilic stains, including the Grimelius method, are usually more sensitive

than argentaffin stains in revealing endocrine cells or tumors. In a recent study, comparison of chromogranin immunoreactivity, with the Grimelius and Masson-Fontana silver stains in a study of carcinoid tumors from the gastrointestinal tract revealed that chromogranin reactivity was the most sensitive method of identifying carcinoid tumors and was only slightly more sensitive than the Grimelius technique. (Table 7-1).[57] Chromogranin was much more sensitive than the Masson-Fontana stain in identifying carcinoid tumors from various locations in the intestine (Table 7-1) (Figs. 7-8,7-9).

NSE is also produced by carcinoid tumors (Fig. 7-10). We have found elevated tissue levels of NSE in carcinoid tumors, although the serum levels were not significantly elevated.[56] Prinz et al found a slightly elevated serum level of NSE in one of five patients with intestinal carcinoid tumors.[50] The concentration of serum levels of NSE may also be related to the presence of metastatic disease.[20,56]

NSE AND CHROMOGRANIN IN OTHER GEP TUMORS

We have localized NSE and chromogranin in goblet cell carcinoid tumors of the appendix and in duodenal paragangliomas (unpublished observations). Other workers have found chromogranin immunoreactivity in pancreatic ductal adenocarcinomas, indicating a mixed endocrine and ductal differentia-

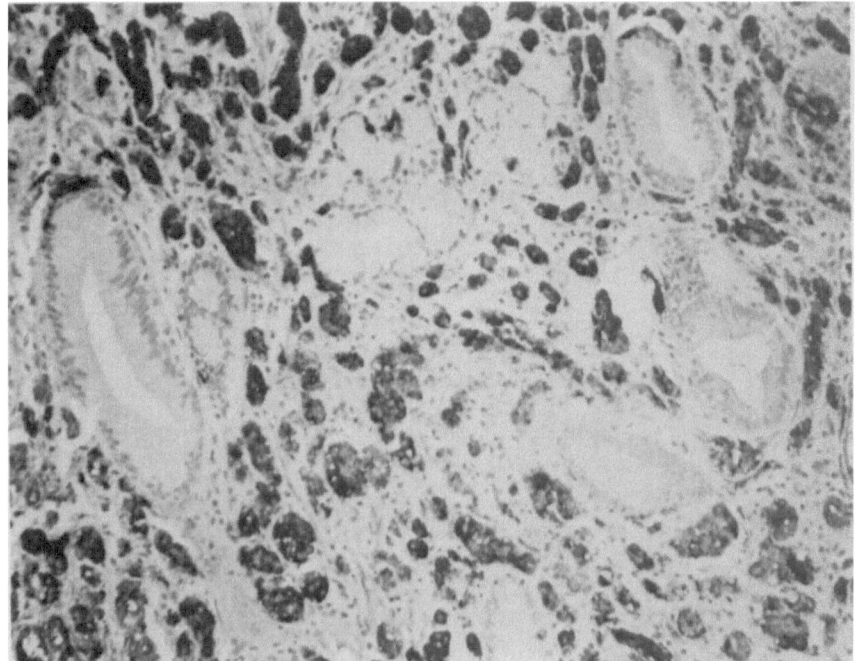

Fig. 7-8. Gastrin-producing carcinoid tumor from stomach showing positive immunostaining for chromogranin in the infiltrating nests of tumor cells (Immunoperoxidase × 208).

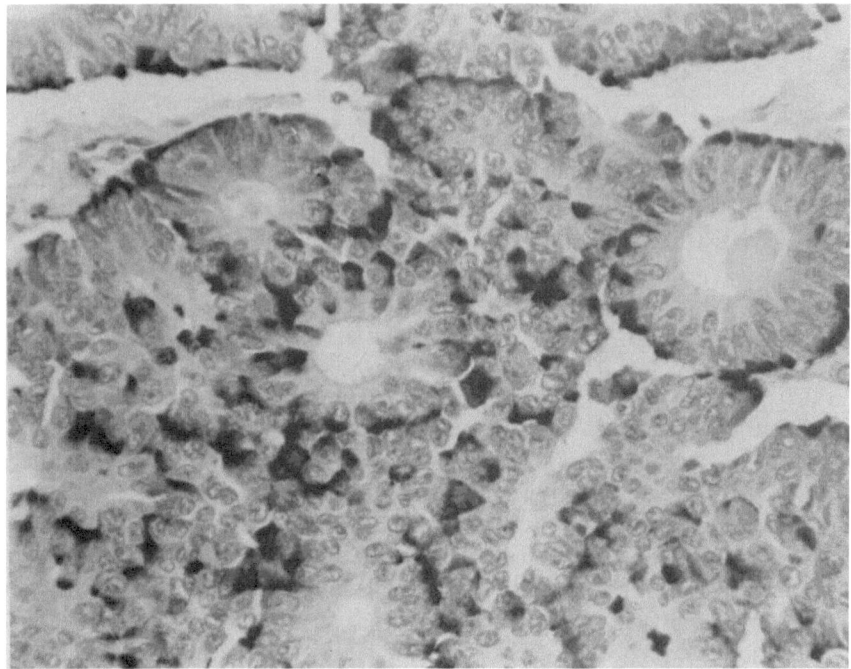

Fig. 7-9. Metastatic carcinoid tumor in liver showing diffuse positive immunostaining for chromogranin in the basal portion of the tumor cells (Immunoperoxidase × 330).

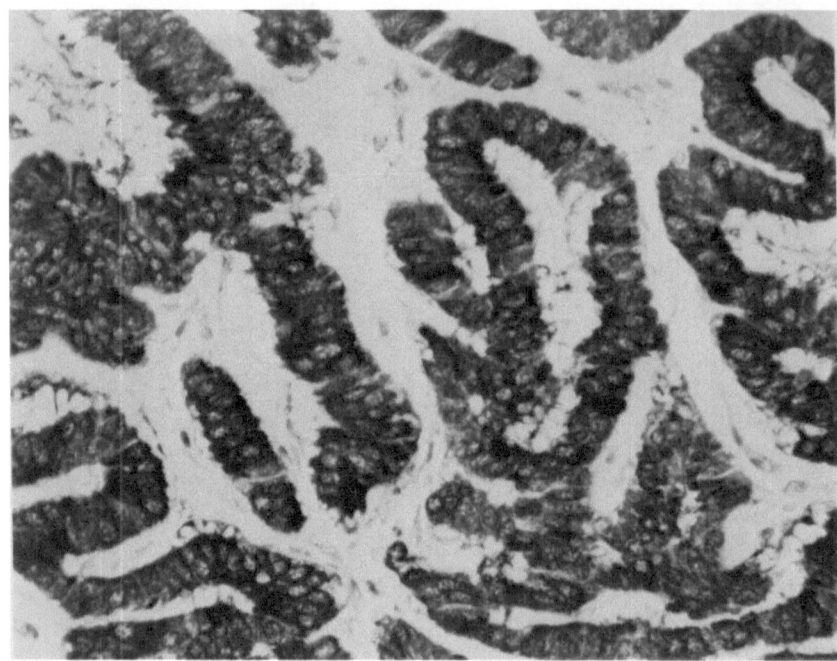

Fig. 7-10. Colonic carcinoid showing intense diffuse positive immunostaining for NSE. (Immunoperoxidase ×330).

tion in these tumors.[58] Chromogranin immunostaining was also more sensitive than the Grimelius technique in localizing neuroendocrine cells in mixed exocrine and endocrine pancreatic tumors.[58]

FUTURE PROSPECTS

The use of NSE and chromogranin to analyze differentiation of endocrine cells, mixed endocrine-exocrine GEP tumors, and hyperplasia of various endocrine cells has not been fully explored. The unique advantage of these broad spectrum markers in studying GEP neuroendocrine tumors is that one can detect endocrine differentiation even if a specific antibody against certain peptides is not available. Thus, the systematic study of normal and neoplastic GEP endocrine cells with NSE and chromogranin may lead to the detection of novel endocrine cells that would not have

been discovered with the use of antisera that react only with known peptides.

SUMMARY

The use of well characterized antibodies against NSE and chromogranin as general markers of endocrine differentiation offers many advantages. Because NSE is a diffuse cytoplasmic marker and chromogranin is localized in secretory granules, these markers are complementary to each other. The use of chromogranin can give some general information about the granule content of endocrine cells and tumors. Chromogranin immunoreactivity and the Grimelius silver stain appear to be closely related, but chromogranin immunoreactivity appears to represent a more sensitive marker for the detection of endocrine differentiation. NSE can be used to study the localization of endocrine cells and nerves within the same tissue, so that the relationship between these two tissues can be visualized simultaneously. The use of NSE and chromogranin as immunohistochemical markers can contribute to the study of endocrine cell and tumor development and differentiation. They also serve as helpful diagnostic aids in pathology.

REFERENCES

1. Moore B.W.: Chemistry and biology of two proteins, S-100 and 14-3-2, specific to the nervous system, in International Review of Neurobiology, Vol 15 C.C. Pfeiffer and J.R. Smythies, (eds) New York, Academic Press, 1972, pp 215–225
2. Moore B.W., McGregor D: Chromatographic and electrophoretic fractionation of soluble proteins of brain and liver. J Biol Chem 146:1647–1653, 1965
3. Marangos P.J., Zomzely-Neurath C., Luk D.C.M., York C.: Isolation and characterization of the nervous system specific protein 14-3-2 from rat brain. J Biol Chem 250:1884–1891, 1975
4. Marangos P.J., Parma A.M., Goodwin F.K.: Functional properties of neuronal and glial isoenzymes of the glycolytic enzyme enolase in brain. J Neurochem 31:727–737, 1978
5. Marangos P.J., Zis A.D., and Clark R.L., Goodwin F.K.: Neuronal, non-neuronal and hybrid forms of enolase in brain: Structural, immunological and functional comparisons. Brain Res 150:113–117, 1978
6. Marangos P.J.: Clinical utility of neuron-specific enolase as a neuroendocrine tumour marker, in Endocrine Tumours. The Pathobiology of Regulatory Peptide-producing Tumours. J.M. Polak and S.R. Bloom (eds). Churchill Livingstone, Edinburgh, 1985, pp 181–192
7. Marangos P.J., Schmechel D.: The neurobiology of the brain enolases, in Essays in Neurochemistry and Neuropharmacology Vol IV. M.B.H. Youdim, W. Lovenberg, D.F. Sharman, Jr. and J.R. Lagnado (eds), Wiley, New York, 1980, pp 211–247
8. Schmechel D.E., Marangos P.J., Zis A.P., Brightman M., Goodwin, F.K.: The brain enolases as specific markers of neuronal and glial cells. Science 199:313–315, 1978
9. Schmechel D.E., Marangos P.J., Brightman M.W.: Neuron specific enolase is a marker for peripheral and central neuroendocrine cells. Nature 276:834–836, 1979
10. Tapia F.J., Barbosa A.J.A., Marangos P.J., Polak J.M., Bloom S.R., Dermody C.: Neuron-specific enolase is produced by neuroendocrine tumours. Lancet i:808–811, 1981
11. Haimoto H., Takahashi Y., Koshikawa T., Nagra H., Kaito K.: Immunohistochemical localization of γ-enolase in normal human tissues other than neurons and neuroendocrine tissues. Lab Invest. 52:257–263, 1983
12. Schmechel D.E.: γ-subunit of the glycolytic enzyme enolase: nonspecific or neuron specific. (Editorial) Lab Invest 52:239–242, 1985
13. Vinores S.A., Bonnin J.H., Rubinstein L.S., Marangos P.J.: Immunohistochemical demonstration of neuron-specific enolase in neoplasms of the CNS and other tissues. Arch Pathol Lab Med 108:536–540, 1984
14. Wick M.R., Scheithauer B.W., Kovacs K.: Neuron specific enolase in neuroendocrine tumors of the thymus, bronchus and skin. Am J Clin Pathol 79:703–707, 1983
15. Tsokos M., Linoila R.I., Chandra R.S., Triche T.J.: Neuron specific enolase in the diagnosis of neuroblastomas and other small round cell tumors in children. Human Pathol 15:575–584, 1984
16. Bishop A.E., Polak J.M., Facer P., Ferri G.L., Marangos P.J., Pearse A.G.E.: Neuron specific enolase: A common marker for the endocrine cells and innervation of the gut and pancreas. Gastroenterol 83:902–915, 1982
17. Asa S.L., Ryan N., Kovacs K., Singer W., Marangos P.J.: Immunohistochemical localization of neuron-specific enolase in the human hypophysis and pituitary adenomas. Arch Pathol Lab Med 108:40–43, 1984
18. Simpson S., Vinik A., Marangos P.J., Lloyd R.V.: Immunohistochemical localization of neuron-specific enolase in gastroenteropancreatic neuroendocrine tumors. Correlation with tissue and serum levels of neuron-specific enolase. Cancer 54:1364–1369, 1984
19. Lloyd R.V., Sisson J.C., Marangos P.J.: Calcitonin, carcinoembryonic antigen and neuron-specific enolase in medullary thyroid carcinoma. An immunohistochemical study. Cancer 51:2234–2239, 1983
20. Lloyd R.V., Warner T.F.: Immunohistochemistry of neuron-specific enolase. In Advances in Immunohistochemistry. R.A. DeLellis (ed), Masson Publishing USA, Inc., 1984, pp 127–140
21. Carney D.D., Ihde D.C., Cohen M.H., Marangos P.J., Bunn P.A., Jr., Minna J.D., Gazder A.F.: Serum neuron-specific enolase: A marker for disease extent and response to therapy of small-cell lung cancer. Lancet i:583–585, 1982
22. Zelter P.M., Marangos P.J., Parma A.M., Sather H., Dalton A., Hammond D., Siegel S.B., Seeger R.C.: Raised neuron specific enolase in serum of children with metastatic neuroblastoma. Lancet ii:361–363, 1983
23. Seshi B., Bell C.E.: Preparation and characterization of monoclonal antibodies to human neuron-specific enolase. Hybridoma 4:13–25, 1985
24. Thomas P., Battifora H., Mandenno C.: Is neuron-specific enolase specific? An immunohistochemical comparison of a monoclonal and a polyclonal antibody against neuron specific enolase. Lab Invest 54:63A, 1986 (Abstract)
25. Vinores S.A., Herman M.M., Rubinstein L.J., Marangos P.J.: Electron microscopic localization of neuron-specific enolase in rat and mouse brain. J Histochem Cytochem 32:1295–1302, 1984
26. Blaschko H., Comline R.S., Schneider F.H., Silver M., Smith A.D.: Secretion of a chromaffin granule protein, chromogranin, from the adrenal medulla after splanchnic nerve stimulation. Nature 215:58–59, 1967
27. Winkler H.: The composition of adrenal chromaffin granules. An assessment of controversial results. Neurosciences 1:65–80, 1976
28. Smith A.D., Winkler H.: Purification and properties of an acidic protein from chromaffin granules on a large scale. Biochem J 103:480–482, 1967

29. Kirschner A.G., Kirschner N.: A specific soluble protein from the catecholamine storage vesicles of bovine adrenal medulla. Biochem Biophys Acta **181**:219–225, 1969

30. O'Connor D.T., Frigon R.P., Sokoloff R.L.: Human chromogranin A. Purification and characterization from catecholamine storage vesicles of human pheochromocytoma. Hypertension **6**:2–12, 1984

31. Hagn C., Schmid K. W., Fischer-Colbvie R., Winkler H. Chromogranin A, B, and C in human adrenal medulla and endocrine tissues. Lab Invest **55**:405–411, 1986.

32. Aunis D., Hesketch J.E., Devilliens G.: Immunohistochemical and immunocytochemical localization of myosin, chromogranin A and dopamine β-hydroxylase in nerve cells in culture and adrenal glands. J Neurocytol **9**:255–274, 1980

33. O'Connor D.J.: Chromogranin: widespread immunoreactivity in polypeptide hormone producing tissues and in serum. Regulatory Peptides **6**:263–280, 1983

34. Lloyd R.V., Wilson B.S.: Specific endocrine marker defined by a monoclonal antibody. Science **222**:628–630, 1983

35. Wilson B.S., Lloyd R.V.: Detection of chromogranin in neuroendocrine cells with a monoclonal antibody. Am J Pathol **115**:458–468, 1984

36. O'Connor D.T., Burton P., Deftos L.J.: Immunoreactive human chromogranin A in diverse polypeptide hormone producing human tumors and normal endocrine tissues. J Clin Endocrinal **57**:1084–1087, 1983.

37. Nolan J.A., Trojanowski J.Q., Hogue-Angeletti R.: Neurons and neuroendocrine cells contain chromogranin: Detection of the molecule in normal bovine tissues by immunochemical and immunohistochemical methods. J Histochem Cytochem **33**:791–798, 1985

38. Somogyi P., Hodgson A.J., Depotter R.W., Fischer-Colbrie R., Schober M., Winkler H., Chubb I.W.: Chromogranin immunoreactivity in the central nervous system. Immunochemical characterization, distribution and relationship to catecholamine and enkephalin pathways. Brain Res Reviews **8**:193–230, 1984

39. Cohn D.V., Elting J.J., Frick M., Elde, R.: Selective localization of the parathyroid secretory protein-I/adrenal medulla chromogranin. A protein family in a wide variety of endocrine cells of the rat. Endocrinology **113**:1963–1974, 1984

40. Varndell I.M., Lloyd R.V., Wilson B.S., Polak J.M.: Ultrastructural localization of chromogranin: A potential marker for the electron microscopical recognition of endocrine cell secretory granules. Histochem J **17**:981–992, 1985

41. Hogue-Angeletti R., Hicker W.F.: A neuroendocrine marker in tissues of the immune system. Science **230**:89–96, 1985

42. Lloyd R.V., Mervak T., Schmidt K., Warner T.F.C.S., Wilson B.S.: Immunohistochemical detection of chromogranin and neuron-specific enolase in pancreatic endocrine neoplasm. Am J Surg Pathol **8**:607–614, 1984

43. Facer P., Bishop A.E., Lloyd R.V., Wilson B.S., Hennessy R.J., Polak J.M.: Chromogranin: A newly recognized marker for endocrine cells of the human gastrointestinal tract. Gastroenterol **89**:1366–1373, 1985

44. DeStephano D.B., Lloyd R.V., Pike A.M., Wilson B.S.: Pituitary adenomas. An immunohistochemical study of hormone production and chromogranin localization. Am J Pathol **116**:464–472, 1984

45. O'Connor D.T., Bernstein K.N.: Radioimmunoassay of chromogranin A in plasma as a measure of exocytotic sympathoadrenal activity in normal subjects and patients with pheochromocytomas. N Engl J Med **311**:764–776, 1984

46. O'Connor D.T., Burton D., Deftos L.J.: Chromogranin A: Immunohistology reveals its universal occurrence in normal polypeptide hormone producing endocrine glands. Life Science **33**:1657–1663, 1983

47. O'Connor D.T., Burton D.W., Parmer R.J., Deftos L.J.: Human chromogranin A: Detection by immunohistochemistry in C cells and diverse polypeptide hormone producing tumors, in Endocrine Control of Bone and Calcium Metabolism. Cohn D.V., Fugita T., Potts, Jr J.J.,Talmage, R.V. (eds). Elsevier Scientific Publications B.V., 1984, pp 187–190

48. Walts A.E., Said J.E., Shintaker P., Lloyd R.V.: Chromogranin as a marker of neuroendocrine cells in cytologic material—an immunocytochemical study. Am J Clin Pathol **84**:273–277, 1985

49. Prinz R.A., Marangos P.J.: Use of neuron-specific enolase as a serum marker for neuroendocrine neoplasms. Surgery **92**:887–889, 1982

50. Prinz R.A., Berme E.W., Kimmel J.R., Marangos P.J.: Serum markers for pancreatic islet cell and intestinal carcinoid tumors: A comparison of neuron-specific enolase, β-human chorionic gonadotropin and pancreatic polypeptide. Surgery **94**:1019–1023, 1983

51. Williams E.D., Sandler M.: The classification of carcinoid tumours, Lancet **1**:238–239, 1963

52. Dayal Y.: Endocrine cells of the gut and their neoplasms. Contemp Issues Surg Pathol **2**:267–302, 1983

53. O'Brian D.S., Tischler A.S., Dayal Y., Beudon R., DeLellis R.A., Wolfe H.J.: Rectal carcinoids as tumors of the hindgut endocrine cells. A morphological and immunohistochemical analysis. Am J Surg Pathol **6**:131–142, 1982

54. Grimelius L., Wilander E.: Silver stains in the study of endocrine cells of the gut and pancreas. Invest Cell Pathol **3**:3–12, 1980

55. Solcia E., Capella C., Buffa R., Frigerio B.: Histochemical and ultrastructural studies on the argentaffin and argyrophil cells of the gut. Chromaffin, Enterochromaffin and Related Cells. Coupland, R.E., Fujita T., (eds) Elsevier Scientific Publishing Company. The Netherlands, 1976, pp 209–225

56. Vinik A.J., Strodel W.E., Lloyd R.V., Thompson N.W.: Unusual gastroenteropancreatic (GEP) tumors and their hormones. In Thompson N.W., Vinik A.I. (eds) Endocrine Surgery Update. Grune & Stratton, New York, 1983, pp 293–320

57. Kumar N.B., Cookingham C.L., Lloyd R.V., Appelman H.: Detection of human chromogranin with a monoclonal antibody in carcinoid secretory granules and its comparison with the generic silver stains and with serotonin. Lab Invest **50**:33A, 1984 (Abstract)

58. Kay D., DeLellis R.A., Dayal Y., Lloyd R.V., Duggan M.A., Tallberg K., Sternberg S.S., Wolfe H.J.: Ductal adenocarcinomas of the pancreas with neuroendocrine cells. An immunohistochemical study. Lab Invest. **52**:33A, 1986 (Abstract).

8

Protein-losing Enteropathy Including Intestinal Lymphangiectasia and Ménétrier's Disease

Hitoshi Asakura M.D.
Akira Morita M.D.
Soichiro Miura M.D.
Masaharu Tsuchiya M.D.
Yasuyoshi Enomoto Ph.D.
Yoonosuke Watanabe M.D.

Protein-losing gastroenteropathy, characterized by an excessive loss of plasma protein into the gastrointestinal lumen, is caused by a wide variety of gastrointestional disorders, which may be classified into three categories:[1] The first category includes disorders that cause an obstruction of intestinal lymphatics. Direct leakage of intestinal lymph into the intestinal lumen is thought to be the mechanism of protein loss. Primary intestinal lymphangiectasia is a typical example of this group.[2,3] Secondary intestinal lymphangiectasia may occur in certain cardiac diseases such as constrictive pericarditis[4] and congestive heart failure, lymphoma, Whipple's disease, Crohn's disease,[5] intestinal tuberculosis, and retroperitoneal fibrosis.[6]

The second group consists of mucosal diseases with erosion or ulceration including ulcerative colitis,[7] Crohn's disease, radiation enteritis, pseudomembranous enterocolitis, and malignant tumors of the gastrointestinal tract.[8] Inflammatory exudation may be the primary cause of protein loss.

The last group includes mucosal disorders without ulceration such as Ménétrier's disease (giant hypertrophy of the gastric rugae),[9] allergic gastroenteropathy,[10] eosinophilic gastroenteritis, sprue syndrome,[11] intestinal bacterial overgrowth[12] and parasitic infections. Loss of proteins into the gastrointestinal lumen is thought to be due to an increased mucosal permeability[13] to protein because of surface cell damage, increased cell loss, and local release of mediators. Vascular permeability may also be an important factor in the gastrointestinal loss of plasms proteins.[14,15] Causes of protein-losing gastroenteropathy are listed in Table 8-1.

DIAGNOSIS OF PROTEIN-LOSING GASTROENTEROPATHY

A major clinical manifestation of protein-losing gastroenteropathy is edema caused by lowered colloidal pressure of plasma and increased transudation of fluid from the capillaries. In addition to the low plasma levels of albumin, the plasma concentrations of

TABLE 8-1
Causes of Protein-losing Gastroenteropathy.

1. Esophagus
   Esophageal carcinoma
2. Stomach
   Giant hypertrophic gastritis
   Ménétrier's disease
   Gastric polyposis (polyp)
   Gastric carcinoma
   Postgastrectomy syndrome
3. Small intestine
   Tropical sprue, nontropical sprue
   Regional enteritis (Crohn's disease)
   Whipple's disease
   Nonspecific granulomatous disease
   Gastrointestinal tuberculosis
   Acute gastrointestinal infection
   Hookworm infection, Trichinosis
   Allergic gastroenteropathy
   Eosinophilic gastroenteritis
   Intestinal lymphangiectasia
   Blind loop syndrome
   Lymphosarcoma, Hodgkin's disease
   Intestinal lymphoma
   Stenosis
4. Colon
   Ulcerative colitis
   Colonic neoplasm
   Polyposis (Cronkhite-Canada syndrome)
5. Heart
   Congestive heart failure
   Constrictive pericarditis
   Interatrial septal defect
   Primary myocardial disease
6. Miscellaneous
   Nephrotic syndrome
   Liver cirrhosis
   Chronic pancreatitis
   Kwashiorkor
   Amyloidosis
   Acute transient gastrointestinal protein loss
   Idiopathic retroperitoneal fibrosis
   Anaphylactoid purpura

gamma globulin, fibrinogen, lipoproteins, alpha 1-antitrypsin, transferrin, and ceruloplasmin are found to be decreased. It is, however, rare that the enteric loss of plasma proteins other than albumin causes clinical problems. Secondary hypogammaglobulinemia and the loss of blood coagulating factors are rarely sufficient, and the depletion of hormone-binding proteins is well compensated by the presence of free hormones. In patients with obstruction of intestinal lymphatics, the leakage and/or impaired absorption of long chain triglyceride and fat-soluble vitamins may be associated with the enteric loss of protein.

The possibility of protein-losing gastroenteropathy should be considered in patients who exhibit hypoproteinemia with or without edema, when other causes for hypoproteinemia, such as liver disease, malabsorption syndrome, and proteinuria are ruled out. Attempts to measure the excretion of protein into the gastrointestinal lumen by direct analysis of aspirated gastrointestinal fluid have been limited by the rapid proteolytic digestion of plasma protein. Therefore, a variety of labeled substances that resist proteolytic digestion and reabsorption have been used for the diagnosis of protein-losing gastroenteropathy. Those include ^{131}I-human serum albumin,[16] ^{131}I-PVP,[17] ^{59}Fe-dextran, [95]Nb-albumin, [67]Cu-ceruloplasmin and ^{51}Cr-albumin.[18] These are still not ideal, however, since they are nonphysiological substances and have a considerably shorter half life in the circulation when compared to that of ^{131}I-albumin. Recently, alpha 1-antitrypsin, a natural plasma protein, has been found to be useful in studying enteric protein loss.[19] Although it is digested in acid gastric juice, it resists proteolytic digestion in the intestinal lumen. It is not selectively secreted into the intestine and its level in plasma and stool can be easily measured. Moreover, the use of radioisotope is not needed in assessment of alpha 1-antitrypsin loss. In addition to the direct methods stated above to detect the loss of plasma protein into the gastrointestinal lumen, kinetic study using radioiodinated human plasma albumin has been widely used to determine if the hypoproteinemia is due to hypercatabolism.

Intestinal Lymphangiectasia of the Small Intestine

Intestinal lymphangiectasia is a disease characterized by a generalized disorder of the lymphatic channels including dilated lym-

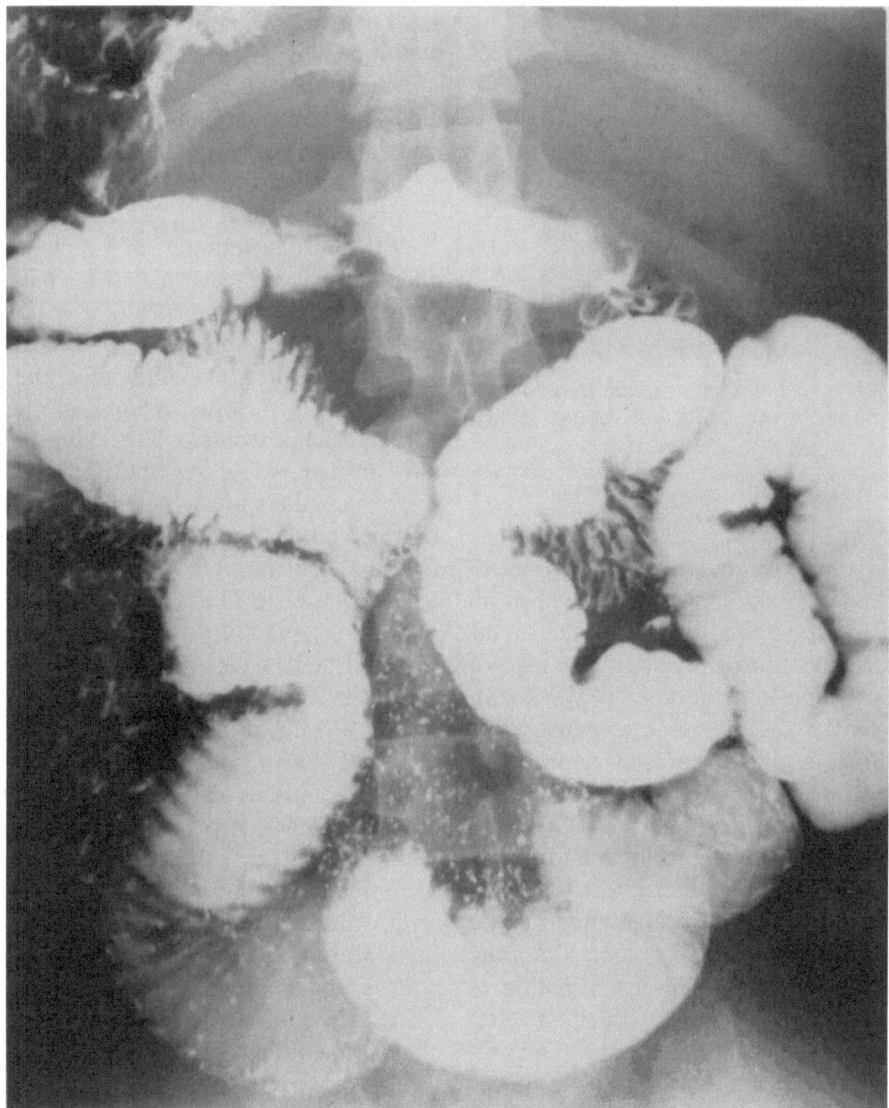

Fig. 8-1. X ray picture of the small intestine in a patient with primary intestinal lymphangiectasia showed thickening of Kerckring's folds and dilatation of bowel lumen.

phatic vessels of the intestinal mucosa and excessive enteric loss of plasma proteins.[2,3] Other important features are hypocalcemia, lymphedema, chyluria, chylothorax, chylous ascites, growth retardation, and lymphocytopenia.[20] This disorder is thought to be caused by mechanical and/or functional obstruction to the flow of lymph from the intestinal lymphatics to the junction of the thoracic duct and subclavian vein. In 1961, Waldmann et al[2] first demonstrated that by using intestinal biopsy and lymphangiography hypoalbumi-

nemia in patients with idiopathic hypoproteinemia was due to the enteric loss of plasma protein and associated with dilated and presumably blocked lymphatic vessels of the intestinal mucosa.

Primary intestinal lymphangiectasia is the manifestation of a generalized disorder in the development of the lymphatic system, which may occur congenitally or by acquired mechanisms. Early onset of peripheral lymphatic edema is often seen in patients with primary intestinal lymphangiectasia. The exact cause

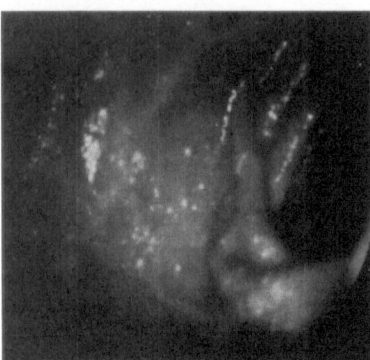

Fig. 8-2. Jejunal endoscopic picture showed scattered white spots and white villi in the jejunal mucosa.

of the lymphatic abnormality, however, has not been fully elucidated. Secondary intestinal lymphangiectasia may occur by obstruction of intestinal and/or mesenteric lymphatic channels and by disturbed drainage of intestinal lymph into the venous system. In case of cardiac diseases such as constrictive pericarditis, it seems that the drainage of lymph into the venous system is deranged by an increased venous pressure.[21]

Thickening of the Kerckring's folds, dilution of the barium column, dilatation of bowel lumen and mucosal nodularity or punctate lucency are the major abnormal findings in the radiographic examination of the small bowel in patients with small intestinal lymphangiectasia (Fig. 8-1).[22] Thickening of the Kerckring's folds appears to be due to the presence of edema and dilated lymphatics in the intestinal mucosa and submucosa. Upper GI X-ray series are usually normal. Diffuse nodular thickening of the intestinal wall with no adenopathy or hepatosplenomegaly and ascites with occasional coexistence of pleural effusion have been noted in body computed tomography (CT) examination in a patient with primary intestinal lymphangiectasia.[23] These small intestinal X-ray and CT findings, however, are not specific for this disorder.

Lymphangiographic studies performed by Kinmonth's method[24] have revealed a variety of abnormalities in intestinal lymphangiecta-

sia. These abnormalities are divided into two conditions; hyperplasia and hypoplasia. Lymphatic blockage at the level of the cisterna chyli, tortuous lymphatic channels, hypoplasia of abdominal lymph nodes in the paraaortic area and obstruction of the thoracic duct may be observed.

With the development of small intestinal endoscopy, it has recently become possible to observe the jejunal mucosa that is 10–40 cm distal to the ligamentum of Treitz.[25] The major small intestinal endoscopic findings in patients with intestinal lymphangiectasia are scattered white spots, white villi and chyle-like substance covering the mucosa.[26] Tiny scattered white spots with a clear margin can be noted on the duodenal and jejunal mucosa (Fig. 8-2). The number of spots observed varied in each case. Those spots are not stained with methylene blue, by which normal intestinal epithelial cells are stained. In addition, they can not be washed or rubbed away. When a magnifying endoscope, Olympus GIF-HM, with the maximal magnifying power of 35 times was used to observe the intestinal mucosa, two types of distribution of white spots, (i.e., solitary or grouped type), were noted (Fig. 8-3). In addition, some villi with white spots were distended and showed an appearance like crabbed fingers. Dissecting microscopic study of biopsied specimens revealed the presence of milky white spots in the stroma of the villi. Further histopathological study demonstrated that the formation of white spots appeared to be due to the markedly dilated lymphatics. Scanning electron microscopic study in Norwegian Lundehunds (puffin dogs) with intestinal lymphangiectasia revealed that some villi were markedly expanded and appeared as coalesced pyramid-shaped structures with a crater-shaped lesion at the villous tip.[27]

In cases of intestinal lymphangiectasia, the degree of dilatation of intestinal lymphatics varies considerably (Fig. 8-4). Dilated lymphatics can be observed in the lamina propria, submucosa and also in the serosa. They may be noted in many villi in some cases or in others only in a few. Edema was observed

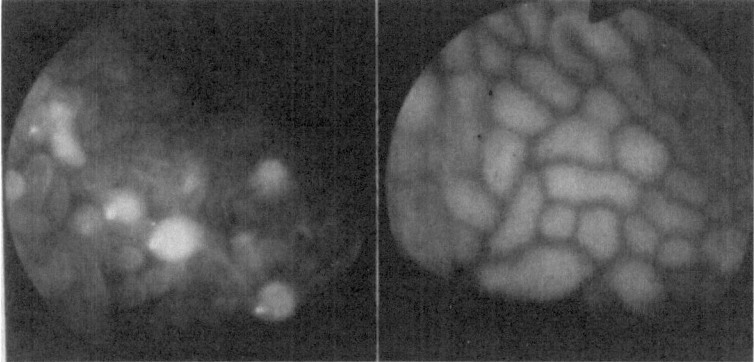

Fig. 8-3. Magnified endoscopic picture revealed each of the mucosal villi white spot (left) and white villi (right) in back of the mucosal villi.

in upper portion of the lamina propria between the epithelial lining and dilated lymphatics (Fig. 8-5). Electron microscopic study revealed that the cavity of the dilated lymphatic vessel was filled with chylomicrons and precipitated lymphprotein (Fig. 8-6). Pinocytotic vesicles containing chylomicron-like substance were noted in the endothelial cells of lymphatic vessel (Fig. 8-7). When the cavity was filled with chylomicron-like substance and precipitated lymphprotein, the thickness of the endothelial cells of intestinal lymphatics in the lamina propria decreased. According to Dobbins, the basal lamina supporting cells, collagen fibers around the lymphatic endothelium and endothelial fibrils were more prominently observed in intestinal lymphangiectasia than in normal subjects (Fig. 8-8).[28]

Since the electron microscopic study demonstrated that the interepithelial spaces and

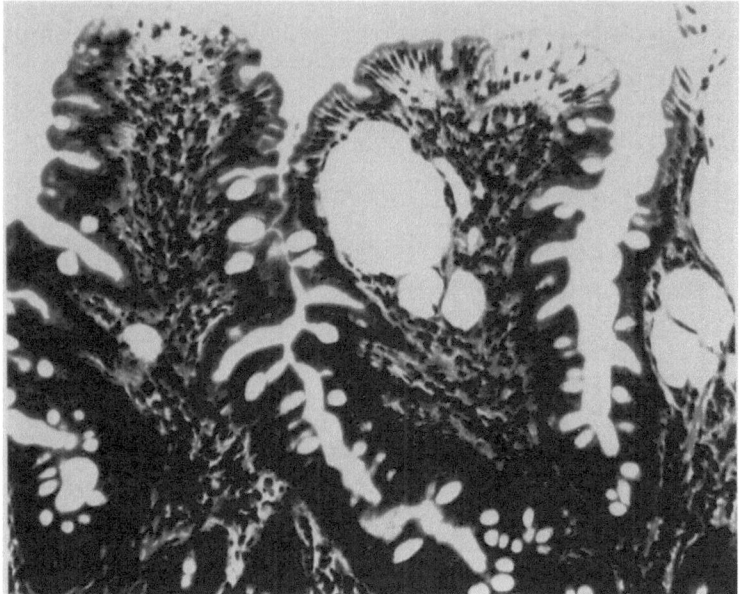

Fig. 8-4. Microscopic picture showed markedly dilated lymphatics in the lamina propria of the jejunal mucosa. ×100, H & E

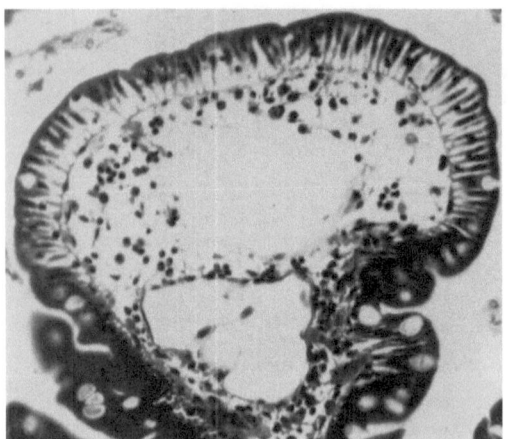

Fig. 8-5. Microscopic picture showed marked edema in the subepithelial space and dilatation of interepithelial spaces. ×200, H & E

stroma were filled with chylomicrons (Figs. 8-9, 8-10) and that the lipoprotein-like substance can be observed in the cavities of endoplasmic reticulum and Golgi apparatus (Fig. 8-11), it is likely that the white color of the villi is due to the mucosal deposition of fats. In the upper portions of villi, a gap between the basal portions of epithelial cells has been observed. Although some enterocytes had prominent microvilli, those of other cells were blunted and decreased in number.[29] Vacuoles containing protein-like material and fat were observed in the cytoplasm of enterocytes and at the intercellular space.

Intestinal lymphangiectasia is frequently seen among Norwegian Lundehunds.[27] In these dogs, vacuolated epithelial cells in the

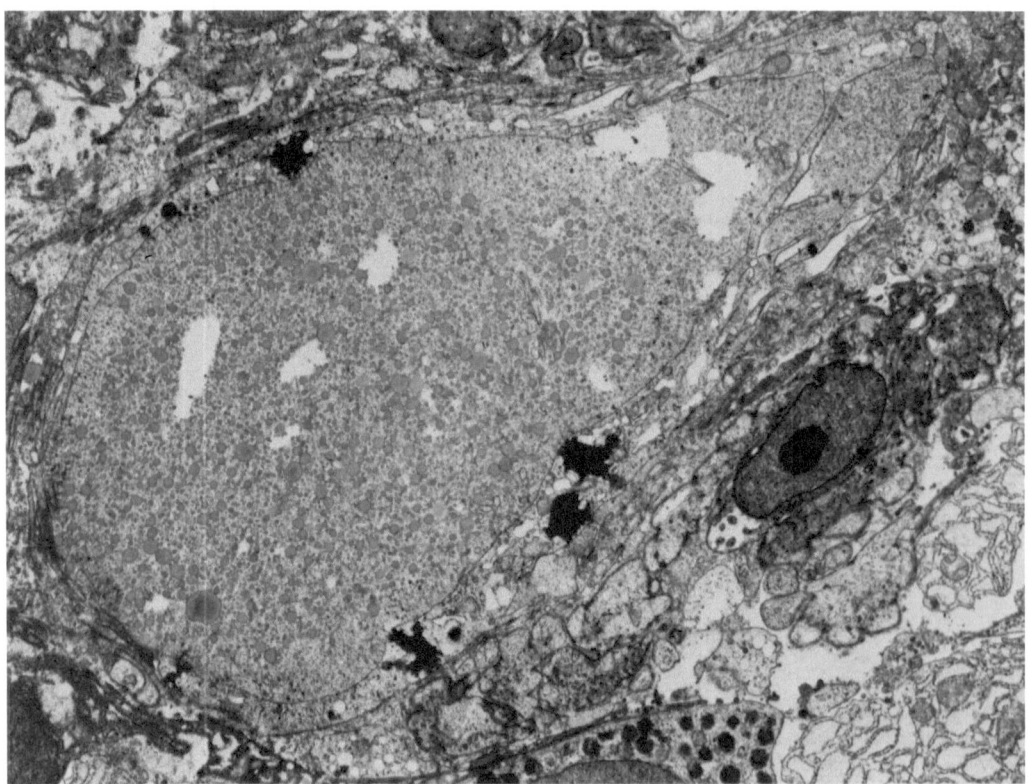

Fig. 8-6. Electron microscopic picture showing large cavity of a dilated lymphatic vessel which was filled with chylomicrons and precipitated lymph proteins. ×5,500

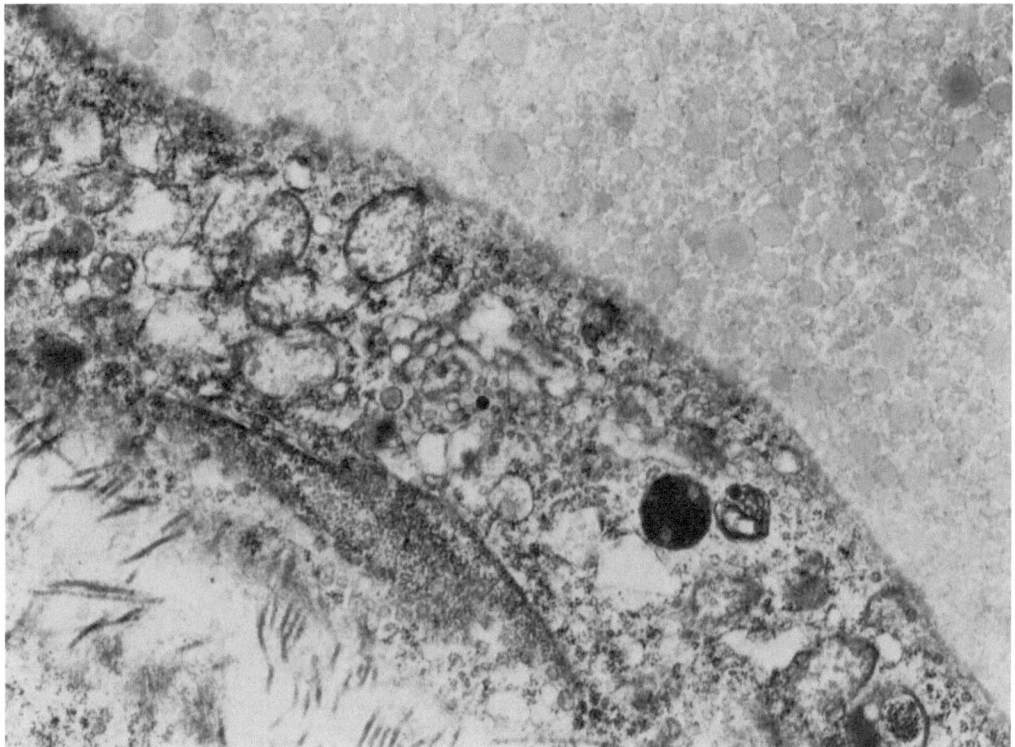

Fig. 8-7. Electron microscopic picture of a lymphatic vessel showed many pinocytotic vesicles containing chylomicron-like substances in its endothelial cells. ×21,000

proximal small intestine have been shown to contain fat detected by oil red staining. The separation of the epithelial cells from the tip of the villi accompanied by a bulging of the epithelial layer is likely to be due to the subepithelial fluid accumulation. Moreover, a snow-white duodenum or white villi was observed in a patient with hypobetalipoproteinemia[30] and in a patient with Whipple's disease.[31]

The diagnosis of intestinal lymphangiectasia is usually established by demonstrating the presence of dilated lymphatics in the intestinal biopsy specimen. Care should be taken, however, since the marked dilatation of intestinal lymphatic vessels has been observed in patients with liver cirrhosis and Behçet's disease who do not exhibit protein-losing gastroenteropathy.[32] It seems important to prove directly the loss of plasma protein into the gut lumen, since it appears that the dilatation of lymphatic vessels of the small intestine is not a sufficient finding to indicate the presence of protein-losing enteropathy.

Chyle-like substances covering the surface of mucosa have been observed at endoscopy examination and surgery (Fig. 8-12) in some cases of intestinal lymphangiectasia. Electron microscopic study has revealed that this substance contains chylomicron-like substances (Fig. 8-13).

Since immunoglobulins and lymphocytes also may be lost into the gut lumen, it is possible that an immunodeficiency state is provoked in patients with this disorder. Serum immunoglobulin levels are decreased in approximately 50% of the patients. We have shown that the number of immunoglobulin-containing cells in the lamina propria of the upper jejunum is markedly decreased in patients with protein-losing enteropathy. Although a count of white blood cells in the peripheral blood is usually normal, the number

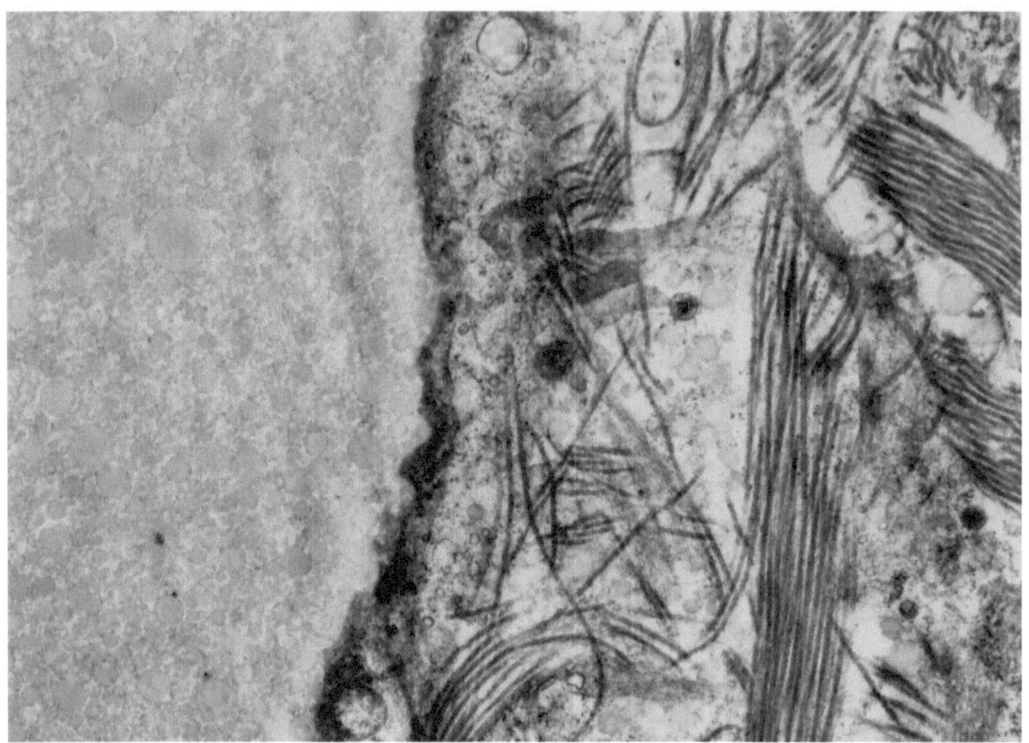

Fig. 8-8. Electron microscopic picture of a lymphatic vessel showed numerous collagen fibers around it. ×21,000

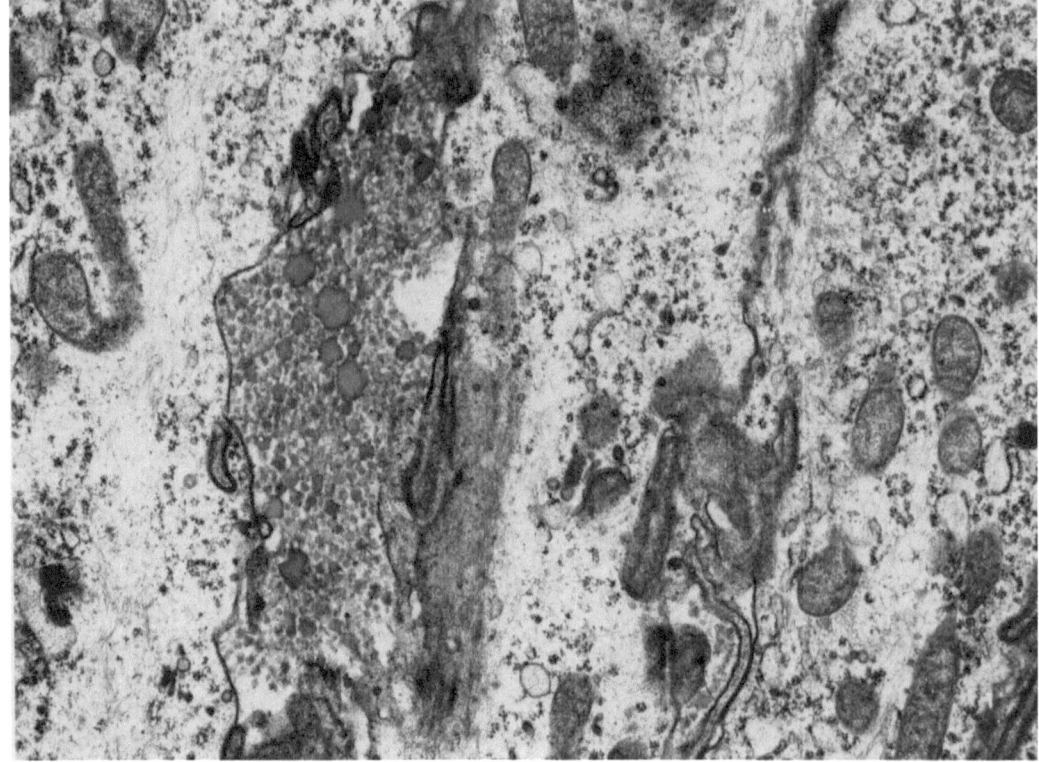

Fig. 8-9. Electron microscopic picture showing lipoprotein-like substances in the interepithelial spaces. ×21,000

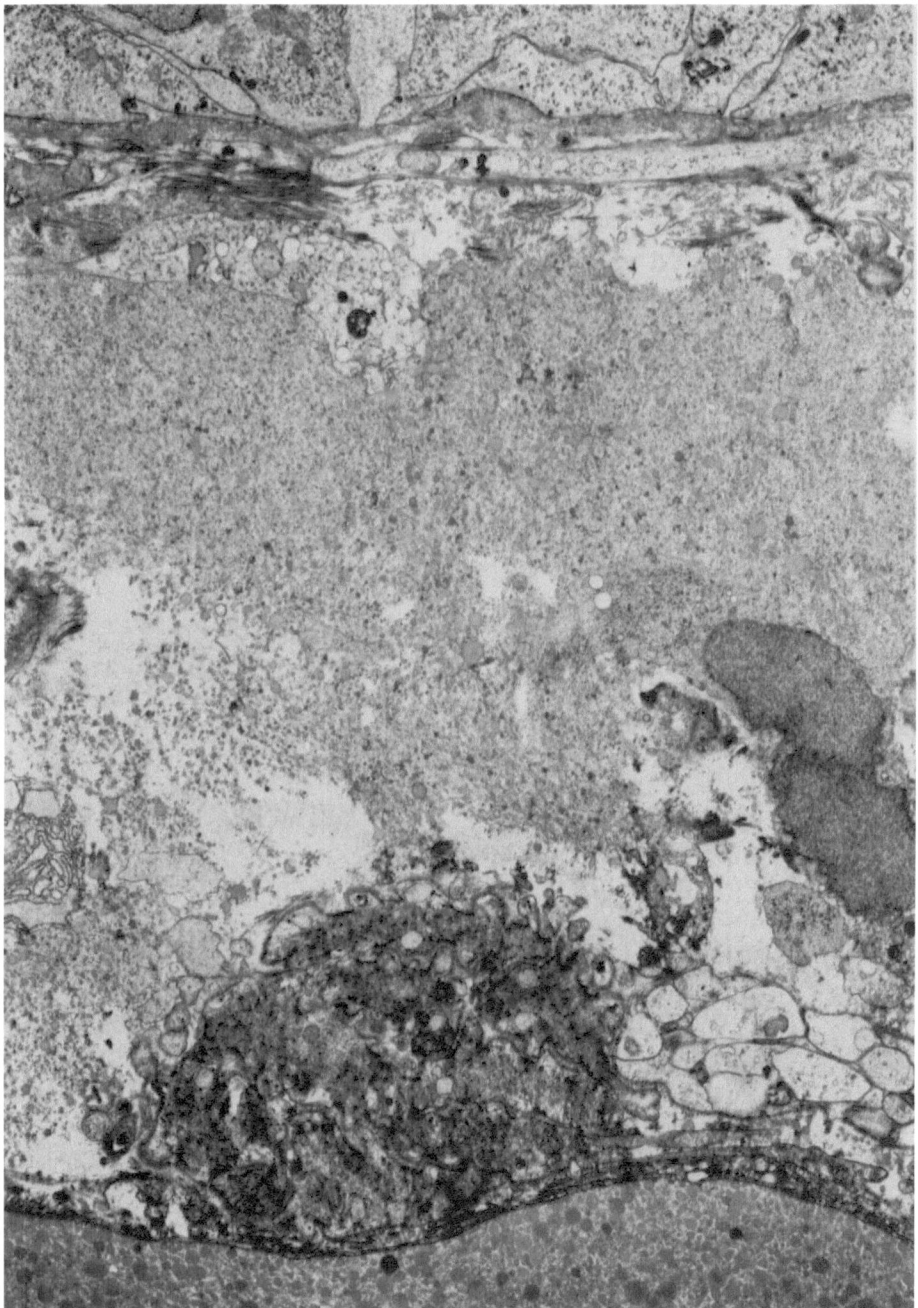

Fig. 8-10. Electron microscopic picture showing numerous chylomicrons and precipitated proteins in the lamina propria of villi of specimens obtained on fasting. ×5,400

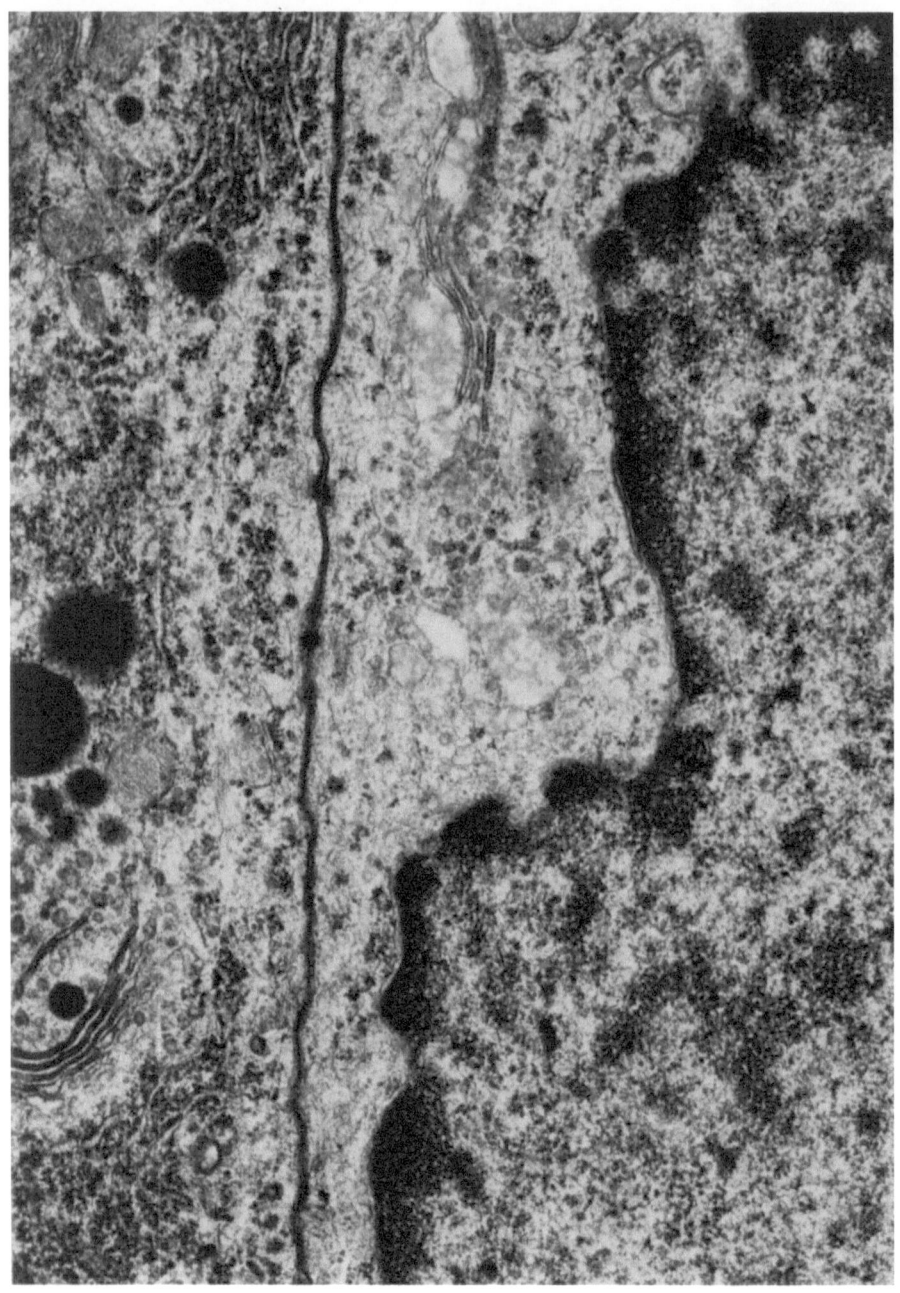

Fig. 8-11. Electron microscopic picture showing lipoprotein-like substances in endoplasmic reticulum and Golgi apparatus. Specimens were obtained in fasting state. ×25,000

of lymphocytes is markedly decreased in many cases. When the subpopulation of lymphocytes is examined, it has been observed that T-cells are decreased, with a relative increase of B-cells (Fig. 8-14). In addition, allergy to skin test antigens and impaired homograft rejection are often noted in patients with intestinal lymphangiectasia.[20,33]

The exact mechanism of the excessive enteric loss of plasma protein in this disease has not been fully elucidated. It is likely that an increased hydrostatic pressure and lymphatic dilatation resulting from the functional or mechanical obstruction of lymph flow may cause a rupture of lacteals concomitant with a loss of chyle into the intestinal lumen.[34] Although this concept is supported by lymphangiographic and endoscopic findings, direct evidence to confirm this hypothesis is not available. According to Landsverk et al,[27] the alteration in the subepithelial hydrostatic tissue pressure may be more important than the mechanism stated above, since an increased tissue pressure may affect the paracellular shunt pathway and permeability of tight junctions. It is thought, however, at this time, that the cellular route is an important pathway for the loss of plasma protein, since epithelial cells have been shown to contain a large number of vacuoles filled with protein-like substance and fat in their cytoplasm.

Low-fat diet is usually effective in treating intestinal lymphangiectasia. This is probably due to a decrease in the pressure within the intestinal lymphatics, since it has been shown that the absorption of long-chain triglycerides increases the flow of intestinal lymph. Medium-chain triglycerides, which are transported to the portal vein, are a good substitute for long-chain triglycerides. A specific drug to treat this disease is not available. However, administration of steroids may be effective in certain cases. Surgical treatment is of limited value, although lymph-enteric fistulas may be resected and lymphatic-venous anastomosis may decrease the pressure within intestinal lymphatics. In cases of secondary intestinal lymphangiectasia, specific treatment should be directed at the primary disease.

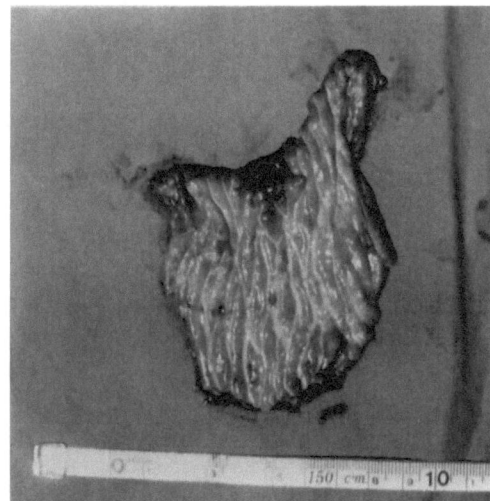

Fig. 8-12. Gross picture of resected specimens obtained from a patient with primary intestinal lymphangiectasia. Milky white material covered the surface of the small intestinal mucosa.

Intestinal Lymphangiectasia of the Large Intestine.

To date, only a few cases of lymphangiectasia of the colon associated with protein-losing enteropathy have been reported by Schaefer et al[35] in 1968, by Ivey et al[36] in 1969, by Griffen et al[37] in 1972, and by Kingham et al[38] in 1982. Cardinal symptoms of this disorder are watery diarrhea, weight loss and edema. Recently we have observed a case of colonic lymphangiectasia with enteric protein loss.[39] In this case, however, edema was not evident for 17 years. Although the mechanism of enteric loss of plasma proteins in this disorder has not been fully understood, it has been shown that the effect of partial colectomy is dramatic in all reported cases. It appears that the treatment and prognosis of this disease are considerably different from those of small intestinal lymphangiectasia.

Slightly different histopathological findings have been obtained in each case. The gross specimens had a pale, glistening and ulcer-free mucosa that contained clear fluid when cut. In other cases, multiple sessile polyps

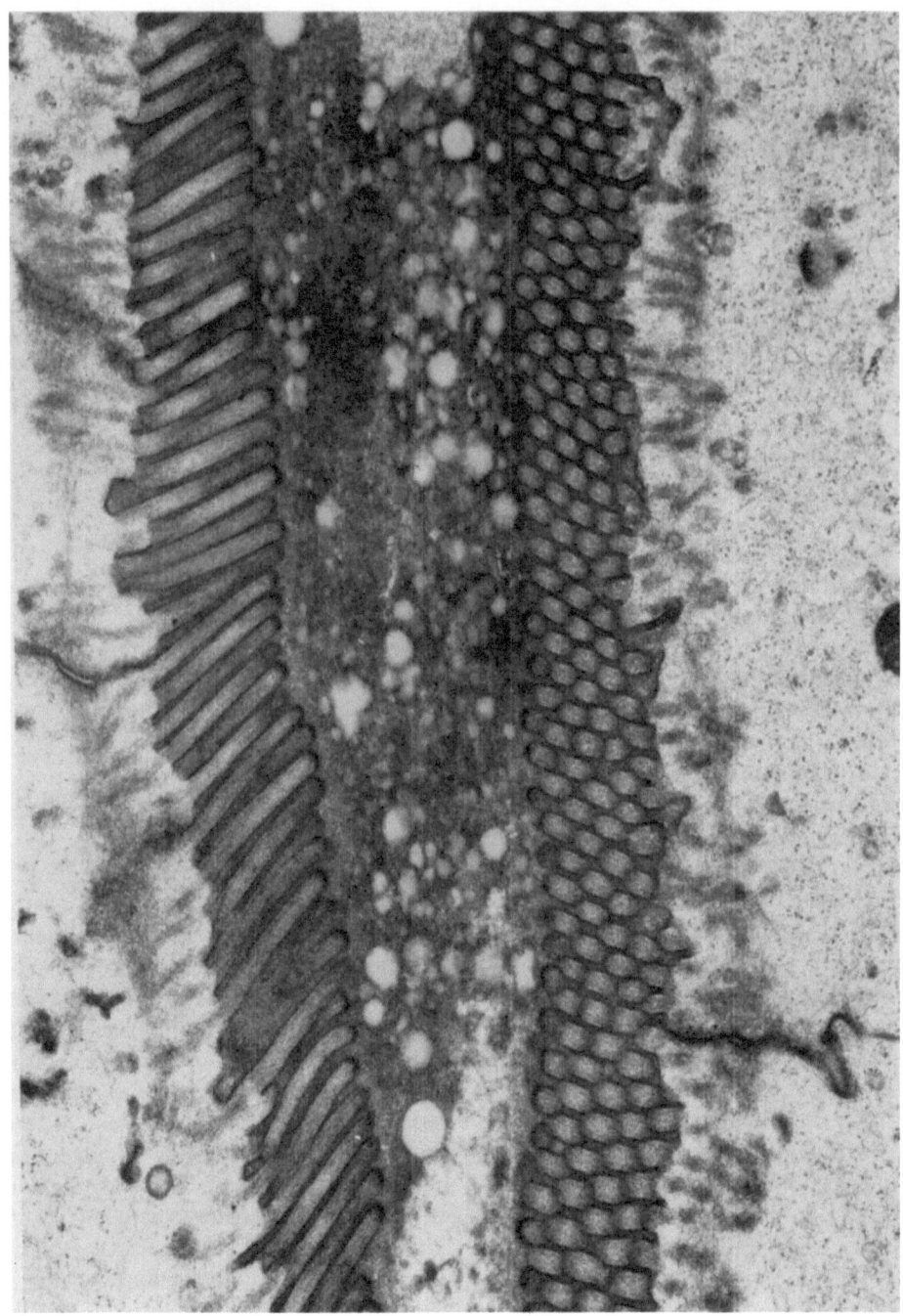

Fig. 8-13. Electron microscopic picture showing that the milky white material contained chylomicron-like substances. ×21,000

174

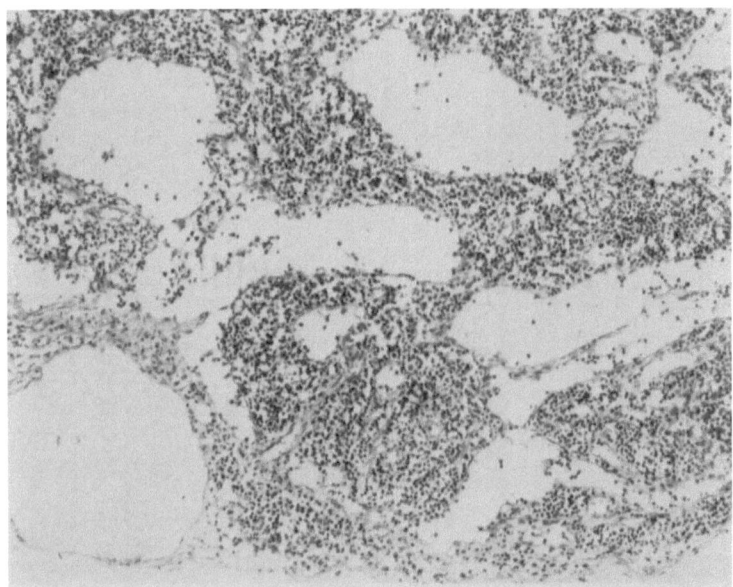

Fig. 8-14. Mesenteric lymph node obtained from a patient with protein-losing enteropathy. Note that paracortical areas (T cell areas) were depleted of lymphocytes. ×100, H & E

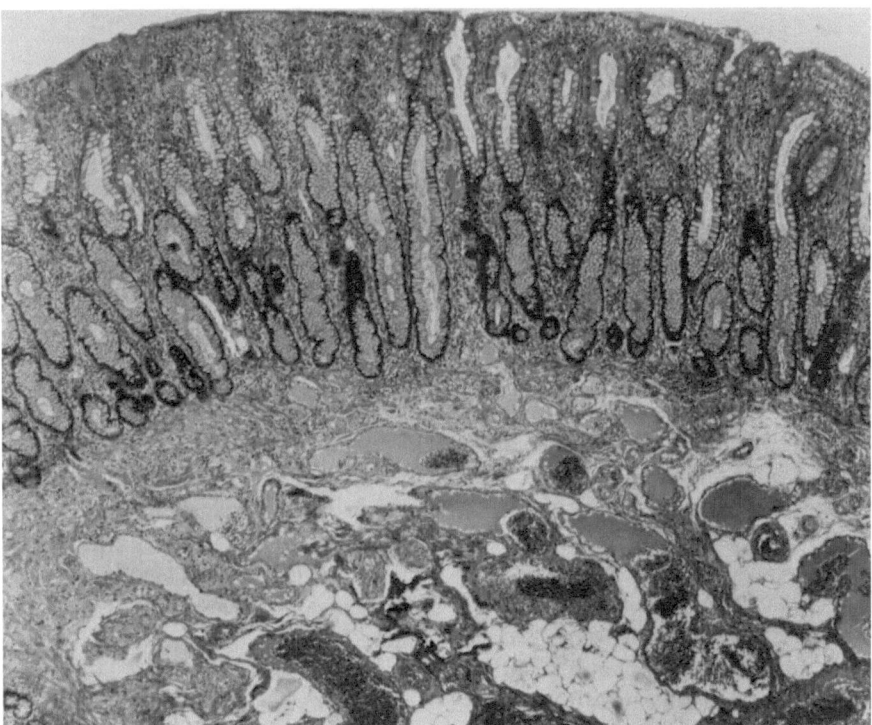

Fig. 8-15. Microscopic picture of resected specimen from a patient with intestinal lymphangiectasia of the large intestine which showed dilated lymphatic vessels in the submucosa and muscularis mucosae. ×40, H & E

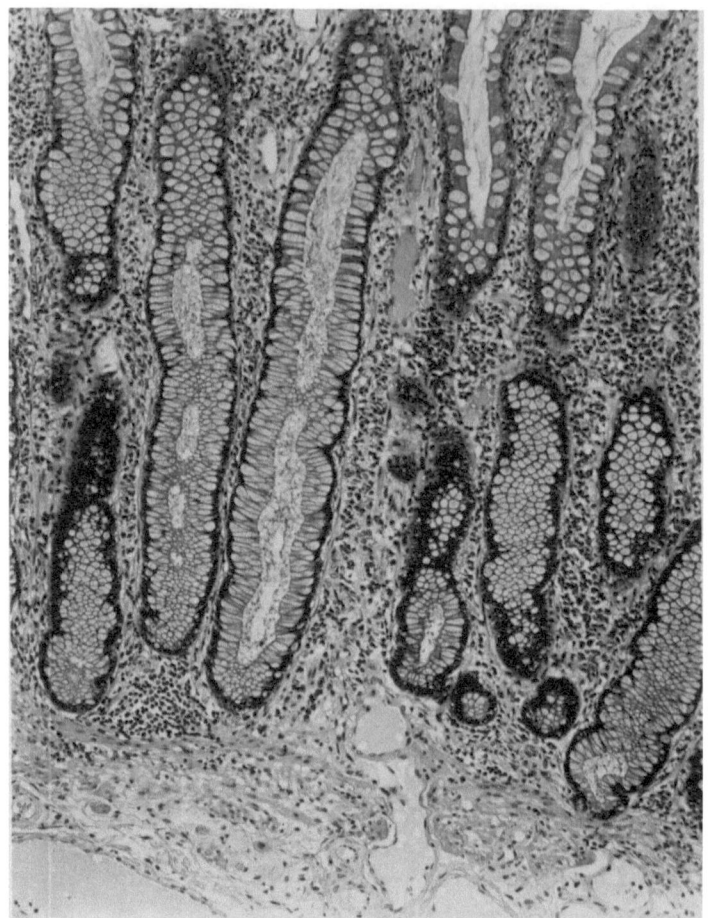

Fig. 8-16. Microscopic picture of lymphangiectasia of the large intestine showing the high location of lymphatics in the lamina propria of the colon. ×100, H & E

were observed in the rectosigmoid area by colonoscopy. Scattered white spots, white villi, and chyle-like substance covering the mucosa, which can be observed in small intestinal lymphangiectasia, are not found in colonic lymphangiectasia. This is probably because fat absorption is not taking place in the colon. Under microscopic examination, commonly observed findings were generalized edema and dilated lymphatic vessels in the submucosa and muscularis mucosae (Fig. 8-15). It has been reported that normally lymphatics are not present in the colonic mucosa except in the lowermost portion next to the muscularis mucosae.[40] In our case, however, the lymphatics could be observed in the higher portion of lamina propria of the colon (Fig. 8-16). Electron microscopic study revealed that there was a dilated lymphatic-like vessel in the lamina propria of the colonic mucosa (Fig. 8-17). There was, however, no chylomicron-like substance except for precipitated lymph protein in its cavity. This finding may support the basic lesion of protein-losing enteropathy.

Schaefer et al[35] observed a fair amount of clear fluid covering the diseased colonic mucosa but failed to detect significant amounts

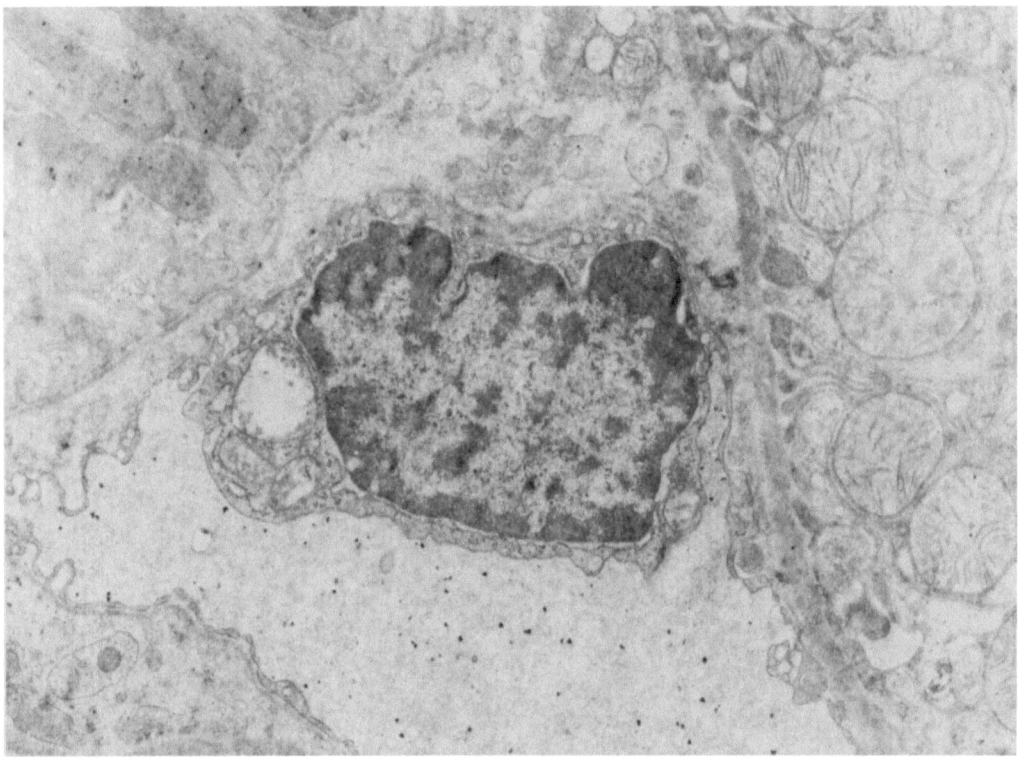

Fig. 8-17. Electron microscopic picture revealed a lymphatic-like vessel in the lamina propria of the colonic mucosa. ×7,000

of protein. Analysis of rectal fluid in our case revealed that the proteins in the fluid were both qualitatively and quantitatively similar to those in the patient's serum, suggesting leakage of serum protein into the colonic lumen.

MÉNÉTRIER'S DISEASE

Giant folds of the stomach can be observed in various diseases including hypertrophic glandular gastritis, Ménétrier's disease, Zollinger-Ellison syndrome, and Bormann type IV gastric cancer.

Diffuse thickening of the gastric wall caused by marked proliferation of the mucosa was first described by Ménétrier[9] in 1888. A number of synonyms for this rare disorder have been used in the literature. These include giant hypertrophic gastritis,[41] tumor-simulating hypertrophic gastritis, gastric polyposis, cystic gastritis, and giant rugal hypertrophy (Fig. 8-18). Ménétrier described two different conditions in his original monograph, namely polyadenomes polypeux and polyadenomes en nappe (sheet-like polyadenomes).[42]

According to Schindler,[43] hypertrophic gastritis can be classified into three forms: chronic hypertrophic interstitial gastritis, chronic hypertrophic proliferative gastritis, and chronic hypertrophic glandular gastritis. The term giant hypertrophic gastritis has been used to describe a variety of microscopic pictures. Detailed histopathological characteristics varied among fourteen cases of giant hypertrophic gastritis reported by Butz.[44] Schindler emphasized that "Ménétrier's disease" should be used only for cases with destruction of glands, tubular overgrowth of

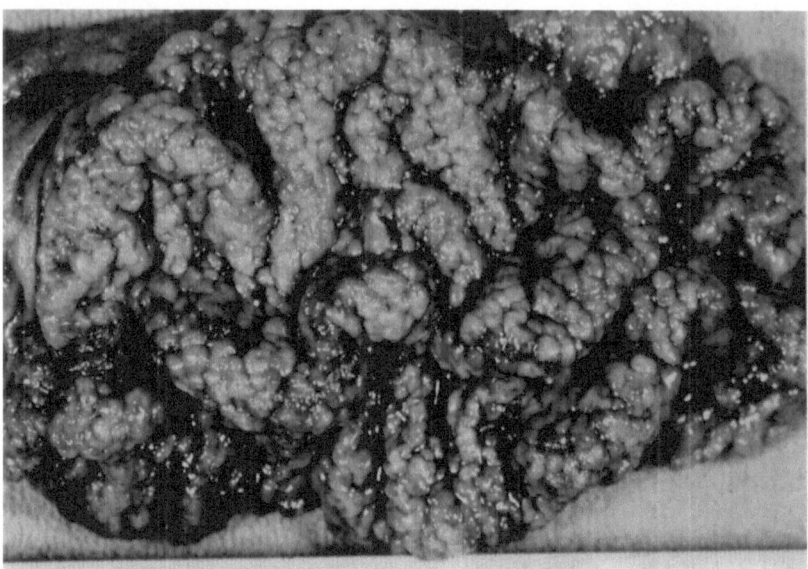

Fig. 8-18. Gross specimen of resected stomach obtained from a patient with Ménétrier's disease.

the surface epithelium, low acid output, and
hypoproteinemia.

We have examined six patients with giant
gastric folds and/or polyposis with protein-
losing gastropathy. Gastroscopy revealed
varying degrees of tortuous giant folds that
were not obliterated by insufflation (Figs. 8-
19, 8-20). The surface of the folds showed irregular and nodular appearances in some

cases, but it was rather smooth in one patient.
Large amounts of white sticky mucus covering the mucosa were noted in all patients. The
active and continuous secretion of gastric
juice, which we call hypersecretion (stalactite
grotto phenomenon), was also observed.

The major histopathological finding in Ménétrier's disease is hyperplasia of the surface
mucous cells, which causes deepening and

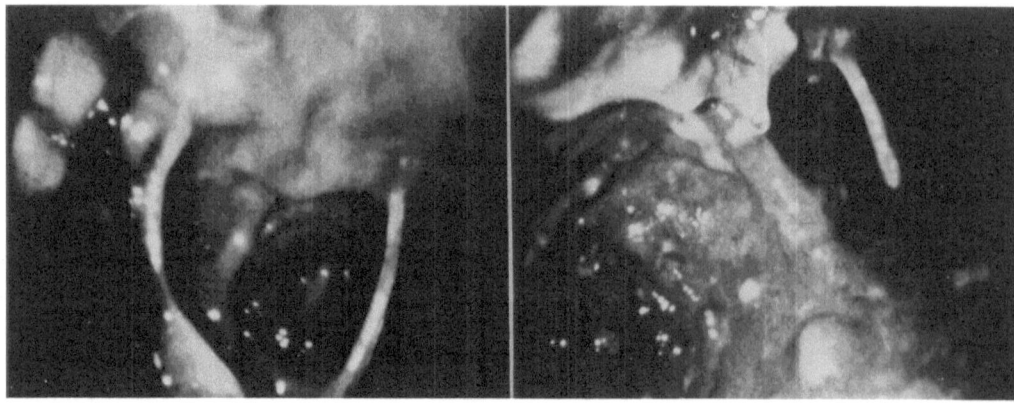

Fig. 8-19. Gastroendoscopy showing giant folds of the stomach. Note hypersecretion and mucus covering the mucosal surface.

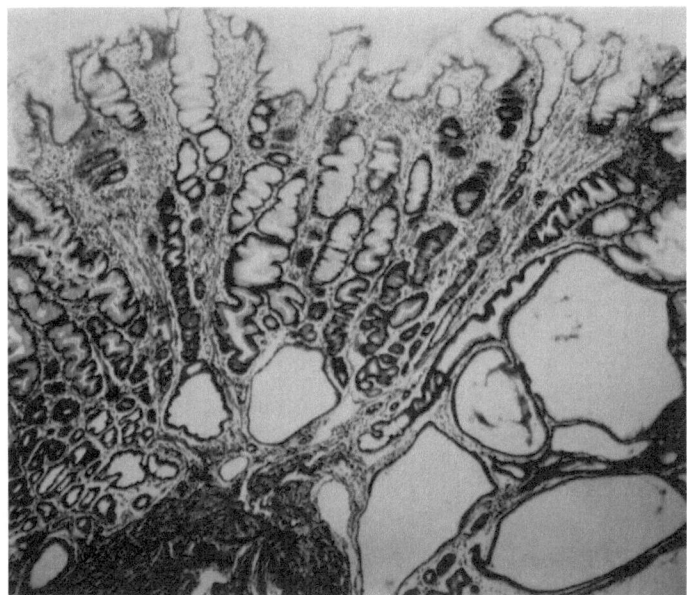

Fig. 8-20. Microscopic picture of the giant folds showed marked proliferation of surface epithelium like a corkscrew. Cystic dilatation of gastric glands was observed. ×40, H & E

tortuosity of the gastric pits. Microscopic pictures of giant folds can be classified into two categories. In one group, the decreased fundic glands with hyperplasia of surface mucous cells are noted. This is accompanied by a complete replacement of parietal cells by mucus-secreting cells (Fig. 8-20). Another type is a hyperplasia of the fundic glands.[45] A varied degree of cystic dilatation of the glands containing eosinophilic substance is observed. Surface epithelial cells of gastric pits secrete a large amount of mucus that is positive for double staining using alcian blue and PAS (Fig. 8-21). In some cases, moderate lymphangiectasia is seen in the submucosa and/or in the lamina propria.[46] It was observed electron microscopically that surface mucous cells were secreting mucous granules into the gastric lumen (Fig. 8-22).

In 1957, Citrin and coworkers[16] first demonstrated loss of plasma protein into the gastric lumen in a patient with giant hypertrophy of gastric mucosa. Although many routes for loss of plasma protein have been postulated in protein-losing gastroenteropathy, the exact

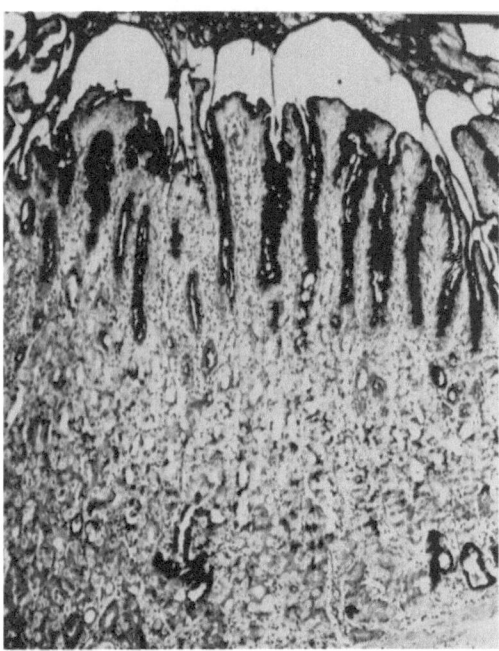

Fig. 8-21. Microscopic picture of gastric giant folds stained with Alcian-blue and PAS showed hyperplasia of mucin-secreting cells and a large amount of mucus. ×120, AB-PAS

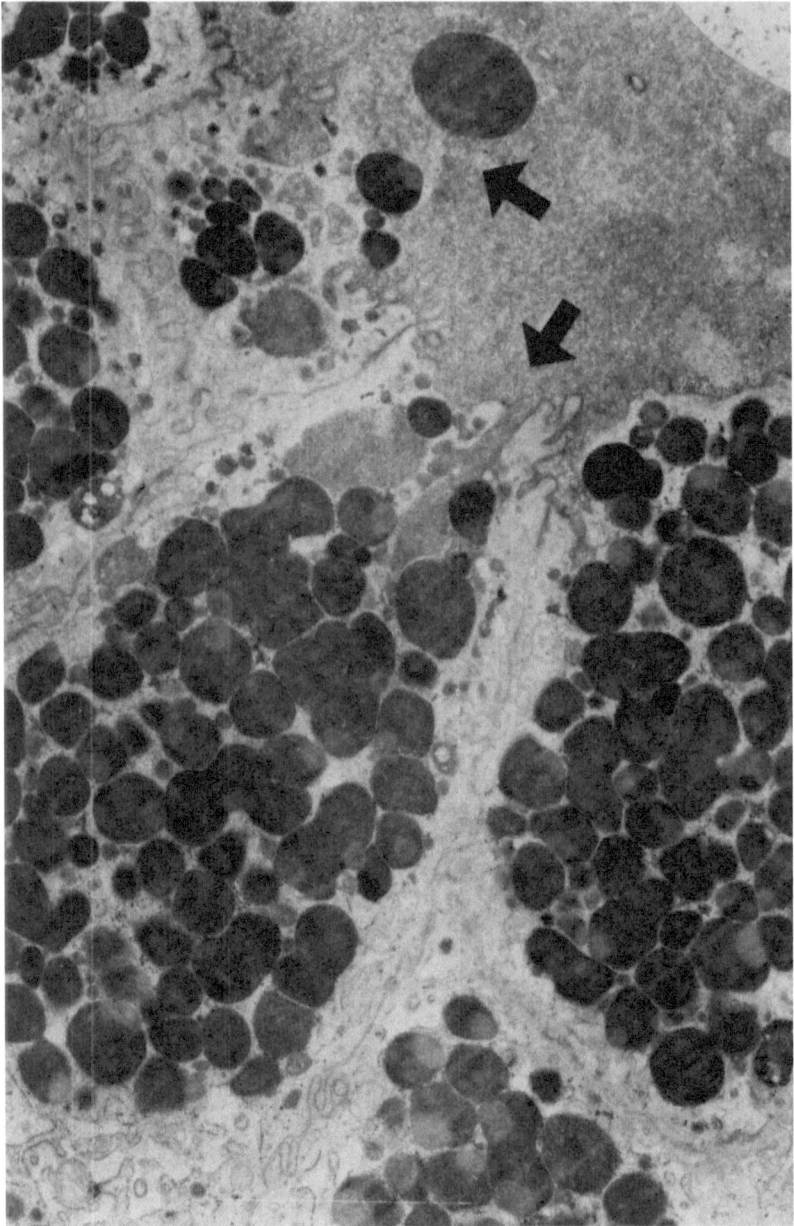

Fig. 8-22. Electron microscopic picture showing that surface mucous cells were secreting their mucus granules into the gastric lumen (arrows). ×3,000

pathway of protein loss through the gastric mucosa has not been clarified. According to Lev and Brus,[47] the transcellular pathway may be a major route for transmucosal efflux of plasma protein, since many intracellular vacuoles containing protein could be observed histochemically in mucosal biopsy specimens obtained from patients with protein-losing gastroenteropathy. However, the importance of an intercellular pathway has been emphasized in experimental protein-losing gastropathy.[48]

In seven patients with hypertrophic gastropathy, Kelly and coworkers performed gastric perfusion and electron microscopic study attempting to elucidate the route of protein loss.[49] Under electron microscopy, tight junctions appeared to be wider than normal in all patients. In addition, acute administration of propantheline bromide reduced leakage of albumin into the gastric lumen and decreased the width of tight junctions. Another antisecretory agent, cimetidine, failed to demonstrate a consistent effect on protein loss and on the width of tight junctions. However, administration of ranitidine, a histamine H_2 receptor antagonist, significantly reduced the gastric protein loss in a few patients with Ménétrier's disease.[50] These results indicate that the paracellular pathway through tight junctions plays an important role in transmucosal efflux of plasma protein. The coexistence of a transcellular pathway, however, cannot be ruled out.

Therapy of hypertrophic gastropathy is still controversial. Total gastrectomy has been reported to be very effective, and an increase in serum albumin level is observed after surgery.[51] Long term administration of anticholinergic agents appeared to be effective for the protein-losing gastropathy.[52]

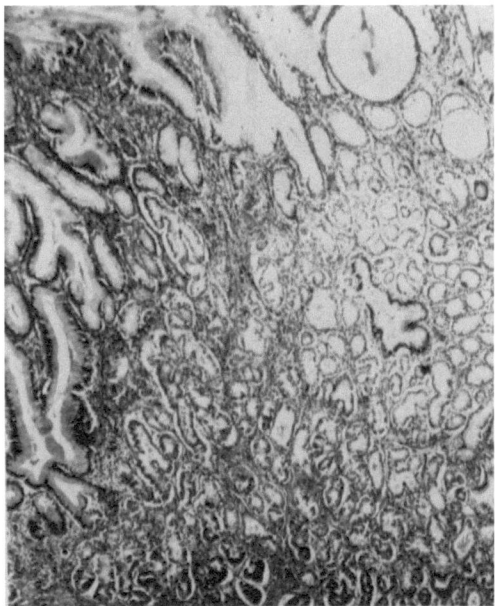

Fig. 8-23. Microscopic picture of gastric lesions from a patient with Cronkhite-Canada syndrome. ×120, H & E

CRONKHITE-CANADA SYNDROME

In Cronkhite-Canada syndrome,[53] the extensive polyposis in the stomach and intestine may be involved, with ectodermal symptoms and hypoproteinemia due to gastrointestinal protein loss. Ectodermal symptoms are alopecia, hyperpigmentation, and dystrophy of the fingernails and toenails. The mechanism of the excessive protein loss in this syndrome is not known. The early reports by Cronkhite and Canada described the polyps as adenomatous in appearance, but recently these polyps were thought to be of the juvenile type. The polyps had cystically dilated glands and an extensive inflammatory reaction similar in some respects to juvenile polyps (Fig. 8-23).

Surface epithelial cells of gastric pits secrete a large amount of mucus that is positive with double staining using alcian blue and PAS (Fig. 8-24). One may think that the mechanism of gastric protein loss in this lesion is similar to that in Ménétrier's disease. The prognosis is poor, but several cases have been reported in which hyperalimentation and prednisolone were effective in clinical improvement.

CONCLUSION

Protein-losing gastroenteropathy is caused by various gastrointestinal disorders. Examination of primary intestinal lymphangiectasia has clarified that the protein loss was caused by direct leakage of intestinal lymph into the intestinal lumen. An increased hydrostatic pressure within the lymphatics may be considered to cause a rupture of lecteals, or an alteration in the subepithelial hydrostatic tissue

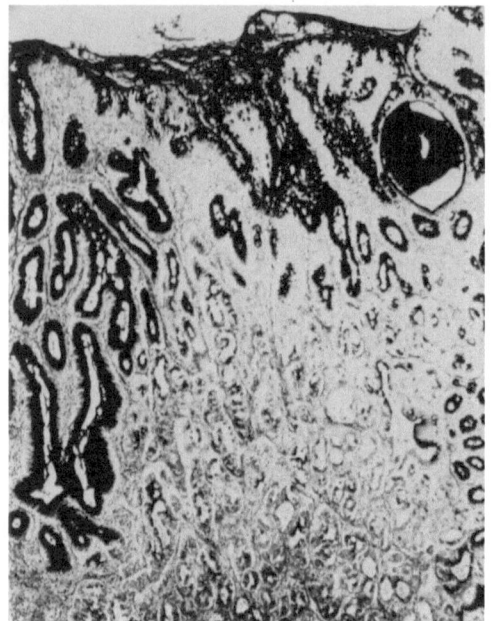

Fig. 8-24. Microscopic picture of the gastric lesions stained with Alcian-blue and PAS. ×120, AB-PAS

pressure, which may be more important. However, ultrastructural study in the present work suggested that the cellular route is an important pathway for the loss of plasma protein.

Rare related disorders, such as lymphangiectasia of the large intestine, Ménétrier's disease, and Cronkhite-Canada syndrome also were briefly described.

REFERENCES

1. Strober W.: Protein-losing enteropathy, In Textbook of Gastroenterology Bouchier I.A.D., Allan R.N., Hodgson H.J.F., et al (eds.). Baillière Tindall, 1984, p 598
2. Waldmann T.A., Steinfeld J.L., Dutcher T.F., Davidson J.D., Gordon R.S.: The role of the gastrointestinal system in idiopathic hypoproteinemia. Gastroenterology **41**:197, 1961
3. Pomerantz M., Waldmann T.A.: Systemic lymphatic abnormalities associated with gastro-intestinal protein loss secondary to intestinal lymphangiectasia. Gastroenterology **45**:703, 1963
4. Petersen V.P., Hastrop J.: Protein-losing enteropathy in constrictive pericarditis, Acta Med Scand **173**:410, 1963
5. Beeker W.L., Busch H.J., Sylvester D.L.: Intestinal protein loss in Crohn's disease. Gastroenterology **62**:207, 1972
6. Chew C.K., Jarzylo S.V., Valberg L.S.: Idiopathic retroperitoneal fibrosis with protein-losing enteropathy and duodenal obstruction successfully treated with corticosteroids. Can Med Assoc J **95**:1183, 1963
7. Steinfield J.L., Davidson J.D., Gordon R.S. Jr., Greene F.E.: The mechanism of hypoproteinemia in patients with regional enteritis and ulcerative colitis. Am J Med **29**:405, 1960
8. Waldmann T.A., Broder S., Strober W.: Protein-losing enteropathies in malignancy. Ann New York Acad Sci **230**:306, 1974
9. Ménétrier P.: Des polyadenomes gastriques et de leurs rapports avec le cancer de l'estomac. Arch Physiol Normale Pathol **4**:32, 1888
10. Waldmann T.A., Wochner R.D., Laster L., Gordon R.S. Jr.: Allergic gastroenteropathy. A cause of excessive gastrointestinal protein loss. New Engl J Med **276**:761, 1967
11. Parkin R.A.: Protein-losing enteropathy in the sprue syndrome. Lancet ii:1366, 1968
12. King C.E., Toskes P.P.: Protein-losing enteropathy in the human and experimental rat blind-loop syndrome. Gastroenterology **80**:504, 1981
13. Kondo M., Bamba T., Hosokawa K., Hosoda S., Kawai K., Masuda M.: Tissue plasminogen activator in the pathogenesis of protein-losing gastroenteropathy. Gastroenterology **70**:1045, 1976
14. Wood J.G., Davenport H.W.: Measurement of canine gastric vascular permeability to plasma proteins in the normal and protein-losing states. Gastroenterology **82**:725, 1982
15. Tsuchiya M., Oshio C., Asakura H., Ishii H., Aoki I., Miyairi M.: Budd-Chiari syndrome associated with protein-losing enteropathy. Gastroenterology **75**:114, 1978
16. Citrin Y., Sterling K., Halsted J.A.: The mechanism of hypoproteinemia associated with giant hypertrophy of the gastric mucosa. N Engl J Med **257**:906, 1957
17. Gordon R.S.: Exudative enteropathy, Abnormal permeability of the gastrointestinal tract demonstrable with labelled P.V.P. Lancet **1**:325, 1959
18. Waldmann T.A., Wochner R.D., Strober W.: The role of the gastrointestinal tract in plasma protein metabolism studies with ^{51}Cr-albumin. Am J Med **46**:775, 1969
19. Florent C., L'Hirondel C., Desmàzures C., Aymes C., Bernier J.J.: Intestinal clearance of α_1-antitrypsin. A sensitive method for the detection of protein-losing enteropathy. Gastroenterology **81**:777, 1981
20. Strober W., Wochner R.D., Carbone P.P., Waldmann T.A.: Intestinal lymphangiectasia: a protein losing enteropathy with hypogammaglobulinemia, lymphopenia and impaired homograft rejection. J Clin Invest **46**:1643, 1967
21. Nelson D.L., Blaese R.M., Strober W., Bruce R.M., Waldmann T.A.: Constrictive pericarditis, intestinal lymphangiectasia, and reversible immunologic deficiency. J Pediatrics **86**:548, 1975
22. Vardy P.A., Lebenthal E., Schwachman H.: Intestinal lymphangiectasia, A reappraisal. Pediatrics **55**:842, 1975
23. Fakhri A., Fishman E.K., Jones B., Kuhajda F., Siegelman S.S.: Primary intestinal lympangiectasia: clinical and CT findings. J Comput Assist Tomogr **9**:767, 1985

24. Kinmonth J.B., Taylor G.W., Harper R.K.: Lymphangiectasia lymphangiography: A technique for its clinical use in the lower limb. Br Med J 1:940, 1955
25. Morishita T., Hibi T., Asakura H., Tsuchiya M., Pescante M., Uylangco C.: Endoscopy of the jejunal mucosa in human cholera. Gastrointest Endosc 24:284, 1978
26. Asakura H., Miura S., Morishita T., Aiso S., Tanaka T., Kitahora T., Tsuchiya M., Enomoto Y., Watanabe Y.: Endoscopic and histopathological study on primary and secondary intestinal lymphangiectasia. Dig Dis Sci 26:423, 1982
27. Landsverk T., Gamlem H.: Intestinal lymphangiectasia in the Lundehund. Acta Path Microbiol Immunol Scand (Sect A)92:353, 1984
28. Dobbins W.O.: Electron microscopic study of the intestinal mucosa in intestinal lymphangiectasia. Gastroenterology 51:1004, 1966
29. Bujanover Y., Liebman W.M., Goodman J.R., Thaler M.M.: Primary intestinal lymphangiectasia. Case report with radiological and ultrastructual study. Digestion 21:107, 1981
30. Mitchell C.J., Scott B.B., Bullen A.W., Lonowsky M.S.: Snow-white duodenum. A new endoscopic sign in a patient with hypobetalipoproteinemia. Gastrointest Endosc 24:123, 1978
31. Volpicelli N.A., Salyer W.R., Milligan F.D., Bayless T.M., Yardley J.H.: The endoscopic appearance of the duodenum in Whipple's disease. Johns Hopkins Med J 138:19, 1976
32. Asakura H., Morita A., Morishita T., Tsuchiya M., Watanabe Y., Enomoto Y.: Histopathological and electron microscopic studies of lymphangiectasia of the small intestine in Behçet's disease. Gut 14:196, 1973
33. Weiden P.L., Blaese R.M., Strober W., Block B.J., Waldmann T.A.: Impaired lymphocyte transformation in intestinal lymphangiectasia: Evidence for at least two functionally distinct lymphocyte populations in man. J Clin Invest 51:1319, 1972
34. Mistilis S.P., Skyring A.P., Stephen D.D.: Intestinal lymphangiectasia: Mechanism of enteric loss of plasma-protein and fat. Lancet, 1:77, 1965
35. Schaefer J.W., Griffen W.O., Dubilier L.D.: Colonic lymphangiectasis associated with a potassium depletion syndrome. Gastroenterology 55:515, 1968
36. Ivey K., DenBesten L., Kent T.H., Clifton J.A.: Lymphangiectasia of the colon with protein loss and malabsorption. Gastroenterology 57:709, 1969
37. Griffen W.O., Belin R.P., Furman R.W., Lieber A., Schaefer J.W., Dubilier L.D.: Colonic lymphangiectasia: Report of two cases. Dis Col Rect 15:49, 1972
38. Kingham J.G.C., Moriarty K.J., Furness M., Levison D.A.: Lymphangiectasia of the colon and small intestine. Brit J Radiol 55:774, 1982
39. Asakura H., Tsuchiya M., Katoh S., Kobayashi K.,

Yonei Y., Yoshida T., Hamada Y., Miura S., Morita A., Kuramochi S., Teramoto T.: Pathological findings of lymphangiectasia of the large intestine in a patient with protein-losing enteropathy. Gastroenterology 91:719, 1986
40. Fenoglio C.M., Kaye G.I., Lane N.: Distribution of human colonic lymphatics in normal, hyperplastic, and adenomatous tissue. Gastroenterology 64:51, 1973
41. Fieber S.S.: Hypertrophic gastritis. Report of two cases and analysis of fifty pathologically verified cases from the literature. Gastroenterology 28:39, 1955
42. Palmer D.: What Ménétrier really said. Gastrointest Endosc 15:83, 1968
43. Schindler R.: On hypertrophic glandular gastritis, hypertrophic gastropathy, and parietal cell mass. Gastroenterology 45:77, 1963
44. Butz W.C.: Giant hypertrophic gastritis. A report of fourteen cases. Gastroenterology 39:183, 1960
45. Brooks A.M., Isenberg J., Goldstein H.: Giant thickening of the gastric mucosa with acid hypersecretion and protein losing gastropathy. Gastroenterology 58:73, 1970
46. Miura S., Asakura H., Tsuchiya M.: Lymphatic abnormalities in protein-losing gastropathy, especially in Ménétrier's disease. Angiology 32:345, 1981
47. Lev R., Brus I.: Morphological and histochemical demonstration of protein in gastric surface epithelium in protein losing gastropathies. Am J Dig Dis 16:589, 1971
48. Munro D.R.: Route of protein losing during a model protein losing gastropathy in dogs. Gastroenterology 66:960, 1974
49. Kelly D.G., Miller L.J., Malagelada J-R., Huizenga K.A., Markowitz H.: Giant hypertrophic gastropathy (Ménétrier's disease): Pharmacologic effects on protein leakage and mucosal ultrastructure. Gastroenterology 83:58, 1982
50. Reinhart W.H., Weigand K., Kappeler M., Roesler H., Halter F.: Comparison of gastrointestinal loss of alpha-1-antitrypsin and chromium-51-albumin in Ménétrier's disease and the influence of ranitidine. Digestion 26:192, 1983
51. Balfour D.C., Hightower N.C., Gambill E.E., Waugh J.M., Dockerty M.B.: Giant hypertrophy of the gastric rugae (Ménétrier's disease) associated with severe hypoproteinemia relieved only by total gastrectomy: report of case. Gastroenterology 16:773, 1950
52. Smith R.L., Powell D.W.: Prolonged treatment of Ménétrier's disease with an oral anticholinergic drug. Gastroenterology 74:903, 1978
53. Cronkhite L.W., Canada W.J.: Generalized gastrointestinal polyposis: An unusual syndrome of polyposis, pigmentation, alopecia and onychotrophia. N Engl J Med 252:1011, 1955

9

Secretory IgA and Mucosal Immune Responses

H. Nagura M.D.
Y. Sumi M.D.

Mucosal immunity is characterized predominantly by a secretory antibody response, involving immunoglobulins of the IgA class. They provide an immunological barrier to foreign matter by preventing absorption of such materials into the mucosal epithelium and penetration into the body. The humoral responses in nonmucosal sites are largely of the IgG class. The cell-mediated immune mechanism is also distinctive in mucosal and nonmucosal lymphoid organs. During the past decade, significant advances have been made in understanding the mucosal immune system. Ontological and physiological relationships between immunocompetent cells in mucosal and nonmucosal sites have been characterized, and the postulation of a common mucosal immune system[1,2] involving the intestinal tract, biliary tract, mammary glands, salivary glands, lacrimal glands, and female genital tract has led to new insights.

The mucosal surface is exposed to a myriad of antigenic substances that have readily demonstrable immunostimulatory or immunomodulatory properties, such as microbes, chemicals, and food, and contact between these antigens, and the mucosal immunological apparatus initiates a diverse series of immunologic events. These include the production of antibodies that are secreted into extracellular body fluids and, in striking contrast, induce hyporesponsiveness of certain nonmucosal (systemic) immunologic reactions.[3,4] The importance of the mucosal immune system in the host-environment interaction and in the pathogenesis of certain diseases of mucosal and nonmucosal tissues has received much appreciation in recent years. A deficiency in mucosal IgA, for example, can severely impair mucosal barrier function, resulting in uptake of noxious substances that could contribute to the pathogenesis of intestinal or systemic diseases.[5] In this review we have summarized the wealth of information about the mucosal immune system, with emphasis on the role of liver in the regulation of the immune responses involving IgA.

PARTICIPATION OF SECRETORY IgA IN THE MUCOSAL IMMUNE SYSTEM IN THE NEONATE

IgG is the only class of antibodies in rat or mouse breast fluid to be transported intact into the offspring circulation across the intestine in substantial quantities, even though these fluids also contain IgA and IgM antibodies.[6,7] The transfer of IgG, however, is sharply limited in time to the first 18 to 21 days of life in the rat.[6,7] Colostrum IgG is

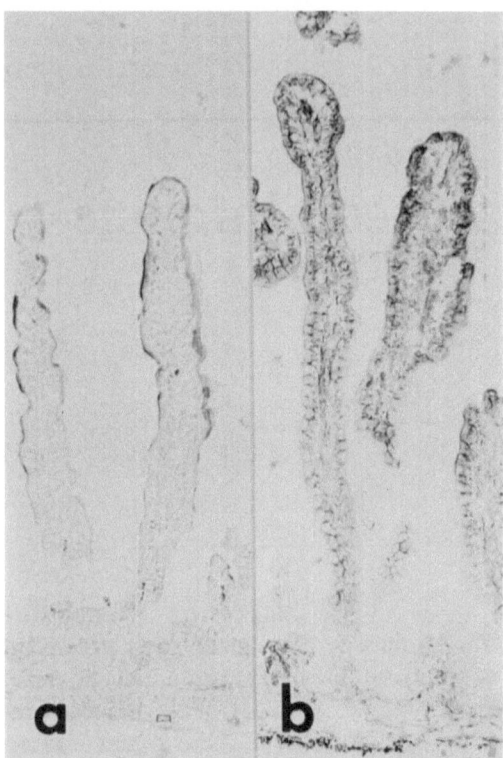

Fig. 9-1. Immunohistochemical localization of IgA (a) and IgG (b) in the proximal intestine of breast-fed neonatal rats. IgA is found on the surface of enterocytes, whereas IgG is localized on the basolateral plasma membranes in addition to the apical surface. No plasma cells are present in the lamina propria.

found in the lower portion of microvilli and intervening apical plasma membranes of proximal enterocytes of breast-fed neonatal rats (Figs. 9-1, 9-2), and is internalized and transported through the cells in cytoplasmic vesicles.[7,8] In the distal small intestine, however, IgG is found in cytoplasmic vacuoles of enterocytes without evidence of transference through the cells.[7,9] Luminal proteolysis is depressed at this age to give the absorptive epithelium in the proximal intestine a chance to remove intact IgG from the other milk proteins and for IgG to be transferred by receptor mediated endocytosis into the circulation. Large quantities of the intact maternal IgG in the circulation may provide passive systemic immunity for the neonates.

In these early days of life in the rat, neither IgA plasma cells in the lamina propria nor IgA in serum can be detected.[7] From the onset of suckling to some time between the 15th and 21st days of life, enterocytes in the proximal small intestine selectively bind colostral IgA (secretory IgA, sIgA) to their surface, and enterocytes in the distal small intestine nonselectively absorb and digest IgA.[7] In suckling calves and piglets, however, much IgA in colostrum is transported into the circulation during the first 24 hours of life, and in man a small amount of breast fluid IgA is transferred across enterocytes for 18 to 24 hours after birth.[10]

Studies of the antibodies in breast milk have shown secretory IgA antibodies against viruses, including polio virus and retrovirus, a series of microbial antigens, such as from E. coli, Salmonella O, Shigella and Vibrio cholerae, and various food proteins such as cow's milk.[11] It is probable that these secretory IgA antibodies on the surface of proximal enterocytes play important roles in the defense of the breast-fed baby against diarrheal infections. It is well documented that such infections are more common in artificially fed than in breast-fed infants.[12] An active response of sIgA antibodies to food proteins also seems to be important as an antigen-exclusion mechanism to prevent allergic diseases in infants.[13]

Breast milk contains many anti-infectious properties other than immunoglobulins, such as lactoferrin, lysozyme, phagocytes, and T- and B-lymphocytes.[12,14,15] When tested separately, lactoferrin or sIgA shows only slight bacteriostatic activity against commensal or enteropathogenic strains of E. coli.[16] Thus the bacteriostatic activity seems to be due to the combined effects of lactoferrin and sIgA, and it was proven that some amounts of lactoferrin are naturally bound to sIgA.[17] Phagocytes in breast milk are composed of lipid-laden neutrophils and macrophages, and they contain large amounts of sIgA. Recently the sIgA secretion from the phagocytes was proven to be initiated by surface membrane stimuli, and to play a role in the immunologic protection of the neonate.[18]

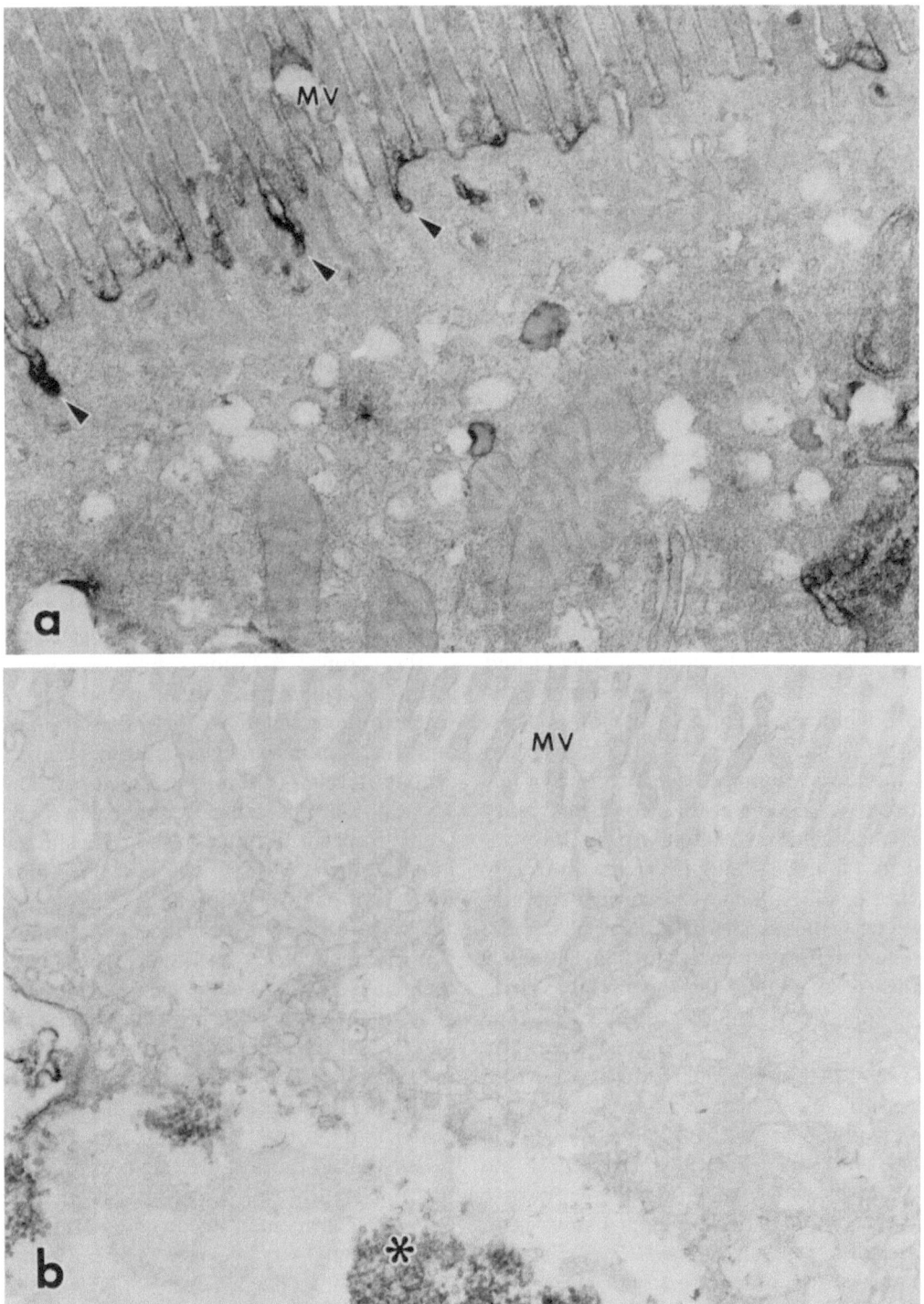

Fig. 9-2. Immunoelectron microscopic localization of IgG in the proximal (a) and distal (b) intestine of breast-fed neonatal rats. IgG is found in the lower portion of microvilli (MV) and apical and lateral plasma membranes of proximal enterocytes. Pinocytotic invaginations of the IgG-containing apical plasma membrane are frequent (◀). In the distal enterocytes, however, IgG is found only in cytoplasmic vacuoles (*) (a, ×30,000 ; b, ×18,000)

DEVELOPMENT AND STRUCTURE OF GUT-ASSOCIATED LYMPHOID TISSUE—ROLE OF ENVIRONMENTAL ANTIGENS IN THE ONTOGENY OF THE MUCOSAL IMMUNE RESPONSES

Structure of Gut-Associated Lymphoid Tissue

The gut-associated lymphoid tissue (GALT) consists of the organized mucosal lymphoid tissues of the gut that comprise Peyer's patches and solitary lymphoid follicles, diffuse collections of lymphocytes and plasma cells within the lamina propria, and the separated lymphocytes between villous epithelial cells. Peyer's patches consist of a collection of lymphoid follicles that occupy the full thickness of the intestinal mucosa and have the specialized patch-associated lymphoepithelium over them. It is now well established that they contain large numbers of B lymphocytes committed to synthesis of IgA antibodies.[19] Peyer's patches consist of a subepithelial dome of comparatively low cell density, follicles that are areas of closely packed small lymphocytes (corona) containing the germinal center with large blast cells, and the interfollicular areas that have been established as thymus-dependent areas with large concentrations of T lymphocytes. The villi overlying the interfollicular areas are known as patch-associated villi (PAV), which have specialized characters and functions for the lymphatic circulation in GALT.

The epithelial cells, which derive from the crypt of the PAV and overlie the Peyer's patch lymphoid tissue, are quite distinct from the absorptive columnar cells. They are more cuboidal and intermingled with specialized cells bearing only a few microvilli on the luminal surface. These cells called "M" cells appear to be specialized to sample the antigenic material present in the lumen of the gut.[20,21] Lymphocytes, mainly T lymphocytes, are abundant in the interepithelial spaces, and some of these lymphocytes may receive antigenic substances from "M" cells and function

to process them.[21] Thus the antigen sampling by "M" cells is supposed to play an important role in the first step of the afferent limb of the mucosal immune response.[22]

The dome region immediately beneath the specialized lymphoepithelial cell layer contains a heterogeneous population of cells,[23] such as large and medium-sized lymphocytes of helper/inducer and suppressor/cytotoxic phenotypes, B lymphocytes, and plasma cells secreting IgM, IgG, and IgA, and macrophages with cell debris and bacterial remnants. Ia antigen-positive dendritic cells are also seen in the dome and the overlying epithelium,[24] and are speculated to function as antigen-presenting cells or as accessory cells for antigen presentation.

The follicles beneath the dome comprise B lymphocyte areas. Most of the recirculating B lymphocytes enter the small lymphocyte zone of the corona.[25,26] Primary follicles without germinal centers are found in the Peyer's patches of neonates and germfree animals, and with stimulation by an antigen, germinal centers develop within the follicle.[27,28] This suggests that the follicle contains cells engaged in specific immune responses. The germinal centers are discrete, well-defined areas where lymphoid blastogenesis takes place. They are composed of large and medium-sized lymphocytes[29] bearing IgM· or IgA on their surfaces.[30] IgM and J chain are appreciated in the perinuclear spaces, Golgi complexes, and the scant endoplasmic reticulum in some lymphocytes.[31] Mitotic figures are common. It is speculated that the germinal center is the site of antigen-specific immune responses and of class switching from IgM to IgA.[32] The processes of follicular dendritic cells are prominent in the germinal center,[29,33] and they might play a role in antigen-trapping. Considerable numbers of T lymphocytes of the helper phenotype[33] and Leu 7-positive human natural killer cells are scattered throughout the corona and germinal centers in human Peyer's patches and solitary lymphoid follicles.[34,35] These cells might collaborate with B lymphocytes in immune responses.

The interfollicular areas, thymus-dependent areas analogous to the paracortex of lymph nodes, contain many venules with unique, tall endothelial cells termed postcapillary venules (PCV),[36] which take origin from venules in the PAV.[37,38] The PCV have been well documented as the sites for traffic of recirculating lymphocytes, as mentioned later. The T lymphocytes are mainly small cells that are in close contact with processes of Ia antigen-positive interdigitating cells.[24] The major populations of T lymphocytes there express the helper phenotype.[34] IgA-secreting plasmablasts are also present in this area.[23] Solitary lymphoid follicles look like small Peyer's patches. They are numerous and distributed in the lamina propria throughout the gastrointestinal tract. The epithelium overlying these structures and the follicles themselves show a similar cellular composition to those of the Peyer's patch.[34,39] Thus, these follicles are supposed to have the same functional abilities as those of the Peyer's patch, and their effect on mucosal immunity must be considerable (Fig. 9-3).

There is a diffuse scattering of immunologically competent cells throughout the lamina propria of villi and crypts, and betwen the epithelial cells where they are known as intraepithelial lymphocytes (Fig. 9-4).[40] The mononuclear cells in the lamina propria consist of mixed populations of T lymphocytes and IgA plasma cells. A majority of T cells there express the helper/inducer phenotype,[41] and are either scattered in the lamina propria or gathered into clusters, mainly along the basement membrane of the epithelium. More than 90% of plasma cells are IgA producers, and the number of IgA plasma cells per unit area of tissue is greater in the lamina propria than anywhere else in the body. Normally, small numbers of plasma cells containing IgM, IgG and IgE can be found. The lamina propria of the PAV surrounding the Peyer's patches contains a higher concentration of plasma cells than is found in villi elsewhere.[23] In addition the PAV have been reported to be selective sites for lodging of alloactivated T lymphocytes.[42] In contrast, most intraepithelial lymphocytes were T cells and expressed the phenotype associated with suppressor/cytotoxic

T cells rather than helper/inducer T cells.[43,44] They are located between and near the basal portion of the epithelial cells,[43,44] and are capable of expressing mitogen-induced cellular cytotoxity, antibody-dependent cellular cytotoxity and natural killer activity.[45]

Development of Gut-Associated Lymphoid Tissue

It is well known that morphologic alterations and distribution of immunologically competent cells in GALT have been correlated with the response to orally presented antigens. The study of germfree mice or rats over the period of conventionalization[46,47] reveals that the exposure of the adult animal to abundant microorganisms resulted in prompt and potent immune responses, which are first observed in the intestinal mucosa and mesenteric lymph nodes at the end of the first week. There exists abundant literature on the hypogammaglobulinemia of germfreè animals and the scarcity of secondary lymphoid follicles in the lamina propria of the villi.[46-50] It is of interest to notice that intraepithelial T lymphocytes and those in the lamina propria are also scanty. By the end of the 3rd or 4th week of conventionalization, these animals have the structure and immunocyte distribution in Peyer's patches or intestinal villi that resemble those of adult conventional animals.[47] This suggests that adult germfree animals are able to respond to external microbial antigens by developing an immunoglobulin-synthesizing tissue, such as GALT, with a potency and a rapidity at least equal to those of conventional animals (Fig. 9-5).

In the study by Hummel,[51] the microscopic anlage of the Peyer's patch first appeared in the wall of fetal rat intestine at 19 to 20 days of gestation. At that time clusters of Ia antigen-positive cells are present beneath the epithelium.[24] In newborn conventional animals, no immunoglobulin-bearing cells are detected in the intestinal lamina propria where aggregates of small lymphocytes have been present. These early lymphocytes are mainly T cells, and Ia antigen-positive dendritic cells are in-

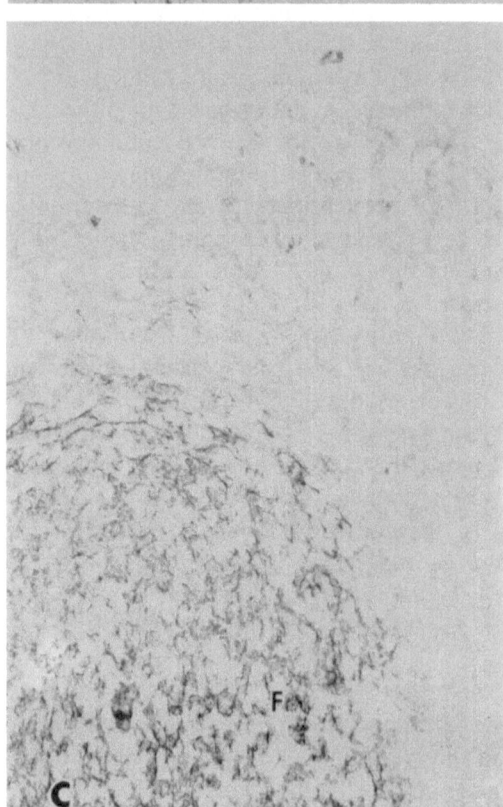

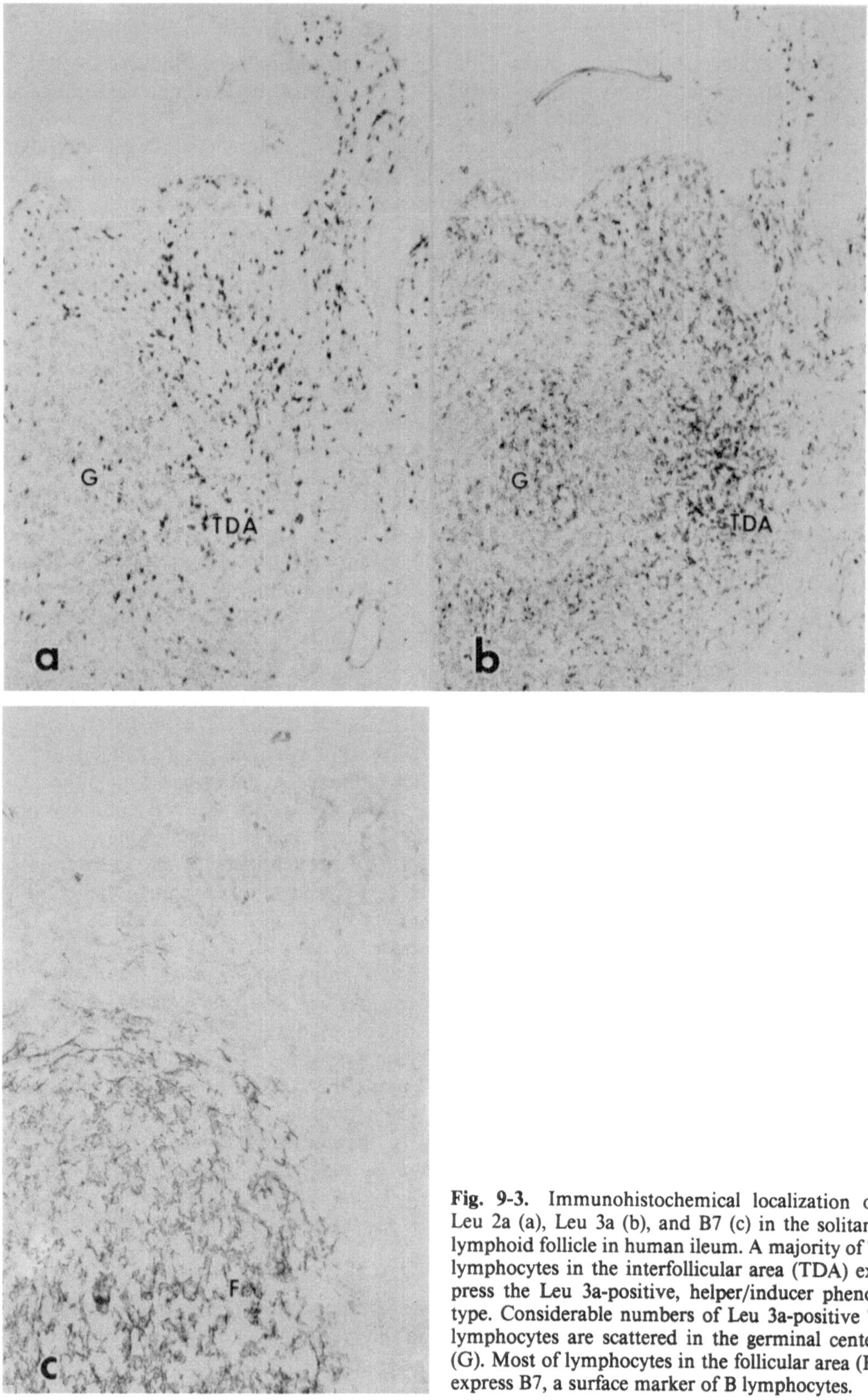

Fig. 9-3. Immunohistochemical localization of Leu 2a (a), Leu 3a (b), and B7 (c) in the solitary lymphoid follicle in human ileum. A majority of T lymphocytes in the interfollicular area (TDA) express the Leu 3a-positive, helper/inducer phenotype. Considerable numbers of Leu 3a-positive T lymphocytes are scattered in the germinal center (G). Most of lymphocytes in the follicular area (F) express B7, a surface marker of B lymphocytes.

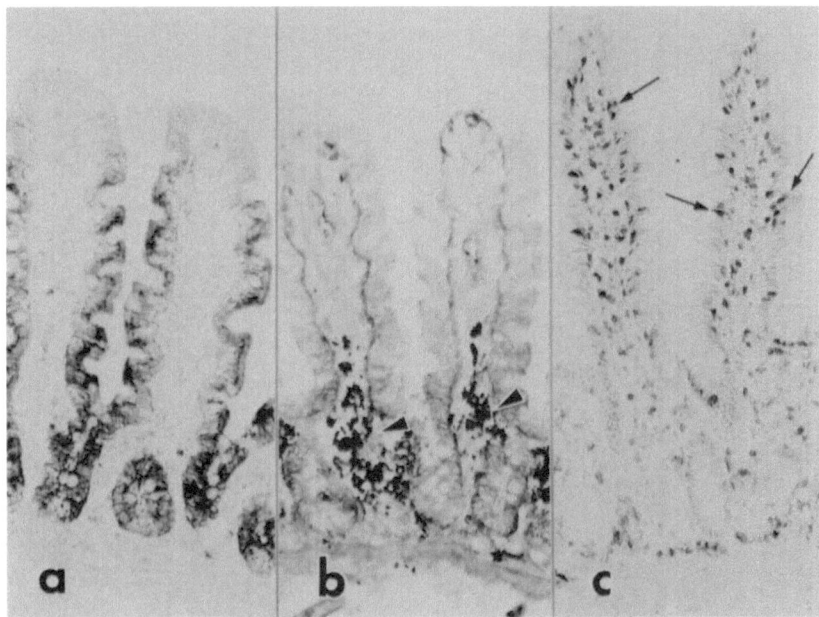

Fig. 9-4 Immunohistochemical localization of SC (a), IgA (b), and Leu 1 (c) in the human ileum. Staining for SC is most prominent in epithelial cells in the crypts with diminished expression by cells on the villi. IgA-staining is also prominent in the epithelial cells in the crypts along the baso-lateral surfaces. There are numerous IgA plasma cells at the base of villi (◄), and numerous Leu 1-positive lymphocytes throughout the lamina propria of villi and crypts and between the epithelial cells (→).

terspersed within the lymphoid aggregates. Mayrhofer et al [24] speculate that it is the prior congregation of Ia antigen-positive cells in the Peyer's patch anlagen, which induces subsequent congregation of lymphocytes at these sites. More recently Spalding et al[52] demonstrated that dendritic cell-T cell mixtures induce polyclonal IgA secretion by Peyer's patch B cells. The first immunoglobulin-bearing cells in young mice and rats are recognized within the first week of life and belong to the IgM class with J chain.[46,47] At that time the Peyer's patch is not yet visible, and the Peyer's patch in the adult develops first between 10 and 14 days after birth in rats.[47]

Cells of the IgA class are first found in significant numbers on day 21 in the intestinal villi and their numbers increase rapidly.[7,46,47] The germinal center develops at four weeks after birth. At six weeks of age, when the rats have been weaned, and the feeding environ-

ment is the same as that of adults, the types and counts of bacteria are almost the same as those in adults.[53] It seems possible that the arrival of IgA plasma cells in the lamina propria and the establishment of microbial flora are intimately related.

DIFFERENTIATION AND MIGRATION OF MUCOSAL LYMPHOID CELLS

It has been well documented that the germinal center of Peyer's patches consists predominantly of B lymphoblasts, and also contains interspersed macrophages, antigen presenting follicular dendritic cells, and small numbers of T lymphocytes of helper phenotype, as mentioned previously. The recent study of Kawanishi et al[32] suggests that the germinal center microenvironment of the

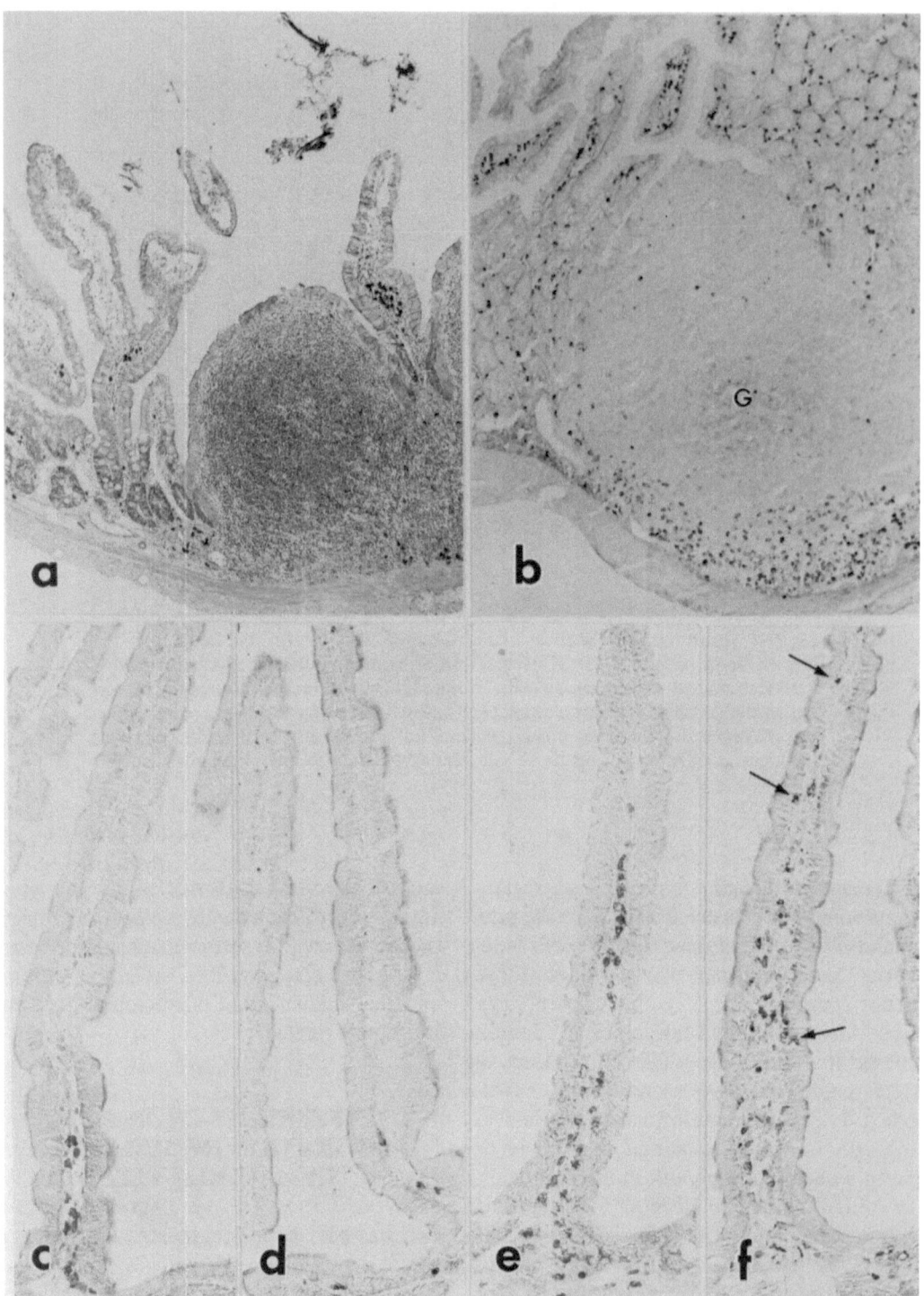

Fig. 9-5. Immunohistochemical localization of IgA plasma cells (a, b, c, e) and T lymphocytes (d, f) in the jejunal mucosa of adult germfree and conventional rats. In the conventional rats lymphoid follicles are well developed, and IgA plasma cells are abundant in the lamina propria of villi and crypts (b, e). Numerous intraepithelial T lymphocytes (→) and others in the lamina propria are also present (f). In germfree rats, however, IgA plasma cells and T lymphocytes are scanty (a, c, d). G:germinal center

Peyer's patch plays an important role in activation, proliferation, and heavy chain class switching during B cell responses, which are largely regulated by several subpopulations of immunoregulatory T lymphocytes and their secreted factors. The primed or activated B lymphoblasts, immediate IgA precursor cells,[19] migrate to the mesenteric lymph nodes, and via the thoracic duct to the general circulation, homing to several external-secreting organs. Some of the cells repopulate the intestinal mucosa, others migrate to the bronchial mucosa, salivary glands, biliary tract, urogenital organs, mammary glands, lacrimal glands, and several other sites in mucous membranes or exocrine glands.[2] Gut T lymphocytes also have migration patterns similar or identical to those described for B cells.

Of particular interest is the suggestion that the organ specificity of lymphocyte migration is determined largely by selective interaction of circulating lymphocytes with endothelial cells of PCV.[54] Parrott and Ferguson[55] described that recirculating lymphocytes also enter PAV from Peyer's patches via anastomosing lymphatic channels, and that this may provide a direct route for migration of lymphoblasts. As previously mentioned, the lamina propria of PAV contains higher concentrations of IgA plasma cells or IgA plasmablasts and is supposed to be a selective site for lodgement of alloactivated T lymphocytes.[42] We have recently made the interesting observation that these mucosal endothelial cells in PCV and PAV share antigens with a peripheral blood monocyte or macrophage subset,[56] capable of presenting soluble antigens and triggering autologous mixed lymphocyte reactions or allogenic T lymphocyte proliferation, associated with HLA-DR and OK-M5 (Fig. 9-6).[57]

Butcher et al[54] suggested that endothelial cells in mucosal and peripheral lymphoid tissues express distinctive determinants or factors for lymphocyte recognition and that lymphocyte migration patterns are programmed by lymphocyte surface receptors complementary to those organ-specific endothelial determinants. Such an organ-specific lymphocyte migration mechanism is largely responsible for the unique feature of the mucosal immune responses.

Figure 9-7 is a schema illustrating the cellular traffic in the mucosal immune system.

TRANSEPITHELIAL TRANSLOCATION OF IMMUNOGLOBULINS INTO EXTERNAL BODY FLUIDS—SC-MEDIATED TRANSPORT MECHANISM

sIgA in the external secretions consists of two molecules of IgA linked by J chain (dimeric IgA, dIgA) in complex with secretory component.[58] These components of sIgA are derived from two different types of cells: plasma cells in the intestinal lamina propria and glandular epithelial cells. Many studies of sIgA origin in mucosal secretions emphasize the role of local production of dIgA molecules by plasma cells underlying the epithelium of mucous membranes and secretory glands.[58-60] The IgA-producing plasma cells in the mucosal sites are responsible for the synthesis of the component proteins of dIgA (the IgA heavy and light chains and the J chain) as well as for the assembly of the components into a dIgA molecule before secretion. However, a significant proportion of IgA in breast milk and bile is serum-derived,[60-62] and in many species the intestine is a site of manufacture of much of the IgA found in blood.[63]

On the other hand, secretory component (SC) is synthesized and expressed on the glandular epithelial cells throughout the entire intestines and biliary ducts as well as in various exocrine glands[34] and, under certain circumstances,[64] the gastric epithelium. The route taken by the IgA across the epithelium has been examined repeatedly by immunohistochemical techniques, most of them involving the gut (Fig. 9-8).[58,65] SC is normally exposed on the basolateral plasma membrane of these epithelial cells. It has been well established that the SC binds dIgA at the basolateral cell surface by noncovalent interactions. The SC-

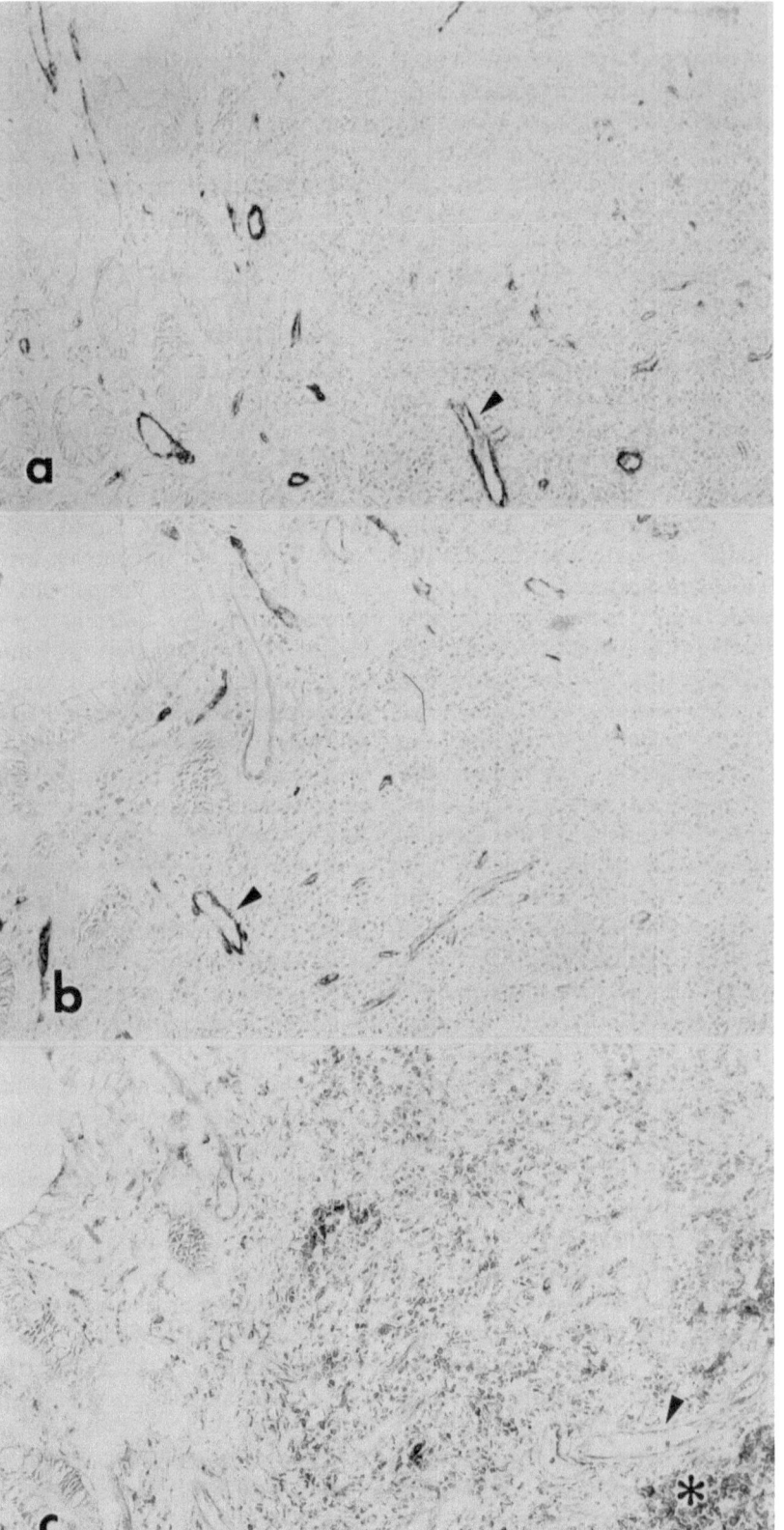

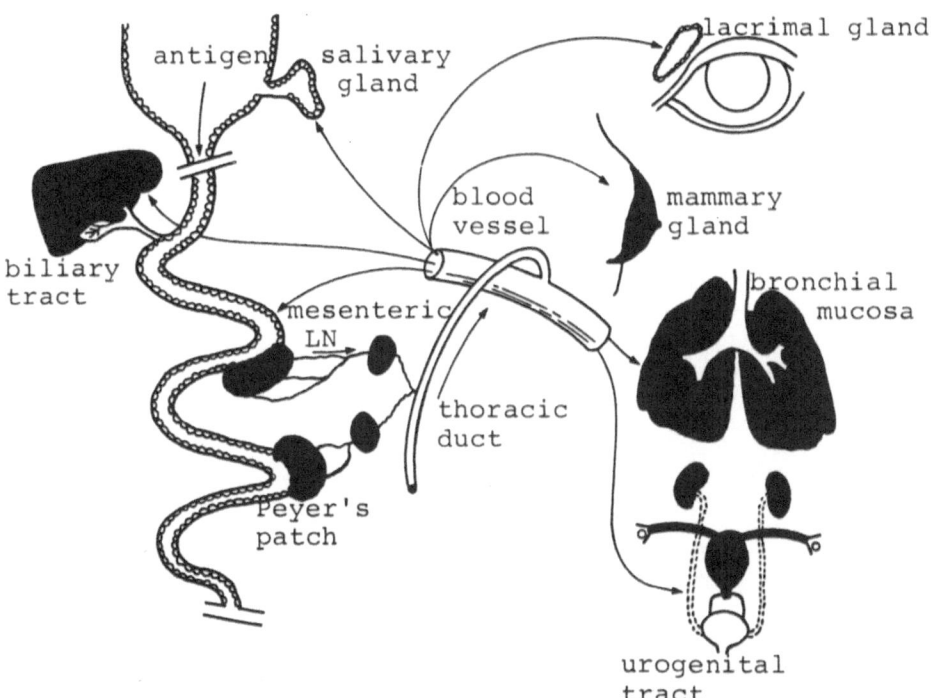

Fig. 9-7. A schematic illustration of the cellular traffic of precursors of IgA plasma cells and T lymphocytes leaving the Peyer's patches after antigenic stimulation (revised from reference 3). The cells home to mucosal sites via mesenteric lymph nodes, thoracic duct and blood circulation.

dIgA complex then undergoes endocytosis, and the complex is transported across the cell to the gland lumen by a microtubule-dependent vesicular transport mechanism and exocytosed at the apical cell surface along with some free SC.

At some point during the transport and secretion, the complex is rendered soluble by proteolytic cleavage of the membrane-associated SC molecule to release the soluble sIgA into the gland lumen. Such a model proposed

← ─────────────────────

Fig. 9-6. Immunohistochemical localization of Factor VIII related antigen (F VIII-RAg) (a), OK-M5 (b), and HLA-DR (c) in the solitary lymphoid follicle of human ileum. Mucosal endothelial cells of capillaries and venules share antigens with peripheral blood monocytes, such as OK-M5 and HLA-DR, as well as an antigen with vascular endothelial cells, F VIII-RAg (◄). Numerous HLA-DR-positive cells are present near the PCV (*).

for SC-mediated epithelial IgA reception and translocation gained strong support from observations made on normal[66] and neoplastic living cells.[67] Pentameric IgM also binds SC. Brandtzaeg[66] reported that a stronger noncovalent interaction was found between pentameric IgM and SC than between dIgA and SC. J chain is detected in dIgA and pentameric IgM,[68] and a role for the J chain is postulated in the SC-binding process. Monomeric IgA and IgG lacking J chain, or sIgA, however, do not bind to the membrane SC. Thus, SC appears to be the cell surface receptor for polymeric immunoglobulins associated with J chain. More recently, Mostov and colleagues[69] clearly demonstrated that SC is not synthesized as a secreted protein but as a much larger transmembrane precursor, and is the proteolytically cleaved, extracellular ligand-binding domain of the polymeric immunoglobin receptor.

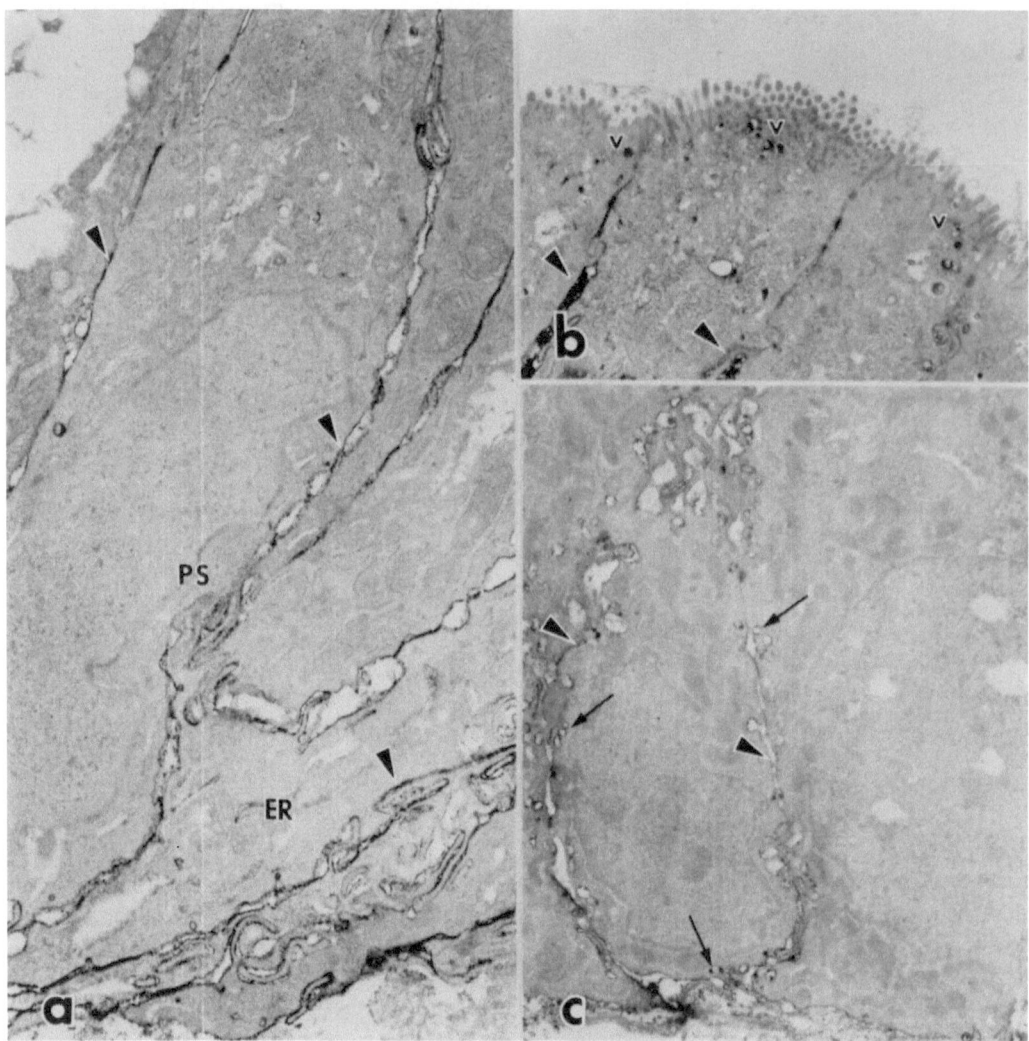

Fig. 9-8. Immunoelectron microscopic localization of SC (a) and IgA (b, c) in human enterocytes. SC is found in the perinuclear spaces (PS), rough endoplasmic reticulum (ER), and along the basolateral plasma membranes (◄). IgA is seen on the external surfaces of the basolateral plasma membranes (◄), which are frequently invaginated by pinocytosis (→). IgA-containing vesicles (V) are numerous in the supranuclear regions. (a, ×8.000 ; b, ×10.000; c, ×9.000)

Moreover, the SC-dIgA pathway diverges from most of other receptor-mediated endocytic pathways. Ahnen et al[58] clearly reviewed the distinctions: (1) the ligand (dIgA) is not ultimately degraded by lysosomes; (2) the receptor on the extracellular membrane (SC) is not recycled to the cell surface for reutilization; (3) the receptor-ligand complex membrane (SC-dIgA) is not dissociated after internalization; (4) the ligand (dIgA) is released from the cell in complex with its receptor (membrane SC) as sIgA. The cellular mechanism responsible for the transport of sIgA is schematically illustrated in Figure 9-9.

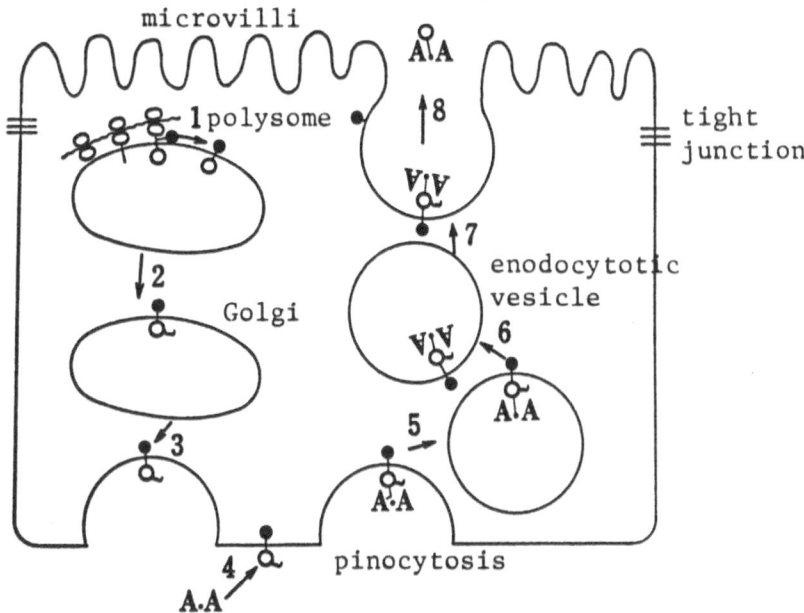

Fig. 9-9. A schematic illustration of the SC-dimeric IgA transport system. See text for explanation of the step numbers.
O:SC (70,000–75,000) — large SC, free SC
●:transport protein (15,000–20,000)
A.A:dimeric IgA
W:terminal sugar

IgA IN LIVER AND BILE—LIVER IS AN INTEGRAL PART OF THE MUCOSAL IMMUNITY

The demonstration of sIgA in normal rat bile has focused attention on the possible relationship of the liver to the mucosal immune system,[70] and the immunological significance of the transport of dimeric IgA by the liver was established soon thereafter. Hepatic bile of man and some other species also contains large amounts of sIgA and perhaps monomeric IgA and dIgA, lacking SC as well.[62,71] In rats, the biliary sIgA is accounted for largely through active transport of dIgA from the circulation to bile. The mechanism is that dIgA combines with SC on the sinusoidal plasma membrane of hepatocytes and the SC-dIgA complexes migrate across the cells by endocytic, vesicular transport to be discharged at the border of the hepatocytic cells that forms

the bile canaliculus.[71,72] In man, however, the earlier authors suggested that translocation of IgA in the liver occurs only across biliary epithelial cells; only these cells, not hepatocytes, contain both SC and IgA (Fig. 9-10).[62]

In addition to the transport of free dIgA, it has been shown that the liver can also function in the removal of antigen from the circulation, in the form of IgA immune complexes.[73–75] The mechanism for transport of IgA immune complexes is the same as that for free dIgA, and therefore SC plays a major role.[73,74] Thus, it is speculated that the hepatic transport of IgA immune complexes from the circulation to the bile represents a unique, noninflammatory mechanism for the disposal of antigens, distinct from the phagocyte-mediated mechanisms that clear conventional complexes.[73] It appears that the function of the hepatic transport mechanism is not only to recover free dIgA from serum and pass it

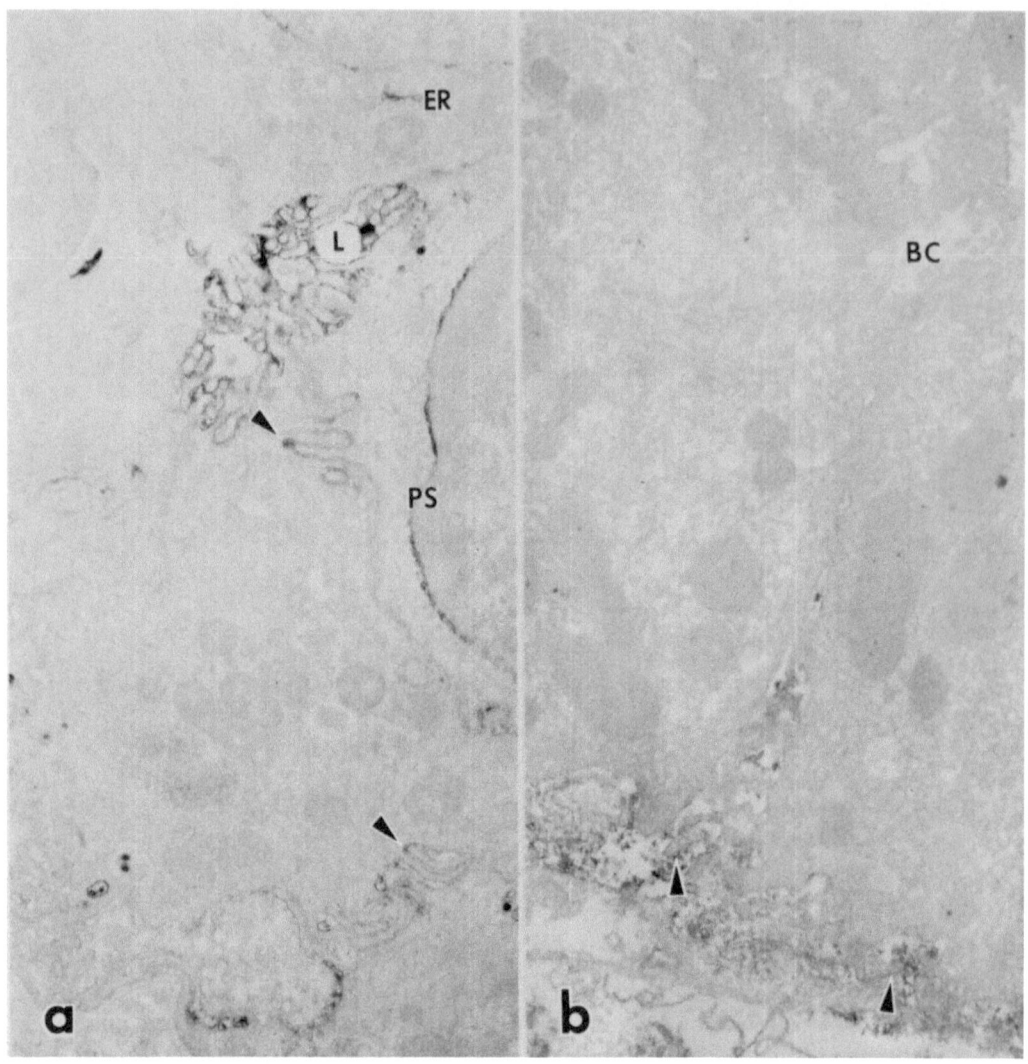

Fig. 9-10. Immunoelectron microscopic localization of SC (a) and IgA (b) in the human liver. SC is seen in the perinuclear spaces (PS), the rough endoplasmic reticulum (ER), the ductal lumen (L), and along the lateral plasma membranes (◀) of ductal epithelial cells. In the case of chronic hepatitis, the external surfaces of the plasma membranes of hepatocytes faced toward the sinusoid and Disse's space have deposits of IgA (◀). No IgA is present in the cytoplasm. (a, ×15,000; b, × 11,000) BC: bile canaliculi

Fig. 9-11. Immunohistochemical localization of OK-M1 (a), OK-M5 (b), HLA-DR (c), and factor VIII related antigen (F VIII-RAg) (d) in the human liver. Sinusoidal endothelial cells show membrane staining for OK-M5 and HLA-DR, but not for OK-M1 and F VIII-RAg. Endothelial cells in the portal areas fail to express OK-M5, but are positively stained for F VIII-RAg (◀) P: portal area

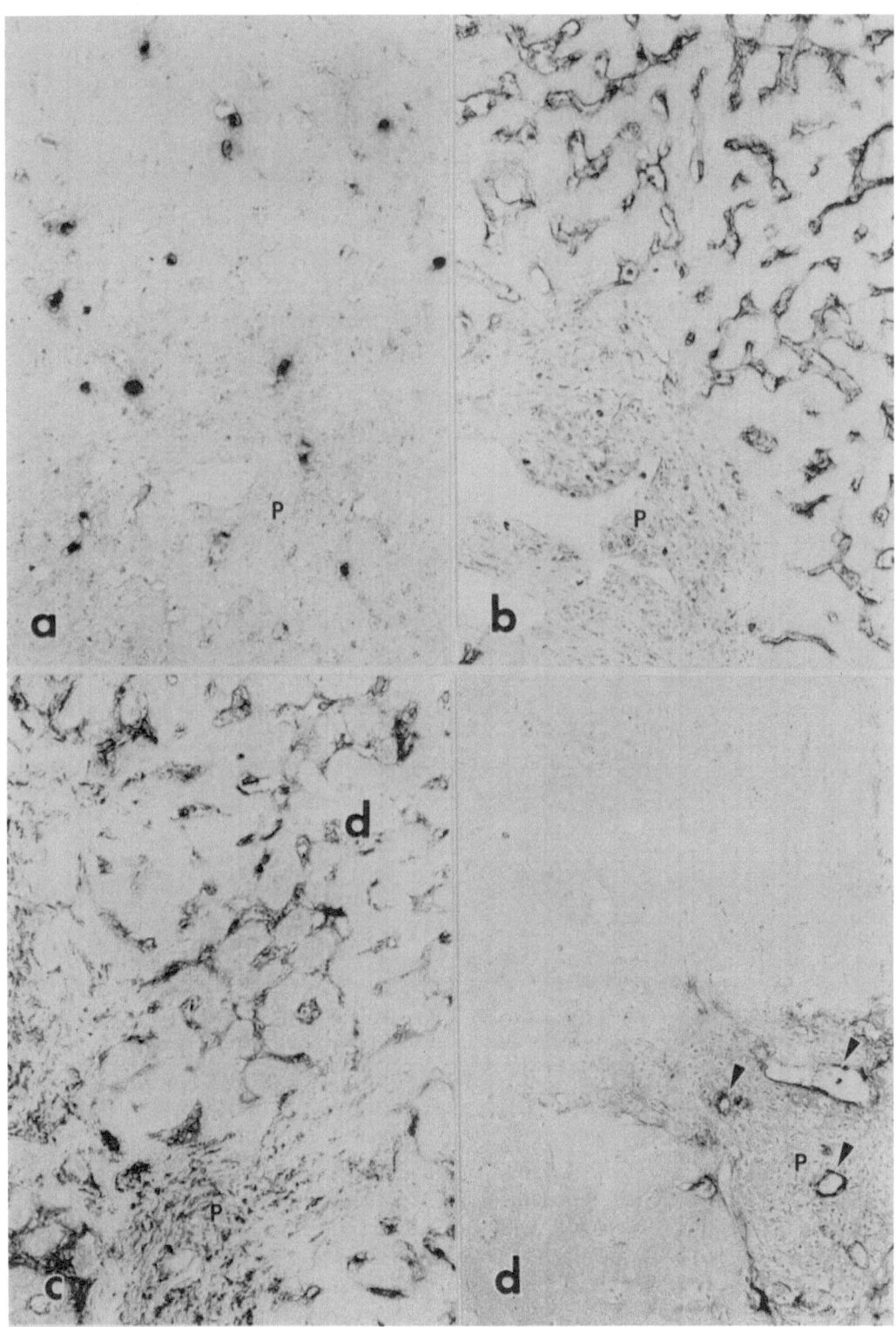

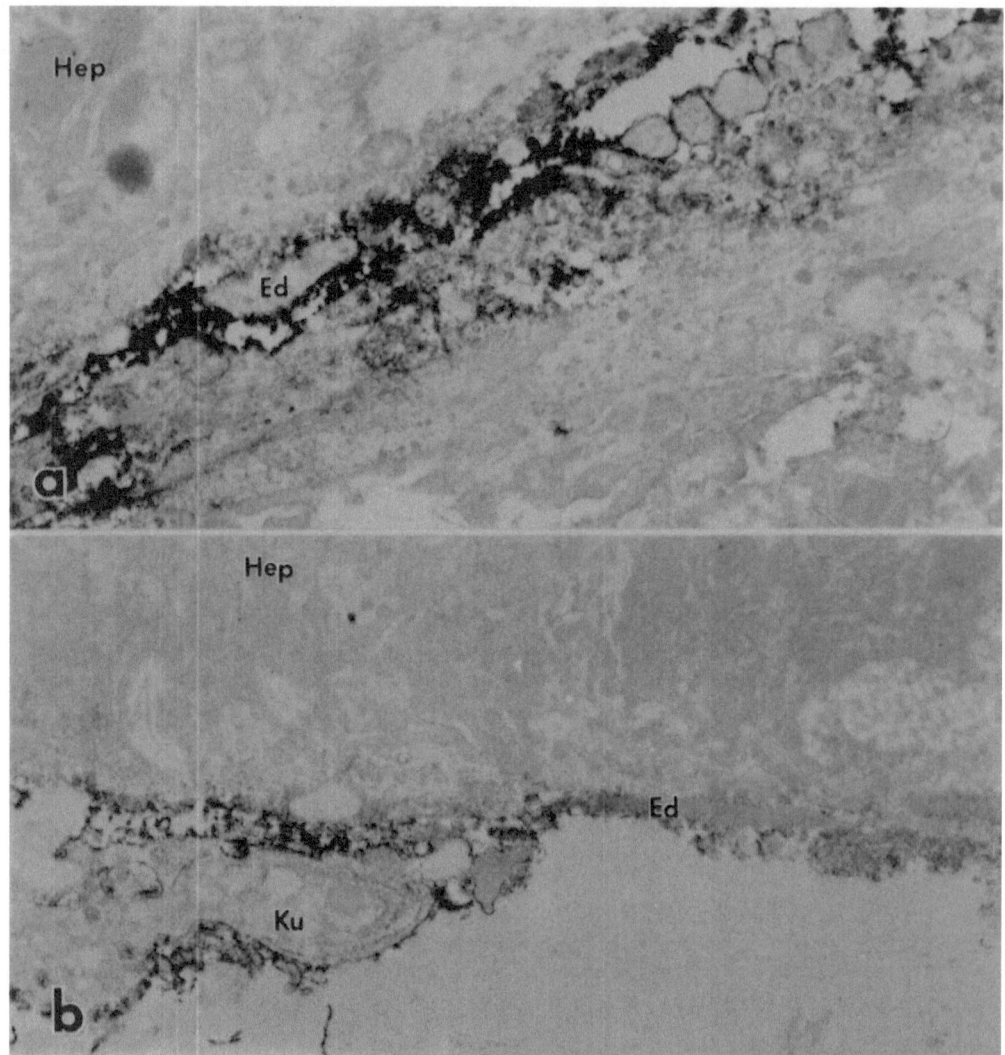

Fig. 9-12. Immunoelectron microscopic localization of OK-M5 (a) and HLA-DR (b) in the human liver. OK-M5 is seen along the plasma membrane of the sinusoidal endothelial cells (Ed). HLA-DR is found on the surface of both endothelial cells and Kupffer cells (Ku). Hep: hepatocytes. (a, ×15,000; b, ×15,000)

into the intestine via the biliary system as an "IgA pump,"[76] but also to clear the circulation of immune complexes that may arise in the gut by the interaction of absorbed food or microbial antigens with locally synthesized IgA antibody as a "scavenger."[53] The latter may be a possible mechanism for returning the IgA immune complexes to the intestine before activating a cascade of immune-mediated inflamatory reactions that occasionally results in tissue damage.

Disruption of the hepatobiliary transport of sIgA and sIgA immune complexes may be implicated in the pathogenesis of several human diseases. A number of diseases have been found in which IgA or IgA immune complexes are deposited in tissues; among these are Berger IgA nephropathy, Henoch-Schoenlein purpura, and dermatitis herpetiformis,[77] as well as alcoholic liver disease and chronic active hepatitis.[78,79] Although the property of the bound IgA has not been fully elucidated, the authors obtained immunohistochemical evidence that IgA and J chain can be found concurrently at the same site of tissues in these diseases, but no SC is identified there (Fig. 9-10).[79] In the liver, IgA and J chain are also found in phagosomes in hepatocytes and Kupffer cells simultaneously with acid phosphatase activity. These results are consistent with the known ability of these cells to bind, take up, and digest dIgA and dIgA immune complexes. Thus, the heavy deposition of IgA on the hepatocytes in alcoholic liver disease and chronic active hepatitis might represent excess IgA in the liver as a result of possible alterations in the sequestering and transport functions of the cells, but it could also be due to increased IgA synthesis.

Impairment of hepatic clearance of IgA by any of these routes could contribute to elevated serum sIgA and/or dIgA. Elevated serum sIgA levels are reported in patients with a broad spectrum of liver diseases, which paralleled classical markers of cholestasis such as serum alkaline phosphatase and biliary polymeric sIgA in blood.[73,80,81] Our recent immunoelectron microscopical observations suggest two routes of regurgitation, first through bile canaliculi, and adjacent hepatocytes into sinusoidal blood; second by extravasation from bile ductules into surrounding portal tract tissues and thence into portal blood vessels.[82] Elevated serum sIgA in patients with surgical portacaval shunts and cirrhosis might be attributable to bypassing both routes of clearance. IgA immune complexes in blood are also found in these diseases.[83]

Recently the authors showed that only the hepatic sinusoidal endothelial cells carry antigens with a peripheral blood macrophage subset capable of presenting soluble antigens and triggering autologous mixed lymphocyte reactions. They showed membrane staining for HLA-DR and OK-M5, but not for OK-M1 (Figs. 9-11,9-12).[84] This suggests that the sinusoidal endothelial cells may play an important role in immune responses or regulations in the liver. Although Kupffer cells are also known to constitute a group of Ia antigen-positive fixed macrophages, and to be responsible for the uptake of circulating antibodies and immune complexes, and for antigen presentation,[85-87] Kupffer cells fail to express OK-M5. Richman et al[88] showed that purified Kupffer cells pulsed with antigen in vitro are fully capable of inducing T cell proliferation. It has been well documented, however, that the liver is an important factor in oral tolerance; food and microbial antigens going to the liver via the portal system induce specific unresponsiveness, and the phagocytic function of Kupffer cells is supposed to be critical to the induction of suppressor responses.[89] Thus, failure by Kupffer cells as well as the sIgA system of an impaired liver to clear such enteric antigens and immune complexes formed in the blood circulation, which may themselves be pathogenic, could result in immune-mediated diseases. Thus, Kleinman et al[83] and the present authors have recognized that the liver is an integral part of the enteric mucosal immune system.[53]

IMMUNOREGULATORY ROLE OF THE MUCOSAL IMMUNE SYSTEM

It is well recognized that the systemic immune response to a specific antigen can be suppressed after the introduction of antigens via the gastrointestinal tract.[89] Recently the mechanism responsible for such important regulatory interactions taking place between the systemic and mucosal systems was extensively explored.[3,4] The anergic state induced by luminal antigens is supposed to be necessary to prevent the occurrence of injurious systemic reactions to antigens that inadvertently cross the mucosal barrier. Although recent studies of the suppression mechanism provide increasing evidence that systemic suppression is due to cellular and/or humoral products of the mucosal immune system, no unifying mechanism responsible for this phenomenon has been elucidated. It is possible that different mechanisms are responsible in different systems. One of the best defined mechanisms for the induction of systemic hyporesponsiveness to orally administered antigens is the introduction of a class-specific regulatory T cell for IgA.[89,90] That reflects the concurrent appearance of T helper cells specific for IgA and T suppressor cells for IgA responses to the antigen fed. Under this condition, oral stimulation may lead to IgG suppression (systemic suppression) associated with IgA enhancement (mucosal enhancement) as stated by Strober et al.[89]

In addition, sIgA antibody is capable of reducing antigen absorption across mucosal surfaces,[91] and hepatobiliary transport of IgA immune complexes provides a means of eliminating antigens that pass the IgA mucosal barrier.[74,75,92] The mucosal antibodies, therefore, may have an important immunoregulatory role. For example, it is well known that patients with selective IgA deficiency have a high incidence of antifood antibodies and an atopic disposition,[93] and patients with chronic liver disease have high titers of antibodies to intestinal microorganisms.[94,95] Experimentally, portacaval shunting in dogs abolishes the tolerogenic effect of feeding dinitrochlorobenzene.[96] Thus, antigen stimulation in the gut can have highly specific and dual immunogenic and/or tolerogenic influence on host immune responses in both intestinal and extraintestinal sites, and the systemic immune unresponsiveness might be very important in the prevention of damaging reactions to antigens that escape the exclusion mechanism at the mucosal surface.

CONCLUSION

The intestinal mucosa provides an extensive surface on which potentially pathogenic microorganisms and food antigens make their initial contact with the body, and the intestine is richly populated with lymphoid tissues capable of initiating and affecting various immune reactions. Of particular interest is the fact that the mucosal lymphoid tissue initiates a diverse series of immunologic events including the production of secretory antibodies at mucosal sites and, in striking contrast, an unresponsiveness of systemic immunological reactions. On the other hand we have focused on the significance of the liver in the immunoregulatory system, particularly the hepatic transport mechanism of sIgA and IgA immune complexes.

As for the movement of the cells within the mucosal immune system, T and B lymphocytes arising in mucosal follicles rapidly leave the follicle and return only to mucosal sites. This leads to the postulation of a common mucosal immune system, involving whole mucosal and exocrine organs. Thus, we have speculated that the mucosal immune system may play a central role in the maintenance of the homeostasis of the total immune system in the body, as well as in the regulation of the systemic immune system.

Until recently, however, mucosal immunity received relatively little attention from both basic and clinical scientists. The challenge for further research in mucosal immune responses is that it may offer the prospect of improved understanding of the immune mechanisms and the pathogenesis of several gastrointestinal and systemic diseases.

ACKNOWLEDGMENTS

The author is very grateful to Professors Keiichi Watanabe and Paul K. Nakane of Tokai University School of Medicine, and to Professor William R. Brown of University of Colorado Health Science Center for helpful discussions.

REFERENCES

1. Bienenstock J.: The physiology of the local immune response and the gastrointestinal tract. In Progress in Immunology 11, vol 4, Brent L, Holborow J. ed. Amsterdam, North-Holland, 1974, p197

2. McDermott M.R., Bienenstock J.: Evidence for a common mucosal immunologic system. I. Migration of B immunoblasts into intestinal, respiratory, and genital tissues. J Immunol 122:1892, 1979

3. Brown W.R.: The central role of the gastrointestinal tract in immunological reactions. Tokai J Exp Clin Med 8:1, 1983

4. Stokes C.R.: Induction and control of intestinal immune responses, in Local Immune Responses of the Gut, Newby T.J., Stokes C.R. (eds). Boca Raton, CRC Press, 1984, p97

5. Hong R., Ammann A.J.: Selective absence of IgA. Autoimmune phenomena and autoimmune disease. Am J Pathol 69:491, 1972

6. Morris B., Morris R.: The absorption of ^{125}I-labelled immunoglobulin G by different regions of the gut in young rats. J Physiol (Lond) 241:761, 1974

7. Nagura H., Nakane P.K., Brown W.R.: Breast milk IgA binds to jejunal epithelium in suckling rats. J Immunol 120:1333, 1978

8. Rodewald R., Kraehenbuhl J.P.: Receptor-mediated transport of IgG. J Cell Biol 99:159s, 1984

9. Rodewald R.: Intestinal transport of antibodies in the newborn rat. J Cell Biol 58:189, 1973

10. Ogra S.S.D., Weintraub D., Ogra P.L.: Immunological aspects of human colostrum and milk. III. Fate and absorption of cellular and soluble components in the gastrointestinal tract of the newborn. J Immunol 119:245, 1977

11. Hanson L.Å., Ahlstedt S., Andersson B., Carlsson B., Dahlgren U., Lidin-Janson G., Mattsby-Baltzer M., Svanborg-Eden C.: The biologic properties of secretory IgA. J Reticuloendothel Soc 28:1s, 1980

12. Hanson L.Å., Winberg J.: Breast milk and defense against infection in the newborn. Arch Dis Child 47:845, 1972

13. Walker W.A.: Antigen penetration across the immature gut: effect of immunologic and maturational factors in colostrum. In Immunology of Breast Milk. Ogra P.L., Dayton D. eds. New York, Raven Press, 1979, p227

14. Diaz-Jouanen E., Williams R.C. Jr.: T and B lymphocytes in human colostrum. Clin Immunol Immunopathol 3:248, 1974

15. Reddy V., Bhaskaram C., Raghuramulu N., Jagadeesan V.: Antimicrobial factors in human milk. Acta Paediatr Scand 66:229, 1977

16. Stephen S., Dolby J.M., Montreuil J., Spik G.: Differences in inhibition of the growth of commensal and enteropathogenic strains of Escherichia coli by lactotransferrin and secretory immunoglobulin A isolated from human milk. Immunology 41:597, 1980

17. Watanabe T., Nagura H., Watanabe K., Brown W.R.: The binding of human milk lactoferrin to immunoglobulin A. FEBS Letters 168:203, 1984

18. Weaver E.A., Rudloff H.E., Goldblum R.M., Davis C.P., Goldman A.S.: Selection of immunoglobulin A by human milk leukocytes initiated by surface membrane stimuli. J Immunol 132:684, 1984

19. Craig S.W., Cebra J.J.: Peyer's patches: an enriched source of precursors for IgA-producing immunocytes in the rabbit. J Exp Med 134:188, 1971

20. Owen R.L., Jones A.L.: Epithelial cell specialization within Peyer's patches: an ultrastructural study of intestinal lymphoid follicles. Gastroenterology 66:189, 1974

21. Owen R.L.: Sequential uptake of horseradish peroxidase by lymphoid follicle epithelium of Peyer's patches in the normal unobstructed mouse intestine.

An ultrastructural study. Gastroenterology 72:440, 1977

22. Bockman D.E., Cooper M.D.: Early lymphoepithelial relationship in human appendix. A combined light and electron-microscopic study. Gastroenterology 68:1160, 1975

23. Simina T., Plesch B.E.C.: An immunohistochemical study of cells with surface and cytoplasmic immunoglobulins in situ in Peyer's patches and lamina propria of rat small intestine. Virchow's Arch B 40:181, 1982

24. Mayrhofer G., Pugh C.W., Barclay A.N.: The distribution, ontogeny and origin in the rat of Ia positive cells with dendritic morphology and Ia antigen in epithelia, with special reference to the intestine. Eur J Immunol 13:112, 1983

25. Howard J.C., Hunt S.V., Gowans J.L.: Identification of marrow-derived and thymus-derived small lymphocytes in the lymphoid tissue and thoracic duct lymph of normal rats. J Exp Med 135:200, 1972

26. Meuwissen H.J., Kaplan G.T., Percy D.Y., Good R.A.: Role of rabbit gut-associated lymphoid tissue in cell replication. The follicular cortex as a primary germinative site. Proc Soc Exp Biol Med 130:300, 1969

27. Cooper G.N., Thonard J.C., Crosby R.L., Dalbow M.H.: Immunological responses in rats following antigenic stimulation of Peyer's patches. II. Histological changes in germ-free animals. Aust J Exp Biol Med Sci 46:407, 1968

28. Pollard M., Sharon N.: Responses of the Peyer's patches in germ-free mice to antigenic stimulation. Infect Immun 2:96, 1970

29. Sobhan P.: The light and electron microscopic studies of Peyer's patches in non-germfree adult mice. J Morphol 135:457, 1971

30. Moore A.R., Hall J.G.: Evidence for a primary association between immunoblast and small gut. Nature (Lond) 239:161, 1972

31. Nagura H., Kohler P.F., Brown W.R.: Immunocytochemical characterization of the lymphocytes in nodular lymphoid hyperplasia of the bowel. Lab Invest 40:66, 1979

32. Kawanishi H., Saltzman L.E., Strober W.: Mechanisms regulating IgA class-specific immunoglobulin production in murine gut-associated lymphoid tissues. I. T cells derived from Peyer's patches that switch sIgM B cells to sIgA B cells in vitro. J Exp Med 157:433, 1983

33. Simina T., Janse E.M., Wilders M.M.: Antigen-trapping cells in Peyer's patches of the rat. Scand J Immunol 16:481, 1982

34. Nagura H., Tsutsumi Y., Shimamura K., Shioda Y., Hasegawa H., Tamaoki K.: Immunohistochemical observation of human solitary lymphoid follicles. Digestive Organ and Immunology 12:89, 1984

35. Shioda Y., Nagura H., Tsutsumi Y., Shimamura K., Tamaoki N.: Distribution of Leu7 (HNK-1) antigen in human digestive organs: an immunohistochemical study with monoclonal antibody. Histochem J 16:843, 1984

36. Gowans J.L., Knight E.J.: The route of recirculation of lymphocytes in the rat. Proc Roy Soc Lond Ser B 159:257, 1964

37. Barclay A.N.: Different reticular elements in rat lymphoid tissue identified by localization of Ia, Thy-1 and MRC OX2 antigens. Immunology 44:727, 1981

38. Bhalla D.K., Murakami T., Owen R.L.: Microcirculation of intestinal lymphoid follicles in rat Peyer's patches. Gastroenterology 81:481, 1981

39. Keren D.F.: Immunology and Immunopathology of the Gastrointestinal Tract. Chicago, American Society of Clinical Pathologists, 1980, p10

40. Ferguson A.: Intraepithelial lymphocytes of the small intestine. Gut 18:921,1977

41. Cerf-Bensussan N., Schneeberger E.E., Bhan A.K.: Immunohistologic and immunoelectron microscopic characterization of the mucosal lymphocytes of human small intestine by the use of monoclonal antibodies. J Immunol 130:2615,1983

42. Sprent J.: Fate of H2-activated T-lymphocytes in syngeneic host. I. Fate in lymphoid tissues and intestines traced with ^{3}H-thymidine, ^{125}I-deoxyuridine and ^{51}chromium. Cell Immunol 21:278,1976

43. Selby W.S., Janossy G., Goldstein G., Jewell D.P.: T lymphocyte subsets in human intestinal mucosa: the distribution and relationship to MHC-derived antigens. Clin Exp Immunol 44:453,1981

44. Shioda Y., Nagura H., Tsutsumi Y., Saito H., Tamaoki K.: Immunohistochemical analysis of intraepithelial lymphocytes of human intestine. Digestive Organ and Immunology 10:149,1983

45. Flexman J.P., Shellam G.R., Mayrhofer G.: Natural cytotoxicity, responsiveness to interferon and morphology of intraepithelial lymphocytes from the small intestine of the rat. Immunology 48:733,1983

46. Crabbe P.A., Nash D.R., Bazin H., Eyssen H., Heremans J.F.: Immunohistochemical observations on lymphoid tissue from conventional and germ-free mice. Lab Invest 22:448,1970

47. Nagura H., Hasegawa H., Yoshimura S., Aihara K., Watanabe K., Ozawa A.: Comparative studies on conventional and germfree rat intestinal mucosa: with special reference to microbial flora and secretory IgA; in Recent Advances in Germfree Research. Sasaki S., Ozawa A., Hashimoto K. (eds). Tokyo, Tokai Univ Press, 1982, p511

48. Gustafsson B.E., Laurell C.B.: Gamma-globulins in germ-free rats. J Exp Med 108:251,1958

49. Miyakawa M., Iijima S., Kobayashi R., Tajima M.: Observations on the lymphoid tissue of the germ-free guinea pig. Acta Pathol Jpn 7:183,1957

50. Wastmann B.S.: Recent studies on the serum proteins of germfree animals. Ann NY Acad Sci 94:272,1961

51. Hummel K.P.: The structure and development of the lymphatic tissue in the intestine of the albino rat. Am J Anat 57:907,1972

52. Spalding D.M., Williamson S.I., Koopman W.J., McGhee J.R.: Preferential induction of polyclonal IgA secretion by murine Peyer's patch dendritic cell-T cell mixture. J Exp Med 160:941,1984

53. Nagura H., Watanabe K.: Mucosal immune system and immune responses in the intestine. In Gastrointestinal Function Regulation and Disturbances, vol.2, Kasuya Y., Tsuchiya M., Nagao F., Matsuo Y. eds. Amsterdam, Excerpta Medica, 1984, p147

54. Butcher E.C., Stevens S.K., Reichert R.A., Scollay R.G., Weissman I.L.: Lymphocyte-endothelial cell recognition in lymphocyte migration and the segregation of mucosal and nonmucosal immunity. In Recent Advances in Mucosal Immunity, Strober W., Hanson L.A., Sell K.W. eds, New York, Raven Press, 1982, p3

55. Parrott D.M., Ferguson A.: Selective migration of lymphocytes within the mouse small intestine. Immunology 26:571,1974

56. Nagura H., Koshikawa T.: Immunocytochemical analysis of the structure and function of Peyer's patches. Jap J Gastroenterol 82:2312,1985

57. Shen H.H., Talle M.A., Goldstein G., Chess L.: Functional subsets of human monocytes defined by monoclonal antibodies: a distinct subset of monocytes contains the cells capable of including the autologous mixed lymphocyte culture. J Immunol 130:698,1983

58. Ahnen D.J., Brown W.R., Kloppel T.M.: Secretory component: the polymeric immunoglobulin receptor. What's in it for the gastroenterologist and hepatologist? Gastroenterology 89:667,1985

59. Nagura H., Brandtzaeg P., Nakane P.K., Brown W.R.: Ultrastructural localization of J chain in human intestinal mucosa. J Immunol 123:1044,1979

60. Nagura H., Tsutsumi Y., Hasegawa H., Watanabe K., Nakane P.K., Brown W.R.: IgA plasma cells in biliary mucosa: a likely source of locally synthesized IgA in human hepatic bile. Clin Exp Immunol 54:671,1983

61. Halsey J.F., Johnson B.H., Cebra J.J.: Transport of immunoglobulin from serum into colostrum. J Exp Med 151:767,1980

62. Nagura H., Smith P.D., Nakane P.K., Brown W.R.: IgA in human bile and liver. J Immunol 126:587,1981

63. Heremans J.F.: Immunoglobulin A. In The Antigens, vol II, Sela Med, New York, Academic Press, 1974, p365

64. Nagura H., Tsutsumi Y., Shioda Y., Watanabe K.: Immunohistochemistry of gastric carcinomas and associated diseases: novel distribution of carcinoembryonic antigen and secretory component on the surface of gastric cancer cells. J Histochem Cytochem 31:193,1983

65. Brandtzaeg P.: Transport models for secretory IgA and IgM. Clin Exp Immunol 44:221,1981

66. Brandtzaeg P.: Polymeric IgA is complexed with secretory component (SC) on the surface of human intestinal epithelial cells. Scand J Immunol 8:39,1978

67. Nagura H., Nakane P.K., Brown W.R.: Translocation of dimeric IgA through neoplastic colon cells in vitro. J Immunol 123:2359,1979

68. Koshland M.E.: Structure and function of the J chain. Adv Immunol 20:41,1975

69. Mostov K.E., Kraehenbuhl J.P., Brobel F.: Receptor-mediated transcellular transport of immunoglobulin: synthesis of secretory component as multiple and larger transmembrane forms. Proc Natl Acad Sci USA 77:7257,1980

70. Lemaitre-Coelho I., Jackson G.D.F., Vaerman J-P.: Rat bile as a convenient source of secretory IgA and free secretory component. Eur J Immunol 8:588,1977

71. Vaerman J-P., Lemaitre-Coelho, I.M., Limet J.N., Delacroix D.L.: Hepatic transfer of polymeric IgA from plasma to bile in rats and other mammals: a survey. In Recent Advances in Mucosal Immunity. Strober W, Hanson LA, Sell KW eds. New York, Raven Press, 1982, p233

72. Takahashi I., Nakane P.K., Brown W.R.: Ultrastructural events in the translocation of polymeric IgA by rat hepatocytes. J Immunol 128:1181,1982

73. Chandy K.G., Hubscher S.G., Elias E., Berg J., Khan M., Burnett D.: Dual role of the liver in regulating circulating polymeric IgA in man: studies on patients with liver disease. Clin Exp Immunol 52:207,1983

74. Brown T.A., Russell M.W., Mestecky J.: Hepatobiliary transport of IgA immune complexes: molecular and cellular aspects. J Immunol 128:2183,1982

75. Peppard J., Orlans E., Payne A.W.R., Andrew E.: The elimination of circulating complexes containing polymeric IgA by excretion in the bile. Immunology 42:83,1981

76. Kraft S.C.: The liver as an "IgA pump." Gastroenterology 80:623,1981

77. Hall R.P., Lawley T.J., Heck J.A.: IgA-containing cir-

culating immune complexes in dermatitis herpetiformis, Henoch-Schoenlein purpura, systemic lupus erythematosus and other diseases. Clin Exp Immunol 40:431,1980

78. Kater L., Jobsis A.C., de la Faille-Kuyper E.H.B., Vogten A.J.M., Grijm R.: Alcoholic hepatic disease. Specificity of IgA deposits in liver. Am J Clin Pathol 71:51,1979

79. Nagura H., Tsutsumi Y., Watanabe K., Hasegawa H., Kobayashi K.: Studies on the relationships of IgA in human liver. Digestive Organ and Immunology 8:315,1982

80. Delacroix D.L., Reymaert M., Pauwels S., Geubel A.P., Vaerman J.P.: High serum levels of secretory IgA in liver disease. Possible liver origin of the circulating secretory component. Dig Dis Sci 27:333,1982

81. Fukuda Y., Imoto M., Hayakawa T.: Serum levels of secretory immunoglobulin A in liver diseases. Am J Gastroenterol 80:237,1985

82. Fukuda Y., Nagura H., Asai J., Satake T.: Possible mechanisms of elevation of serum immunoglobulin A in liver diseases. Am J Gastroenterol 81:315,1986

83. Kleinman R.E., Harmatz P.R., Walker W.A.: The liver: an integral part of the enteric mucosal immune system. Hepatology 2:379,1982

84. Nagura H., Koshikawa T., Fukuda Y., Asai J.: Hepatic vascular endothelial cells heterogeneously express surface antigens associated with monocytes, macrophages and T lymphocytes. Virchows Arch A 409:407,1985

85. Berzofsky J.A., Richman L.K., Strober W.: Determinant-specific antigen presentation by liver Kupffer cells under control of H-2-linked Ir genes. In Recent Advances in Mucosal Immunity. Strober W., Hanson L.A., Sell K.W. eds, New York, Raven Press, 1982, p215

86. Praaning-van Dalen D.P., Brouwer A., Knook D.L.: Clearance capacity of rat liver Kupffer, endothelial, and parenchymal cells. Gastroenterology 81:1036,1981

87. Souhami R.L.: The effect of colloidal carbon on the organ distribution of sheep red blood cells and the immune response. Immunology 22:685,1972

88. Richman L.K., Klingenstein R.J., Richman J.A., Strober W., Berzofsky J.A.: The murine Kupffer cell. I. Characterization of the cell serving accessory function in antigen-specific T cell proliferation. J Immunol 123:2602,1980

89. Strober W., Richman L.K., Elson C.O.: The regulation of gastrointestinal immune responses. Immunology Today, August:156,1981

90. Richman L.K., Graeff A.S., Yarchoan R., Strober W.: Simultaneous induction of antigen-specific IgA helper T cells and IgG suppressor T cells in the murine Peyer's patch after protein feeding. J Immunol 126:2079,1981

91. Andre C., Lambert R., Bazin H.: Interference of oral immunization with the intestinal absorption of heterologous albumin. Eur J Immunol 4:701,1974

92. Stokes C.R., Swarbrick E.T., Soothill J.F.: Immune elimination and enhanced antibody responses: functions of circulating IgA. Immunology 40:455,1980

93. Cunningham-Rundles C., Brandeis W.E., Good R.A., Day N.K.: Bovine antigens and the formation of circulating immune complexes in selective immunoglobulin A deficiency. J Clin Invest 64:272,1979

94. Thomas H.C., Derilliers D., Potter B.J., Hodgson H., Jain S., Jewell D.P., Sherlock S.: Immune complexes in acute and chronic liver disease. Clin Exp Immunol 31:150,1978

95. Triger D.R., Alp M.H., Wright R.: Bacterial and dietary antibodies in liver disease. Lancet 1:60,1972

96. Cantor H.M., Dumont A.H.: Hepatic suppression of sensitization to antigen absorbed into the portal system. Nature (London) 215:744,1967

10

Crohn's Disease in Japan—A Clinicopathologic Study

Haruki Wakasa, M.D.
Hidemasa Ishikawa, M.D.
Hikaru Watanabe, M.D.

There have been an increasing number of reports[1-10] describing morphologic features of inflammatory bowel disease (IBD), particularly Crohn's disease, in recent years. Previously, there were thought to be two forms of Crohn's disease, acute and chronic; the acute form has been excluded by the finding that it was induced by Yersinia[11-13] or Anisakis.[14] Actually, the term Crohn's disease[15] includes regional granulomatous ulcerative colitis,[16] right-sided (regional) colitis,[17,18] regional colitis[19] and regional segmental colitis.[20]

Crohn's disease has long been considered a rather rare disease in Japan. To clarify the state of Crohn's disease in Japan, a research committee concerned with this disease was organized under the auspices of the Japanese Gastroenterological Society. This committee has consulted on cases on a nationwide scale and selected cases that were unmistakably Crohn's disease. Of course, during the course of this work, the development of endoscopic procedures and X-ray examination yielded much useful information.

Herein, we describe some characteristic clinicopathologic features of Japanese Crohn's disease, which were seen during the course of the study.

CRITERIA FOR DIAGNOSIS PROPOSED BY THE COMMITTEE

The Japanese Research Committee[23,24] proposed the criteria composed of six key findings as follows: (1) discontinuity of lesions, (2) cobblestone-like appearance and/or longitudinal ulcers, (3) transmural inflammation, (4) noncaseous epithelioid cell granulomas, (5) fissures and/or fistulae, and (6) anal lesions. These diagnostic criteria were based on the descriptions of Evans and Acheson,[23] Lennard-Jones,[24,25] Fahrländer and Baerlocher[26] and Korelitz et al.[27] The committee consulted on cases of Crohn's disease and allied disorders on the basis of these criteria, and diagnosed each case according to the steps shown in Table 10-1, ranging from clinical examination to diagnostic biopsy and surgical specimen.

In diagnosis of Crohn's disease, however, intestinal tuberculosis, ulcerative colitis, ischemic enterocolitis, radiation (entero-) colitis, intestinal Behçet's disease, simple (nonspecific) ulcer of the small or large intestine, "nonspecific multiple ulcers of the small intestine" and acute terminal ileitis, etc., should be excluded beforehand, even when a combi-

TABLE 10-1
Diagnostic Criteria for Crohn's Disease (Japanese Research Committee)

	Examination	X-ray	Endoscopy	Biopsy	Surgical specimen
Discontinuity of lesion		+	+	+	+
Cobblestone appearance and/or longitudinal ulcer		+	+		+
Transmural inflammation	+ (tumor)	+ (stenosis)	+ (stenosis)		+
Granuloma				⊕	⊕
Fissures and/or fistulae	+'	+'	+'	+'	+'
Anal lesion	+'				+'

Crohn's disease diagnosis requires findings of at least + + ⊕ or + + + +'.

nation of all six of the above-mentioned findings is noted.

During the period from 1978 to 1982, the committee was able to select 102 cases consisting of 75 surgically resected cases and 27 biopsied cases of the disease according to the criteria.

MATERIALS AND METHODS

These findings are based on data from 102 cases in which there was consultation, 11 cases that involved surgical resection, and 10 cases in which biopsy was done.

Clinical observation of 113 cases consisting of the cases in which there was consultation and those that involved resection was carried out. For morphologic study, biopsy and surgical specimens from 10 cases were processed for light microscopic, immunohistochemical, and electronmicroscopic observation as standard procedure.

Sections from paraffin blocks were stained with hematoxylin-eosin, Masson's trichrome, Gram, Ziehl-Neelsen, and Grocott's silver, and for immunohistochemical procedures sections were processed for lysozyme, α_1-antitrypsin, α_1-antichymotrypsin and S-100 protein according to the peroxidase antiperoxidase method (PAP method). In some cases, monoclonal antibodies for T or B cell aggregates were used to clarify the characterization of lymphoid cell aggregates in the intestinal wall.

For electronmicroscopic observation, fresh specimens were fixed with glutaraldehyde-formalin and then postfixed with osmium. After embedding with Epon, thin sections were made using an LKB ultramicrotome and stained with uranyl-lead.

CLINICAL FEATURES

Age and sex distributions are shown in Figure 10-1. About 60% of the patients were in their third decade at the time of diagnosis, followed by those in their second decade. Males outnumbered females. Regarding lesion site, 26 patients had lesions in the small intestine only, and 38 patients had them in the large intestine. In 59 cases, lesions were found in both the small and large intestines (Table 10-2). Among these 113 cases, surgery was performed in 86, the rate of surgical procedure for each type of lesion being 88.5% for ileitis, 76.5% for ileocolitis, and 47.5% for colitis. With regard to symptoms, abdominal pain was the most common complaint at the onset, followed by diarrhea, fever, bloody stools, anemia, abdominal discomfort, emaciation, nausea, and vomiting. As to the relation of symptoms to lesion sites, there was a tendency for cases with small intestinal lesions to have fever and anemia, and for those with

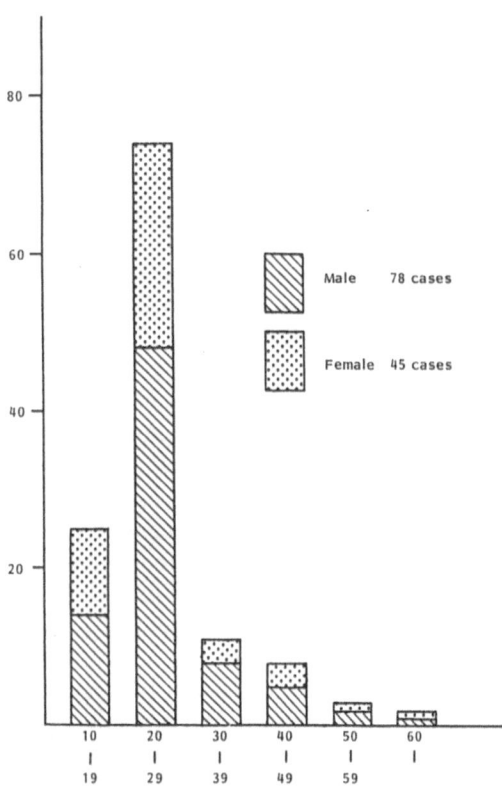

Fig. 10-1. Age distribution in patients with Crohn's disease. Abscissa: year range, Ordinate: number of cases.

Male 78 cases

Female 45 cases

TABLE 10-2
Site of Lesion

Small intestine	26 cases
Small and large intestines	59
Large intestine	38
Total	123

by malabsorption syndrome, fistulae, massive hemorrhage, disturbance of growth, and arthralgia.

PATHOLOGIC FEATURES

Macroscopic findings: It is very important to observe the endoscopical finding and/or gross appearance of resected intestine when diagnosing Crohn's disease. In typical Crohn's disease, macroscopic findings are usually characteristic, and therefore, a definite diagnosis of Crohn's disease should not be made when the gross appearance is atypical. It is well known that the terminal ileum and the right-sided colon are more frequently involved than the left-sided colon in Crohn's disease. Resected small intestine is usually covered with mesenteric fibroadipose tissue throughout its entire length. Fibroadipose tissue becomes irregularly nodular, a condition induced by granulomatous infiltration characteristic of the disease. The segmental and/or discontinuous lesions characterized by intestinal wall thickening accompanying consequent obstructive symptoms, cobblestone-like appearance, and ulceration are often compared to the lesions of ulcerative colitis in which the rectum and the left colon are diffusely affected, which then spread throughout the entire colon.[28] Cobblestone-like appearance is characterized by edematous swelling of mucosa, which is surrounded by intercommunicating and fissuring ulceration.

In surgically resected specimens of the small intestine in cases of Crohn's disease, intestinal wall thickening was the most frequent feature, followed by longitudinal ulcers and

large intestinal lesions to have bloody stools in addition to abdominal pain and diarrhea.

Symptoms at diagnosis were also similar to those at onset. Cases with small intestinal lesions seem to show more symptoms of obstruction in comparison to those with large intestinal lesions.

With regard to laboratory data, an increased erythrocyte sedimentation rate was found in 86% of the males and 94% of the females. Anemia, characteristically hypochromic anemia, was more frequently observed in the females than in the males. Decreased serum iron and leukocytosis were also observed in connection with hypoproteinemia with decreased A/G ratio. An increased serum α_2-globulin was found in 70% of the cases.

The most frequently observed complication was protein-losing enteropathy, followed

TABLE 10-3

Macroscopic Findings of Resected Samples

	Small Intestinal Lesion	Large Intestinal Lesion
Longitudinal ulcer	51 (82)*	28 (52)
Cobblestone appearance	29 (47)	44 (81)
Thickening of intestinal wall	55 (89)	46 (85)
Stenosis	23 (37)	12 (22)
Fistulae	11 (18)	13 (24)
Aphthoid ulcer	18 (29)	9 (17)
Total	62	54

* Percent in parenthesis.

cobblestone-like appearance (Table 10-3). On the other hand, in cases with large intestinal lesions intestinal wall thickening and cobblestone-like appearance were almost equally observed (Table 10-3). Gross observation shows cobblestone-like mucosal appearance with intestinal wall thickening to be the most common morphologic feature of Crohn's disease in Western countries,[29] but such cases are rather less prominent in Japan.

Among Japanese cases, the most characteristic feature of resected intestine is the existence of longitudinal ulcers located on the side of mesenteric attachment. Such ulcers were observed in 82.3% of the cases with small intestinal lesions (Table 10-3; Figs. 10-2, 10-3). This observation was also supported by other studies of cases in Japan.[5] It is not infrequent that the length of longitudinal ulcers in the terminal ileum is as great as 50 cm accompanied by edematous swelling in the surrounding mucosa. The mesenteric attachment opposite the longitudinal ulcer site, that is, the side with Peyer's patches, is usually intact, covered with normal appearing mucosa. A mild to moderate inflammatory cell infiltration, however, is usually present in the mucosa proper and the submucosal layer. In cases with short ulcers, sequential cobblestone-like swelling is found in the mucosa surrounding the ulcer in the terminal ileum, and short stick-like inflammatory polyps are also observed in the lesion.

Aphthoid ulcers, considered to be early lesions of Crohn's disease and probable extensions of longitudinal ulcers, were found in one-third of the cases with small intestinal lesions and one-fifth of those with large intestinal lesions.

The occurrence of longitudinal ulcers in

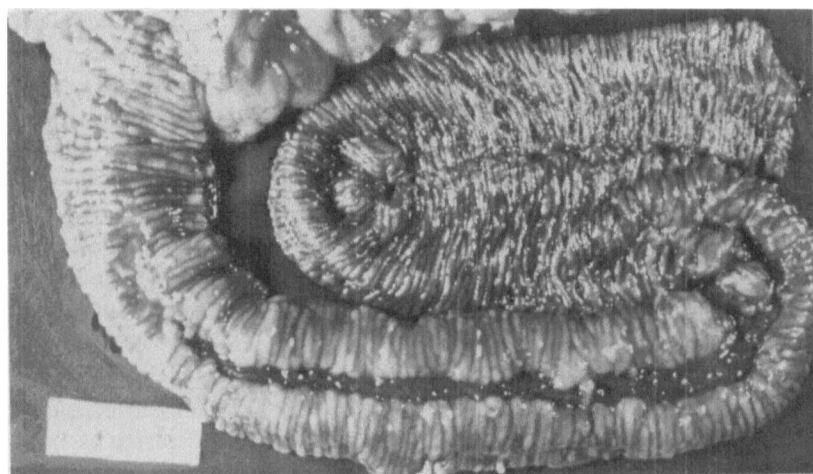

Fig. 10-2. This case, from a 19-year-old female, shows a longitudinal ulcer surrounded by edematous mucosa of the small intestine (Iwaki City Hospital case).

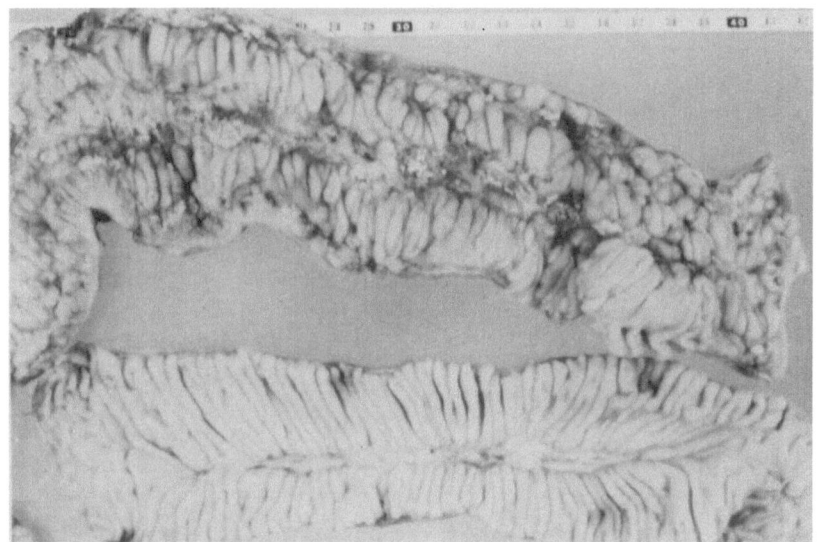

Fig. 10-3. In this case, from a 27-year-old male, longitudinal ulcer and serpiginous and irregularly shaped long ulcers are observed in the small intestine (Ōgaki Municipal Hospital case).

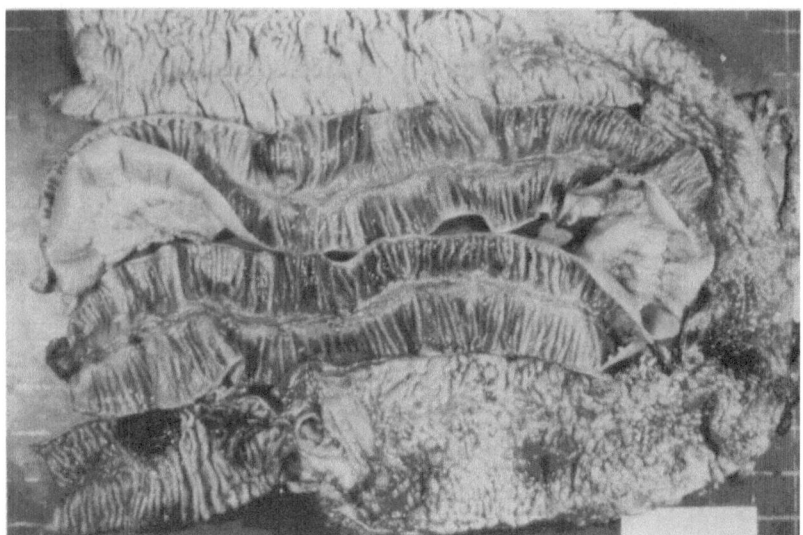

Fig. 10-4. This case, from a 22-year-old male, has both longitudinal ulcer in the ileum and cobblestone-like appearance in the colon (Yokohama City University case).

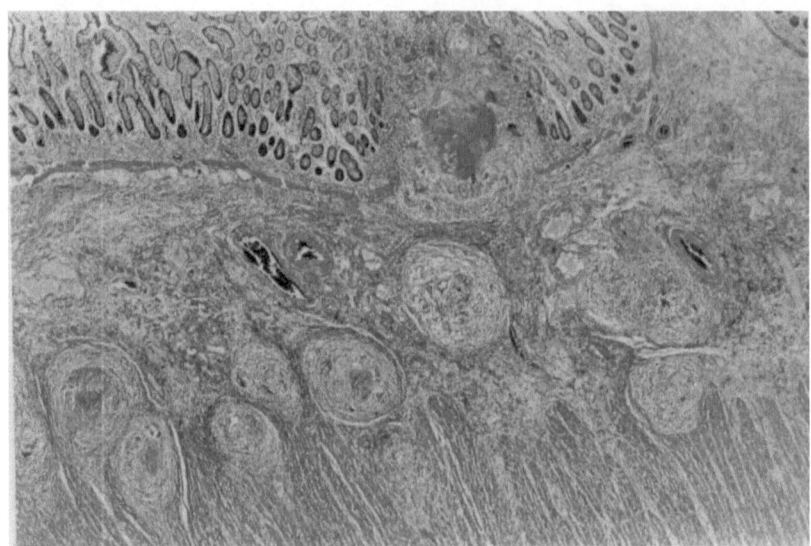

Fig. 10-5. Caseous tubercle in mucosa proper and several tubercles are formed in the submucosal and muscular layers. H&E × 20

cases with large intestinal lesions was observed in 57% of the cases, which is markedly lower than the rate of occurrence in the terminal ileum (Table 10-3). Regarding these ulcers observed in the large intestine, there were usually 2 or 3 in line, and they were short and irregular in shape and mainly observed at the site of colonic teniae.

In very rare cases, longitudinal ulcers in the ileum and a prominent cobblestone-like appearance in the large intestine with several fissures were both seen (Fig. 10-4). Such a finding suggests that both longitudinal ulcers and a cobblestone-like appearance are recognized as morphologic characteristics of Crohn's disease. Fissures and/or fistulae, having a reddish inflammatory mucosal appearance with necrotic tissue, were often present in resected intestines.

GENERAL HISTOLOGICAL FEATURES

It is rather difficult to make a definite diagnosis of Crohn's disease when only histologic slides are used in the absence of infor-

mation on gross appearance. In addition, it is also necessary to obtain clinical information such as that provided by X-ray, endoscopical findings and clinical history for proper diagnosis of the disease.

The diagnostic criteria used in Japan are very strict compared to those of Western countries, because of the need to differentiate this disease from other diseases, particularly intestinal tuberculosis (Fig. 10-5).[30,31] With routine endoscopic biopsy specimens of the intestine, diagnosis has to be based on microscopic observation of the mucosal and upper portion of submucosal layers. In addition to gross appearance, disproportionate findings, for example, a more intense inflammatory process in the submucosal layer than in the mucosal layer, are very helpful for diagnosing Crohn's disease.

The following findings are histological features of resected specimens of Crohn's disease: (1) transmural inflammatory process, (2) sarcoidlike noncaseous granuloma formation, (3) lymphoid aggregates in the intestinal wall, (4) ulceration, fissures and/or fistula formation, (5) fibrosis in the submucosal layer, (6) lymphangiectasia of the intestinal wall, and

TABLE 10-4

Microscopic Findings of Resected Samples

	Small Intestinal Lesion	Large Intestinal Lesion
Transmural inflammation	62 (100)*	51 (96)
Granuloma	56 (90)	44 (83)
Fissures	48 (77)	42 (98)
Lymphangiectasia	41 (66)	32 (60)
Total	62	53

* Percent in parenthesis.

(7) longitudinal ulcers with formation of subsequent amputation neuroma at the ulcer base.

There were also some differences in histological features between cases with small intestinal lesions and with large intestinal lesions. Thickening of intestinal wall and ulceration with subsequent formation of amputation neuroma at the ulcer base were more prominent in the small intestine than in the large intestine (Table 10-4).

As described above, longitudinal ulcers are characteristically found in the ileum in 80–90% of the cases of Crohn's disease (Table 10-4). These ulcers usually extend to the submucosal layer (Fig. 10-6), but in rare instances, the muscle layers are involved (Fig. 10-7). Aphthoid ulcers usually develop over lymphoid aggregates and contain a small number of granulocytes. In rare cases it is also observed that aphthoid ulcers detected by endoscopy extend to the longitudinal ulcers after some time. It is also possible that longitudinal ulcers may arise from aphthoid ulcers in some instances. It is difficult, however, to explain why ulcers of the small intestine with Crohn's disease are always formed on the mesenteric side. There is no direct correlation between granuloma formation and longitudinal ulceration based on our observations. At the ulcer base, extensive fibrosis and formation of so-called traumatic or amputation neuromas are usually present indicating that the ulcer is old.

As inflammatory cells, plasma cells, lymphocytes, eosinophils, and some mast cells are observed in the lesion. Granulocytes usually appear in the central portion of fissures and/or fistulae. Lymphocytic infiltration showing some aggregation is not so prominent in the mucosal layer, but it is rather prominent in the submucosal and subserosal layers.[32] These lymphocytes are mainly helper

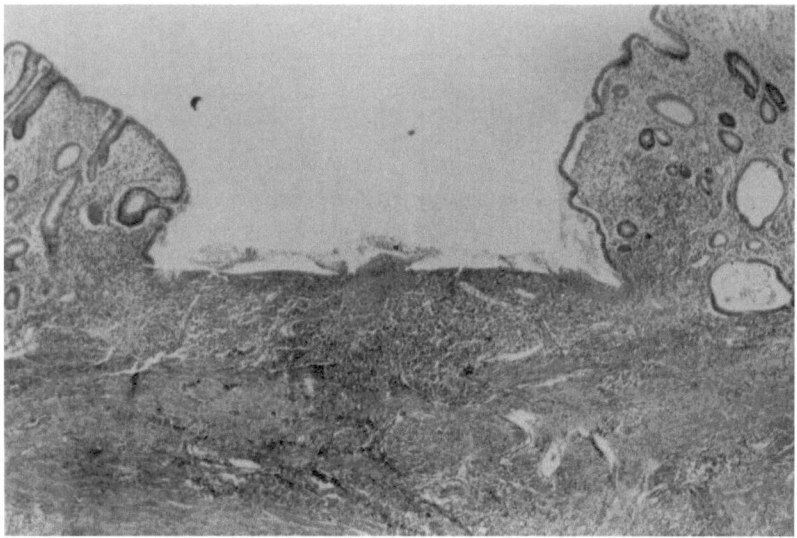

Fig. 10-6. Histologic low power view of longitudinal ulcer. H&E × 40

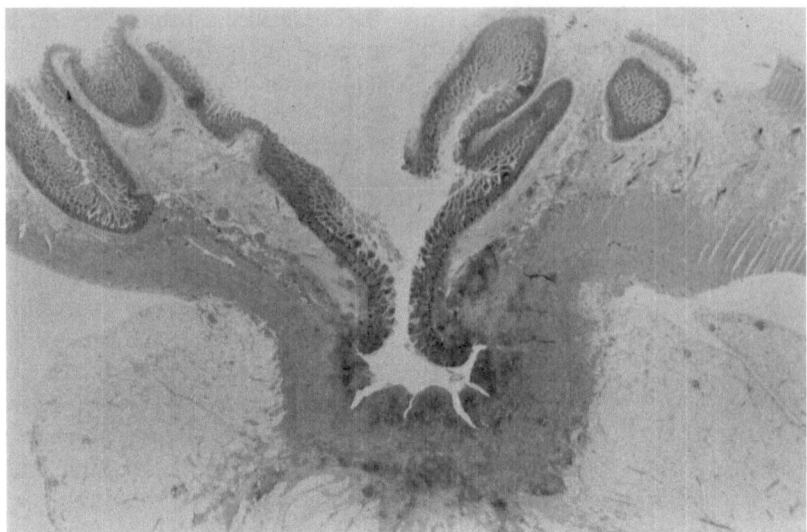

Fig. 10-7. Deep longitudinal ulcer and several fissures are distinctly formed on the side of mesenteric attachment. H&E × 5

T-lymphocytes as analyzed by monoclonal antibodies of Leu-series using frozen sections of fresh biopsy specimens. In the mucosa proper, small lymphocytes surround periglandular tissue, and they are also mainly helper T-lymphocytes (Fig. 10-8).[33] In regenerating mucosa, pseudopyloric glands are often observed.

Fibrosis is histologically more extensive than expected from macroscopic appearances. Peyer's patches usually contain an active hyperplastic germinal center in which nu-

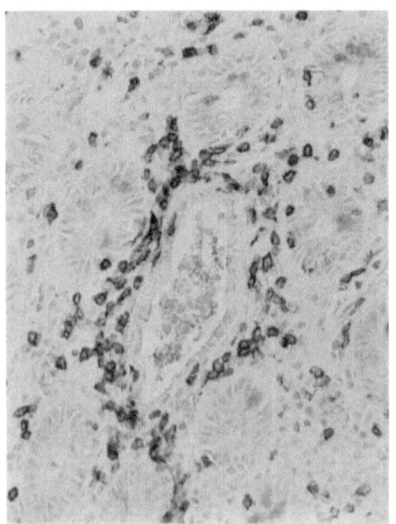
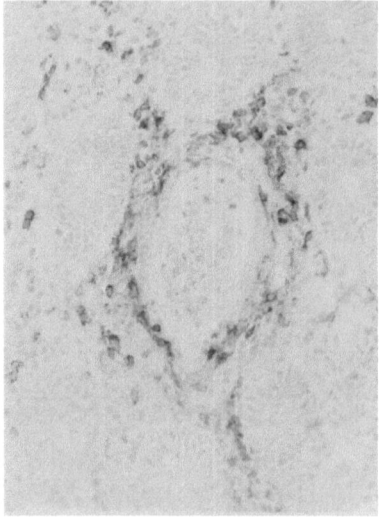

Fig. 10-8. Lymphocytes surrounding glandular epithelium are mainly helper T lymphocytes, analyzed by a) Leu 4 (Pan T) and b) Leu 3a (helper) monoclonal antibodies. PAP, × 250

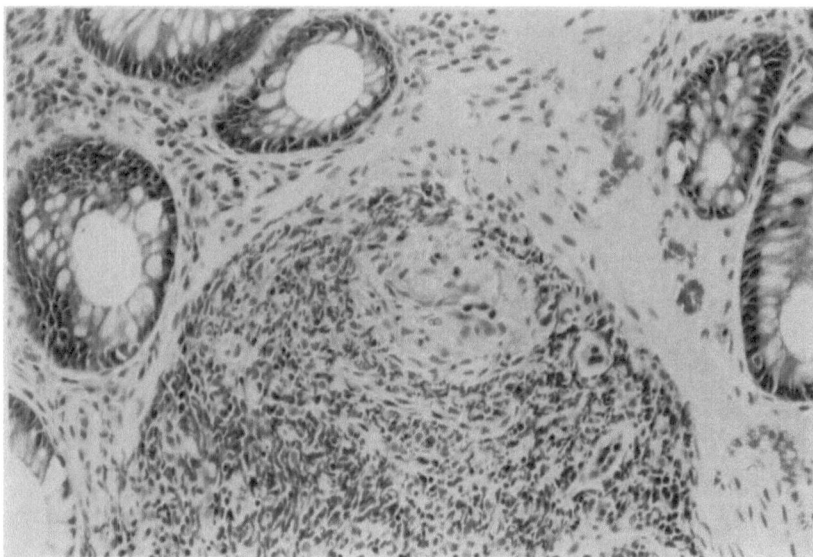

Fig. 10-9. Granuloma observed in rectal biopsy from normal appearing mucosa of the patient with active Crohn's disease in the small intestine. H&E × 200

merous tingible body macrophages appear. It is very useful to examine mesenteric lymph nodes in order to differentiate Crohn's disease from tuberculosis and Yersinia enterocolitica. In tuberculous infection, epithelioid granulomas in the lymph nodes are usually characterized by caseous necrosis, and tend to fuse with each other, usually resulting in large tubercles. Yersinia enterocolitica is characterized by the occurrence of granulocytes in the granuloma centers. On the other hand, granulomas in Crohn's disease are similar in size and have no tendency to fuse with each other.

MORPHOLOGIC FEATURES OF EPITHELIOID CELL GRANULOMA—HISTOLOGIC AND ELECTRONMICROSCOPIC OBSERVATION

Although it is well recognized that epithelioid granulomas, which are considered to be a diagnostic clue, are found in the intestinal wall with varying incidence, their occurrence varies. Especially in biopsy specimens, the existence of granulomas is very helpful in correctly diagnosing the disease. In our study,

granulomas were found in 90% of the cases in which there were small intestinal lesions and in over 80% of the cases in which there were large intestinal lesions. The occurrence of granulomas in Crohn's disease in Western countries, however, is usually encountered in 50–70% of the cases.[34] Even in cases without evidence of granulomas in one histologic slide only, granulomas are almost always found if serial sections are made, and it is sometimes necessary to make over 300 sections.

It is possible to find granulomas in rectal biopsy specimens even when the rectal mucosa appears to be normal in cases that are in the active phase of Crohn's disease. Watanabe[35] examined up to 2040 serial sections in an attempt to find granulomas and found such granulomas in 3 cases out of 4 with ileocolonic lesion and 3 out of 3 with large intestinal lesion (Fig. 10-9). The rate of occurrence of granuloma detected by serial sections is markedly higher than in those studies performed in Western countries.[36–40] The difference in frequency of granulomas in cases of Crohn's disease between Japan and Western countries is probably based on some difference in diagnostic clues. In our study granulomas were found to form not only in lymphatic tissue of

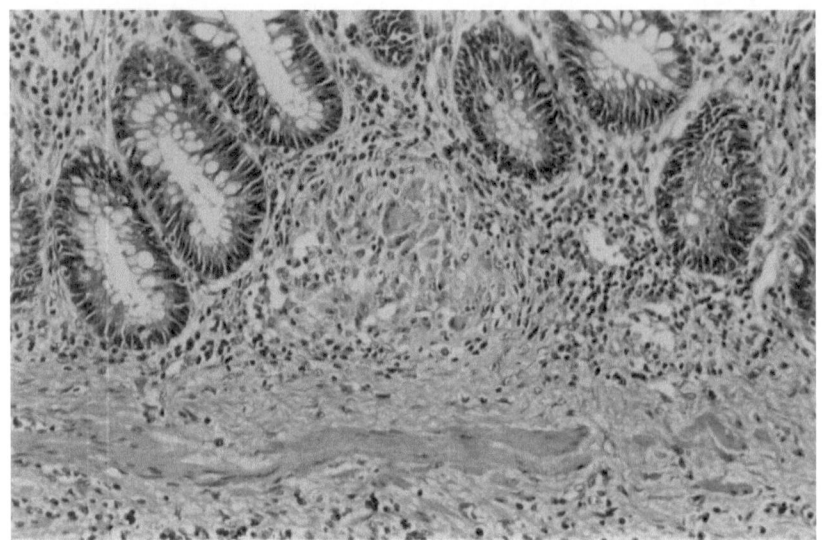

Fig. 10-10. Granuloma in mucosa proper. Epithelioid cells with formation of Langhans type giant cells are observed. H&E × 150

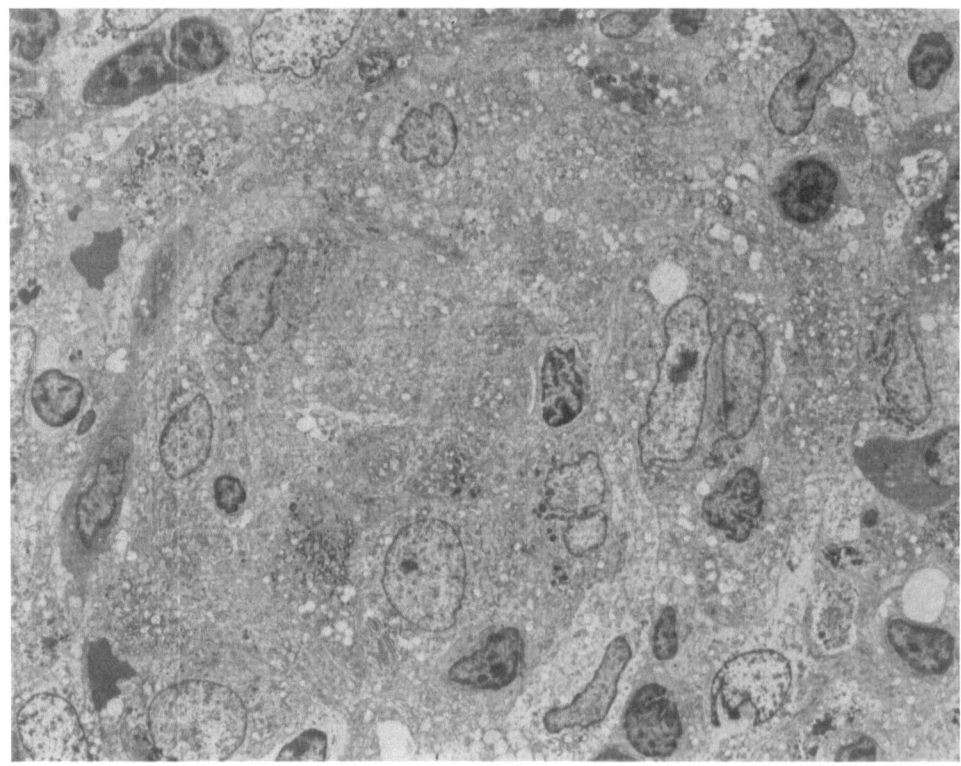

Fig. 10-11 Electronmicroscopic appearance of granuloma. Epithelioid cells have abundant cytoplasm with or without lysosomes. ×1,800

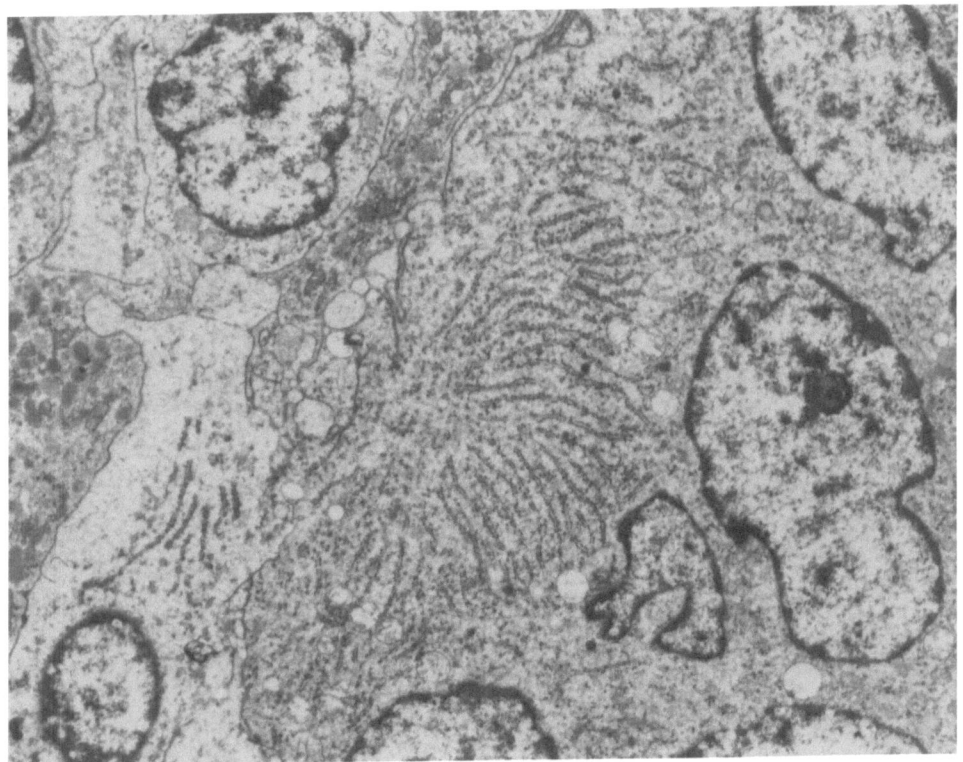

Fig. 10-12. Well developed rough endoplasmic reticulum arranged parallel in peripheral portion of Langhans type giant cell. ×2,700

the mucosal layer, but in all layers of the intestine. This observation was previously described by Rappaport.[41]

Cellular component of granuloma: Granulomas observed in mucosal and submucosal layers are composed of numerous epithelioid cells characterized by abundant cytoplasm and oval nuclei (Fig. 10-10). Epithelioid cells in granulomas of the mucosal and submucosal layers are rather compactly arranged in comparison to those found in other layers. Epithelioid cell granulomas often contain Langhans-type giant cells that are smaller in size and have fewer nuclei in comparison to those of tuberculous granulomas. Foreign body type giant cells phagocytizing calcified material are sometimes found in the subserosal layer, but they are not specific for the disease and might be formed as a reaction of

macrophages to necrotic tissue caused by ulceration. With PAP method, lysozyme, α_1-antitrypsin, and α_1-antichymotrypsin are always positively stained in epithelioid cells,[42] and are especially intensely positive in Langhans-type giant cells. Electronmicroscopic observation reveals that epithelioid cells have abundant cytoplasm containing many organelles and lysosomes (Fig. 10-11). Cell nuclei are usually round to oval with distinct small nucleoli. Langhans-type giant cells usually contain numerous mitochondria and parallel arrangement of the endoplasmic reticulum is observed in the peripheral portion of the cytoplasm (Fig. 10-12).

Size and frequency of granulomas in each layer: The size of granulomas and the frequency of occurrence in each layer of the intestinal wall were calculated to differentiate epithelioid granulomas of Crohn's disease

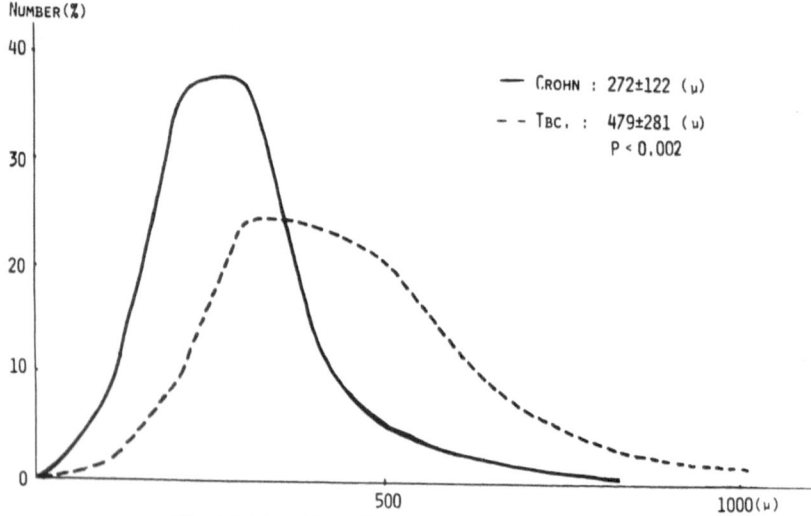

Fig. 10-13. Size of granulomas in each layer.

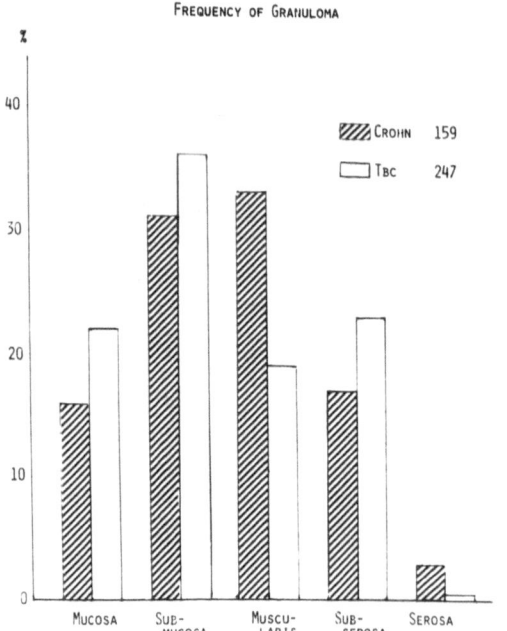

Fig. 10-14. Frequency of granulomas.

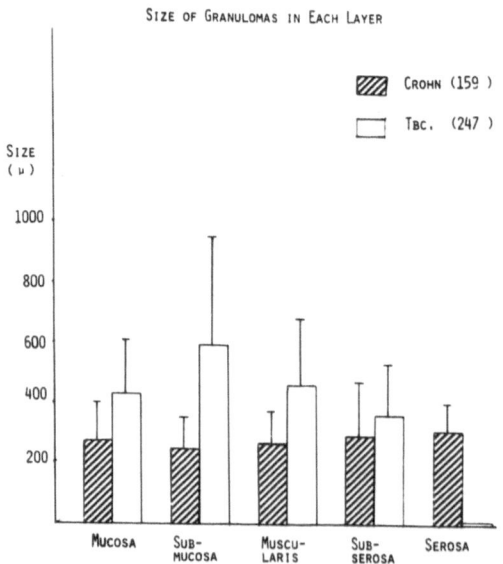

Fig. 10-15. Size of granulomas: TBC vs Crohn's disease.

218

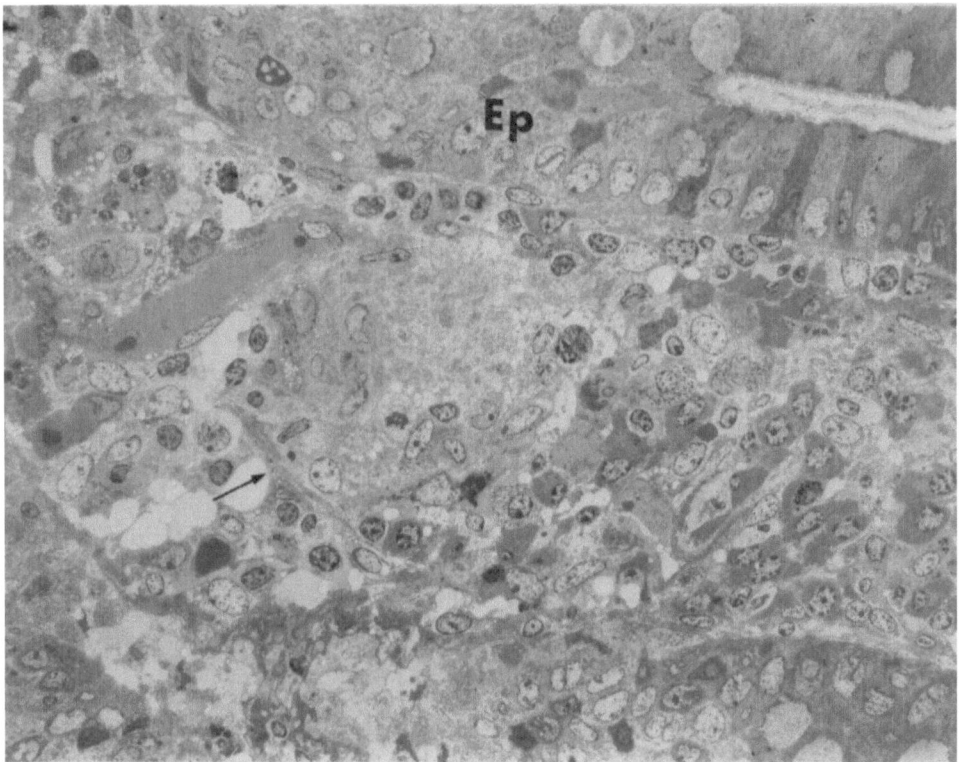

Fig. 10-16. A tiny granuloma (arrow), considered to be early, is formed in pericapillary area beneath the epithelial cells. ×930

from those of tuberculosis. The data based on the calculation for 159 granulomas of Crohn's disease and 247 of tuberculosis are summarized in Figures 10-13 and 10-14. Granuloma size as calculated by diameter is similar in all layers in Crohn's disease, but different in different layers in the case of tuberculosis. The size of tuberculous granulomas in the submucosal layer is larger than those of other layers because of the confluent tendency of granulomas. The relation between the size of granulomas and frequency in two diseases is shown in Fig. 10-15, and the mean size in Crohn's disease is $272 \pm 122 \ \mu$ and that in tuberculosis is $479 \pm 281 \ \mu$.

With regard to the frequency of granulomas in each layer, it is not so different between the two diseases, except that it was slightly higher in the muscular layer in Crohn's disease. Electronmicroscopic observation indicates that

early granulomas are formed in the pericapillary area of the mucosal layer proper just beneath the surface epithelium (Fig. 10-16). These tiny distinct granulomas composed of a small number of epithelioid cells are observed to be sharply demarcated from surrounding cells. On the basis of electronmicroscopic observation, it is difficult to determine whether granuloma formation in the mucosal layer is closely related to lymphatics, because lymphatics are not distinct in this area. Electronmicroscopic observation using a wide hole mesh was performed to define the relation of granulomas to lymphatics, and it was found that granulomas were distinctly formed in perilymphatic tissue and/or intralymphatic spaces. Epithelioid granulomas intermingled with small lymphocytes are clearly formed in the lumina of lymphatics (Fig. 10-17). Even in histologic slides, granulomas are often found

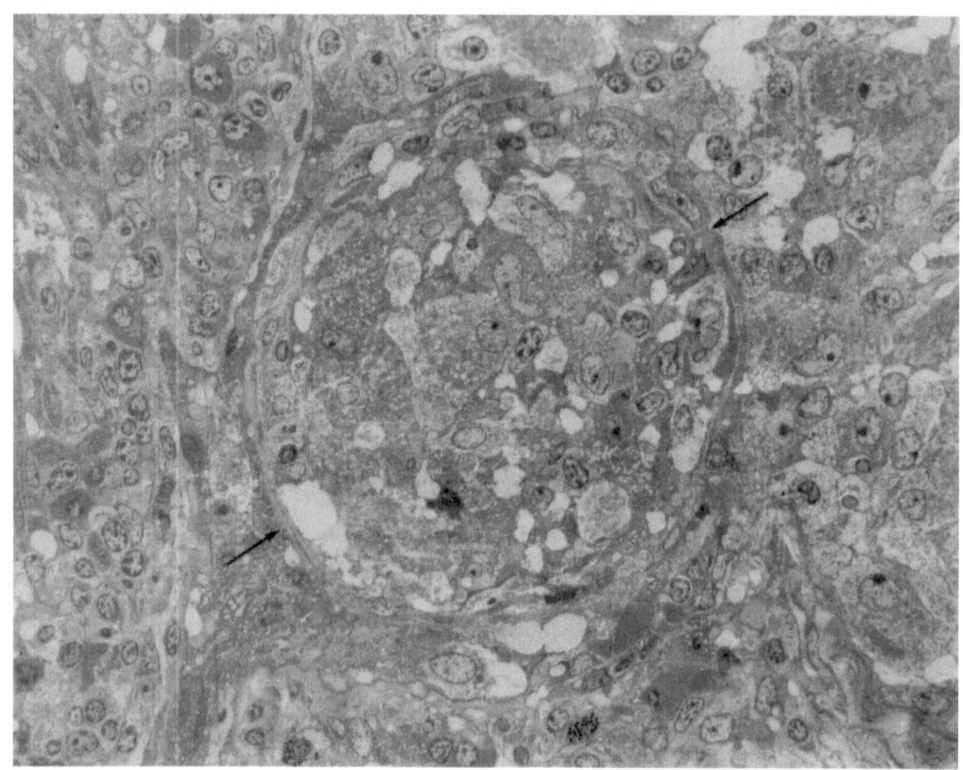

Fig. 10-17. Cluster of epithelioid cells intermingled with small lymphocytes are clearly present in lymphatic lumen (arrows). ×830

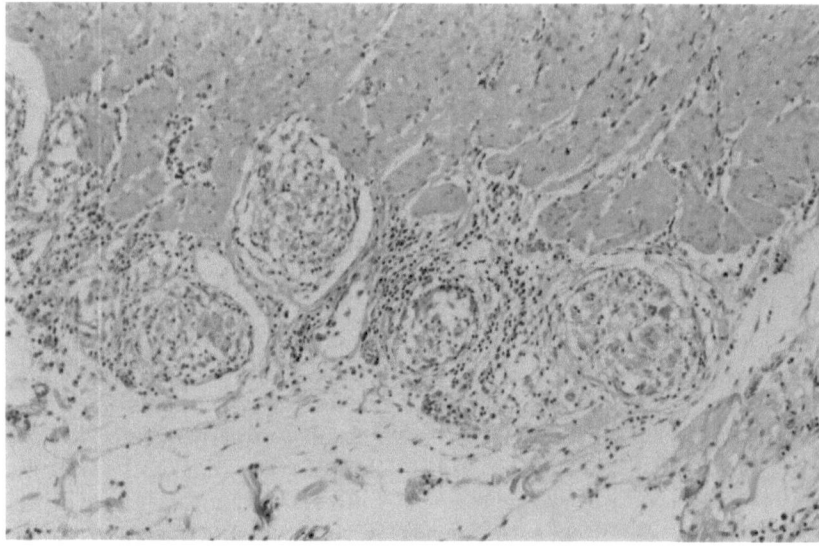

Fig. 10-18. Granulomas in the subserosal layer are present in the lymphatics showing luminal obstruction. H&E × 100

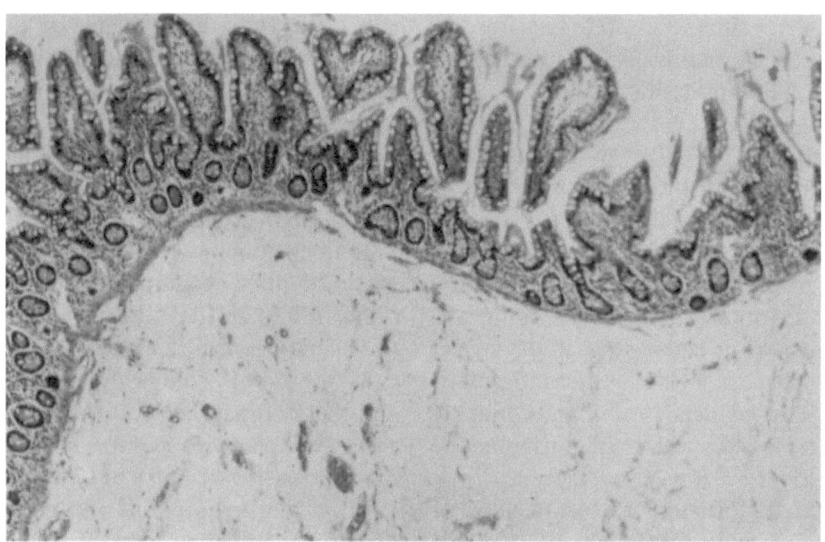

Fig. 10-19. Marked submucosal edema, probably in accord with cobblestone-like swelling, is formed by the obstruction of the lymphatics by granuloma. H&E × 40

in dilated lymphatics and in the perineural space of Auerbach's plexus of muscular layers.

Similar findings show that granulomas are even more intimately related to lymphatics in the subserosal layer (Fig. 10-18) and outside the serosa where lymphangitis or perilym-

in the submucosal layer (Fig 10-19). Such edematous swelling of mucosal and submucosal layers might be correlated with the cobblestone-like gross appearance. It is reasonably recognized that in case of longstanding cobphangitis might obstructively induce lymphangiectasia with consequent lymphedema

MN   I9 F

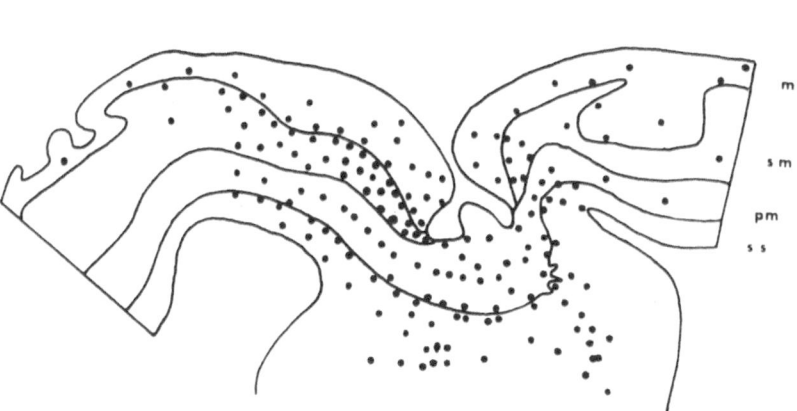

Fig. 10-20. This schema shows the distribution of granulomas revealed by serial sections from a 19 year old female. m = mucosa, sm = submucosa, pm = pars muscularis, ss = subserosa.

blestone-like edematous swelling, fibrosis may finally occur mainly in the submucosal layer on the mesenteric side.

Distribution of granulomas: Light microscopic observation of serial sections of histologic specimens shows the frequency of granulomas to be quite different from case to case. Granulomas are scattered in the submucosal layer, but were observed in clusters in the area surrounding Peyer's patches and in the deeper mucosal layer close to the lamina muscularis mucosae. The tendency of granulomas to cluster was also observed in the muscular and subserosal layers.

Schematic distribution and extension of granulomas are shown in Figure 10-20. From our morphologic observations, it is concluded that lymphatics have a close relationship to the formation and extension of granulomas in the intestinal wall.

DISCUSSION

Inflammatory bowel disease is a disorder in which immunological background is necessary for understanding.[43, 44]

Crohn's disease has been considered rare in Japan, because there have been no definite diagnostic criteria. However, cases have been increasing in number since the establishment of clinicopathologic criteria proposed by the Japanese Research Committee for Crohn's Disease. This committee, composed of clinicians and pathologists, consulted on cases of intestinal disorders suspected of being Crohn's disease on a nationwide scale and diagnosed each case. In Japan, it is necessary to differentiate cases of Crohn's disease from tuberculosis, but in recent years cases of tuberculosis have been decreasing markedly.

In Western countries, there are two peaks in age distribution, but in the Japanese cases of the present series, there is no such tendency. The data in the present study were obtained at time of diagnosis, not at onset.

The most prominent feature of Crohn's disease in Japan is the existence of longitudinal ulcers in the small intestine exclusively on the side of the mesenteric attachment. On the other hand, ulcers in the large intestine are usually irregular in shape and are seen in short lines at the sites of colonic teniae.

Cases in Western countries reveal a marked wall thickening with a cobblestone-like appearance, often accompanied by stenosis. It is rather infrequent to observe cases with such classic morphologic features in Japan. The occurrence of both cobblestone-like appearance and longitudinal ulcers in the same case suggests that these two features should be recognized as basic attributes of Crohn's disease.

Regarding longitudinal ulcers, it was confirmed in only one case of our series that aphthoid ulcers definitely extended to the ulcer after some time. In most cases, however, no such clinicopathologic finding was obtained. It is also suggested that the site of longitudinal ulcers in Crohn's disease is similar to that of ischemic enteritis frequently occurring in cases with cardiac disorder or in elderly persons.

Morphometric data on the thickness of intestinal arteries in Crohn's disease show an increase in thickness of the arterial wall outside of the intestine, which may indicate that ischemic change previously existed in the wall.[45] It is also suggested that blood flow is decreased in intestinal arteries of Crohn's disease.[46] In Western countries, the frequency of longitudinal ulcers is low, even sometimes showing railtrack-like appearance in figures. At present, it is speculated that an inflammatory process including granulomatous lesions develops around the lymphatics and involves blood vascularity, and then the occurrence of ischemic change.

Epithelioid cell granulomas, which are noncaseous, rather smaller and more similar in size compared with those of tuberculosis, are formed in all layers of the intestine and lymph nodes. Among Japanese cases, epithelioid cell granulomas are highly useful for diagnostic purposes, because of their frequency, which is high compared with that in Western countries. Examination of 300 serial sections revealed granulomas not only in the overt lesion but also in the biopsy specimens from normal appearing rectal mucosa of cases in the active phase of Crohn's disease. Such a finding showing granulomas and inflammatory process in rectal mucosa apart from any grossly visible lesion confirms that the intestine may be involved extensively,[47, 48] even when it is covered with normal looking mucosa. Therefore, wide surgical resection is sometimes ineffective in preventing recurrence.[8]

As described above, epithelioid cells are formed from macrophages, which are positive for lysozyme, α_1-antitrypsin and α_1-antichymotrypsin as shown by the PAP method. It is thought that macrophages may appear first and that granulomas are then formed as the result of early reaction in the intestinal wall. With electronmicroscopic observation, early tiny granulomas are seen to be formed in the pericapillary area of the upper mucosal layer just beneath the surface epithelium. They eventually extend to the deeper layers through the lymphatics. Granulomas formed in or around lymphatics in the subserosal layer may induce the obstruction of lymphatics with subsequent submucosal edema of the intestinal wall. Lymphangiectasia and cobblestone-like appearance may ensue in accord with intestinal edema induced by the obstruction of lymphatics in the subserosal layer and outside the intestine. Ultrastructural abnormalities of intestinal lymphatics in Crohn's disease, reported by Kovi,[49] who found no gaps in lymphatic walls, may also play a role in intestinal edema. It is suggested that granulomas formed with relation to lymphatics may be an important factor in the etiopathogenesis of Crohn's disease.

SUMMARY

Morphological study of cases of Crohn's disease in Japan revealed a high frequency of longitudinal ulcers in the terminal ileum and epithelioid cell granuloma formation in the intestinal wall. The pathogenesis of longitudinal ulcers is still uncertain, but the location of such ulcers is similar to that of ischemic change suggesting that the inflammatory process may induce vascular change.

Epithelioid cell granulomas found in the lesion of the mucosal layer proper may be considered as an early cellular reaction in Crohn's disease, and these granulomas are closely related to lymphatics as shown by electron- and light-microscopic observation. No definitive causative agent was confirmed by our intensive observation.

ACKNOWLEDGMENTS

We are very grateful to the members of the Japanese Research Committee for Crohn's Disease (Chairman: Prof. S. Yamagata). We express our appreciation to Mr. T. Ito and Mr. Y. Sasaki for their technical assistance and to Mrs. M. Hangai for the preparation of the manuscript.

REFERENCES

1. Morson B.C., Dawson I.M.P.: Gastrointestinal Pathology, Blackwell, Oxford, London, Edinburgh and Melbourne, 1979
2. Dvorak A.M., Dickersin R.: Crohn's disease: Transmission electron microscopic studies. I. Barrier function. Possible changes related to alterations of cell coat, mucous coat, epithelial cells, and Paneth cells. Human Pathol 11:561, 1980
3. Dvorak A.M., Monahan R.A., Osage J.E., Dickersin R.: Crohn's disease: Transmission electron microscopic studies. II. Immunologic inflammatory response. Alterations of mast cells, basophils, eosinophils and the microvasculature. Human Pathol 11:606, 1980
4. Dvorak A.M., Monahan R.A., Osage J.E., Dickersin R.: Crohn's disease: Transmission electron microscopic studies. III. Target tissues. Proliferation of and injury to smooth muscle and the autonomic nervous system. Human Pathol 11:620, 1980
5. Watanabe H.: Histopathological diagnosis of inflammatory bowel disease of the large intestine. Clinical Radiology 25:789, 1980 (in Japanese)
6. Wakasa H., Yamazaki T.: Pathology of inflammatory bowel disease. Naika Mook 14:35, 1980 (in Japanese)
7. Rowland R., Pounder D.J.: Crohn's colitis. Pathol Annu 17 (Pt 1), 267, 1982
8. Hamilton S.R.: Pathologic features of Crohn's disease associated with recrudescence after resection. Pathol Annu 18, 191, 1983
9. Wakasa H., Ishikawa H., Asano S.: Crohn's disease, morphologic features. J Jpn Soc Colo-Proctol 36:472, 1983 (in Japanese)

10. Saito K.: Crohn's disease; some problems on histopathological diagnosis. Pathology & Clinical Medicine 2:163, 1984 (in Japanese)
11. Winblad S., Niléhn B., Sternby N.H.: Yersinia enterocolitica (Pasteurella X) in human enteric infections. Brit Med J 2:1363, 1966
12. Sjöström B.: Acute terminal ileitis and its relation to Crohn's disease. In "Regional Enteritis (Crohn's Disease)" Engel A, Larsson T (eds), Nordiska Bokhandelns Förlag, Stockholm, p 73, 1971
13. Kato Y., Hattori T., Oh-ya H., Suzuki T., Yoshino S., Kato H., Nishikawa H.: A case of acute terminal ileitis by Yersinia enterocolitica. Jap Gastroenterology 73:56, 1976 (in Japanese)
14. Ishikura H., Hayasaka H., Kikuchi Y.: Acute regional ileitis at Iwanai Kokkaido. With special reference to intestinal Anisakiasis. Sapporo Med J 12:183, 1967
15. Diseases of the gastrointestinal tract. Vol III, Provisional International Nomenclature. ed. Btesh S, CIOMS, Geneva, 1973
16. Bargen J.A., Weber H.M.: Regional migratory chronic ulcerative colitis. Surg Gynec Obstet 50:964, 1930
17. Crohn B.B., Ginzburg L., Oppenheimer G.D.: Regional ileitis. A pathologic and clinical entity. JAMA 99:1323, 1932
18. Crohn B.B., Berg A.A.: Right-sided (regional) colitis. JAMA 110:32, 1938
19. Dubins J.A.: Regional colitis (with report of two cases). Rev Gastroenterol 6:293, 1939
20. Castro Barbosa J. de, Bargen J.A., Dixon C.F.: Regional segmental colitis. Proc Staff Meet Mayo Clin 20:134, 1945
21. The Japanese Research Committee for Crohn's Disease (Chairman: Yamagata S.): Diagnostic criteria for Crohn's disease. Jap Gastroenterology 73:1467, 1976 (in Japanese)
22. The Japanese Research Committee for Crohn's Disease (Chairman: Yamagata S.): Crohn's disease in Japan. Gastroenterol Jpn 14:366, 1979
23. Evans J.G., Achsen E.D.: An epidemiological study of ulcerative colitis and regional enteritis in the Oxford area. Gut 6:311, 1965
24. Lennard-Jones J.E.: Definition and diagnosis. In "Regional Enteritis (Crohn's Disease)", ed. Engel A., Larsson T., Nordiska, Bokhandelns Förlag, Stockholm, p 105, 1971
25. Lennard-Jones J.E.: Etiology and epidemiology of Crohn's disease. Canad J Surg 17:379, 1974
26. Fahrländer H., Baerlocher C.H.: Clinical features and epidemiological data in the Basle area. In "Regional Enteritis (Crohn's Disease)", ed. Engel A., Larsson T., Nordiska, Bokhandelns Förlag, Stockholm, p 131, 1971
27. Korelitz B.I., Present D.H., Alpert L.I. Marshak R.H., Janowitz, H.D.: Recurrent regional ileitis after ileostomy and colectomy for granulomatous colitis. N Engl J Med 287:110, 1972
28. Lockhart-Mummery H.E., Morson B.C.: Crohn's disease (regional enteritis) of the large intestine and its distinction from ulcerative colitis. Gut 1:87, 1960
29. Muto T.: Comparative appearances of Crohn's disease in England and Japan: A preliminary personal experience. Stomach and Intestine 13:385, 1978 (in Japanese)
30. Watanabe H., Enjoji M., Yao T.: Histopathology of intestinal tuberculosis. Stomach and Intestine 12:1481, 1977 (in Japanese)
31. Yao T.: Current state of intestinal tuberculosis. Naika Mook 14:165, 1980 (in Japanese)
32. Meuwissen S.G.M.: Analysis of the lymphoplasmacytic infiltrate in Crohn's disease with special reference to identification of lymphocyte populations. Gut 17:770, 1976
33. Ishikawa H.: Macroscopical, microscopical and immunohistological studies on intestinal lesion of Crohn's disease. Fukushima J Med Sci 37 (1) [in press] (in Japanese)
34. Schachter H., Kirsner J.B.: Crohn's Disease of the Gastrointestinal Tract. John Wiley & Sons, New York, 1980
35. Watanabe H., Endo K., Sato T., Unoura A., Okata T., Namiki T., Nakamura K., Ôto T., Kobayashi M.: Identification of granulomas by rectal biopsies from patients with active Crohn's disease. Annual Research Committee Report for Inflammatory Bowel Disease p. 269 from Ministry of Health and Welfare, 1983 (in Japanese)
36. Korelitz B.I., Sommers S.C.: Rectal biopsy in patients with Crohn's disease. JAMA 237:2742, 1977
37. Rotterdam H., Korelitz B.I., Sommers S.C.: Microgranulomas in grossly normal rectal mucosa in Crohn's disease. Amer J Clin Pathol 67:550, 1977
38. Goodman M.J., Kirsner J.B., Riddell R.H.: Usefulness of rectal biopsy in inflammatory bowel disease. Gastroenterology 72:952, 1977
39. Hill R.B., Kent T.H., Hansen R.N.: Clinical usefulness of rectal biopsy in Crohn's disease. Gastroenterology 77:938, 1979
40. Iliffe G.D., Owen D.A.: Rectal biopsy in Crohn's disease. Digest Dis Sci 26:321, 1981
41. Rappaport H., Burgoyne F.H., Smetana H.F.: The pathology of regional enteritis. Milit Surgeon 109:463, 1951
42. Wakasa H., Ishikawa H.: Crohn's disease; special reference to granulomas. Annual Research Committee Report on Inflammatory Bowel Disease, p. 369, from Ministry of Health and Welfare, 1984 (in Japanese)
43. Shorter R.G., Huizenga K.A., Spencer R.J.: A working hypothesis for the etiology and pathogenesis of non-specific inflammatory bowel disease. Am J Dig Dis 17:1024, 1972
44. Kobayashi J.: Crohn's disease. Medicina 20:220, 1983 (in Japanese)
45. Sasaki I., Funayama Y., Imamura M., Konno Y., Sato T.: Morphometric analysis of intestinal arteries in Crohn's disease. Annual Research Committee Report on Inflammatory Bowel Disease, p. 387, from Ministry of Health and Welfare, 1984 (in Japanese)
46. Hultén L., Lindhagen J., Lundgren O,. Fasth S., Åhrén C.: Regional intestinal blood flow in ulcerative colitis and Crohn's disease. Gastroenterology 72:388, 1977
47. Goodman M.J., Skinner J.M., Truelove S.C.: Abnormalities in the apparently normal bowel mucosa in Crohn's disease. Lancet I: 275, 1976
48. Dunne W.T., Cooke T.W., Allan R.N.: Enzymatic and morphometric evidence for Crohn's disease as a diffuse lesion of the gastrointestinal tract. Gut 18:290, 1977
49. Kovi J.: Ultrastructure of intestinal lymphatics in Crohn's disease. Am J Clin Pathol 76:385, 1981

Index

Numerals in *italics* indicate a figure, "t" following a page number indicates tabular matter.

225